Praise for *R*

I have had the privilege of working with and learning from many top health and performance experts. Chris's teaching and his new book **REST EAT MOVE** *is in a league of its own and something I follow to feel and be my best.*

—**Mel Tucker**, Head Football Coach, Michigan State University

REST EAT MOVE *is an inspiring and practical masterpiece for a healthy and satisfying life from a master of wellness training. With a distillation of research and personal experience, Chris Johnson shares his mastery of vitality, wellness, and joyfulness. This is the one book on wellness that expertly covers all the bases. It will motivate you, make you laugh, and provide you with in-depth and accurate knowledge for your own wellness journey. In short, this is one incredible book!*

—**Phil Nuernberger,** PhD, President, Strategic Intelligence Skills, author of *Strong and Fearless*

Chris Johnson's latest book **REST EAT MOVE** *contains the essential ingredients for living your best life. In all areas of my professional career, as a college president, CEO of a bank, and a state director for a 1.3-million-member nonprofit organization, On Target Living has been a part of my journey both professionally and personally. Bringing them into our organization was one of the smartest decisions I've ever made. Their approach doesn't require gimmicks or artificial supplements. It simply requires knowing and understanding how to live our best life. This book reinforces the philosophy of Chris Johnson and his professionalism, passion, and purpose to create a healthier world. It is a must read for anyone looking to feel and be their best!*

—**Paula Cunningham**, Director, AARP Michigan

Chris Johnson has once again hit the mark with his extensive new book, **REST EAT MOVE**, *bringing forward new data and thoughts on the importance of diet, sleep, and exercise to performance on the job and a long and healthy life. Chris is one of my personal heroes. His team made a marked and dramatic difference on our entire 250,000 employee body at AT&T over the past decade, changing and in some instances saving lives with their groundbreaking insights. Anyone or any organization interested in improved health and productivity would be well served to read Chris's latest book.*

—**Bill Blasé**, Retired EVP of Human Resources, AT&T

The tactics covered **REST EAT MOVE** *are proven and sustainable ingredients for high performance. It is not a fad! It is based on experience and daily methods of successful outcomes lived by the author. He is my go-to for all things health- and fitness-related to sustain optimal performance as a CEO, wife, mother, and community member.*

—**Molly Fletcher**, Professional speaker, former sports agent, and author of *The Energy Clock*

As a cardiothoracic surgeon, I treat so many diseases that are either directly caused by or are deeply impacted by lifestyle and eating choices we all make in our modern society. Having a positive effect on those choices is difficult. Habits are hard to break. My advice has always been to make the diet and exercise regimen simple, inexpensive, and healthy. Then I met Chris Johnson and learned of his system and his three basic tenets: sleep better, eat healthy, and move more. With **REST EAT MOVE**, *Chris has prepared a logical and reproducible method for achieving goals of healthy living, and they are grounded in his exercise physiology training, his abiding interest and study of source dietary benefits, and his extensive work in the health and fitness world for more than 30 years. Where Chris's program shines is in his power of positive energy, encouragement, and enthusiasm which makes all this come together. His absolute love of helping people become healthier is the unadorned crown on the head of his program.*

—**Walter Halloran, MD**, Cardiothoracic Surgeon, Beacon Medical Group

I was at a hotel in Kentucky getting ready to present to a large group of successful financial advisors in the Southeast. Prior to my presentation, I happened to peek in the room to see who was presenting before me. I noticed a sharp looking guy, who looked as fit as a fiddle up in front of the room. The entire audience was mesmerized. I stopped my preparation and immediately started listening. To this day, I'm thankful I did! The moment I saw Chris Johnson speak, I knew I needed more of On Target Living in my life, the lives of my teams, and the lives of all those I love. His common sense, yet elegant approach to better ways of eating, exercising, and resting, enables us to consistently perform at a higher level. It's been 12 years since and so many of his nutritional suggestions, movement recommendations and rest tips have consistently made me a better husband, a better father, a better leader, and an overall better human being.

—**Colin C. Lake**. CIMA®, Founder/President, Developing the Next Leaders

We have worked with Chris and his team for over 15 years on these concepts and tactics, and the results are outstanding. Not just losing weight, but game- changing outcomes in other areas like sleep, vitality, and overall quality of life. And unlike other approaches it's simple to get started and see meaningful results. Do yourself a favor – read this book and get started today!

—**David Patchen**, Senior Vice President, Advisor Education and Practice Management, Raymond James

Other Titles by Chris Johnson

Meal Patterning

Fitness "Fore" Golf

On Target Living Nutrition

On Target Living Cooking

On Target Living: Your Guide to a Life of Balance, Energy, and Vitality

Capacity

REST
EAT
MOVE

you have the power to feel your best

CHRIS JOHNSON

First Edition

Published by On Target Living, LLC, Okemos, MI 48864
http://ontargetliving.com

Editor and Project Coordinator: Paula Johnson
Book Design/Layout: Design 2
Graphic Design/Images: Lauren Brumbach
Copy editor: Bonney Mayers
Cover Design: Lauren Brumbach, Steven Glynn
Photography: Steven Glynn

ISBN 978-0-9727281-9-5

Printed in the United States of America

10 9 8 7 6 5 4 3 2 1

Table of Contents

Introduction

My own journey to better health began with challenges, as it may for many of you. The pursuit of better health has been a very rewarding journey for myself and for my family. It became a meaningful career and life's work. All my experience and knowledge have led me to a mission of sharing what I have learned along the way to help people like you learn how to achieve the "Power of Feeling Your Best!" I hope you are excited to take your own journey to your best health.

Growing up in Michigan I loved my childhood. My parents Jean and Gary were great, but like many Baby Boomers I did not get a lot of guidance or supervision. "Just come home when the streetlights come on."

I was raised on a diet of Captain Crunch cereal, whole milk, white bread, bologna and Miracle Whip sandwiches, Beefaroni, and Hostess pies and cupcakes. Kool-Aid and Pepsi were my drinks of choice. I had skin and digestive problems from age 8 to 20, was prescribed cortisone cream along with oral medications for over 10 years, and was told by my doctors that my problems were due to sensitive skin.

In 1978 I stopped drinking cow's milk on the advice from my economics professor Dr. Louis Junker. Dr. Junker had a shaved head, rode his bike to work, dug his own well, was fit looking, and was extremely passionate about his health and well-being. It was Dr. Junker who first opened my eyes to the power of food, that food is truly medicine. Dr. Junker was a gift to Western Michigan University and its students, and I will be forever grateful for his guidance and inspiration.

My first job after graduating from college with a business and economics degree was with Butternut Bread. I was hired as a route salesperson delivering white bread along with Dolly Madison cakes. I would wake up at 2:30 a.m. and work until 6 p.m., putting in 75-80 hours per week, and running the entire day. I was sleep deprived. As I look back on it, my adrenal glands must have been shot! After one year with Butternut Bread, I went to work for Frito-Lay on the recommendation from one of my lifelong friends, Rick Norris, again as a route salesperson delivering Doritos, Ruffles, Lays, Fritos, Tostitos, and Cheetos. Frito-Lay was a great job with reasonable hours, and I stayed for six years. For over seven years I lived in grocery stores watching and learning how the stores get you to buy, but most of all, watching and observing the people and what they were putting in their grocery carts.

Two years into working with Frito-Lay I knew I wanted to pursue a different path, but what? I looked into physical therapy and sports medicine.

I loved working out and got interested in body building and eating healthier. What really changed my life was a two-hour talk with Dr. Kwok Ho, an exercise physiology professor at Michigan State University. Dr. Ho asked all the right questions. As I stood up and started to leave his office that day, he said something that I will never forget. "Chris, you are a prevention guy, so go out in the world and help people get and stay healthy!" So, in the fall of 1985 I entered graduate school at Michigan State University and Dr. Ho became my academic advisor.

After going to graduate school and acquiring a master's degree in exercise physiology, I went to work for Butterworth/Metropolitan Wellness Center in Grand Rapids, Michigan. On a typical day I would spend the first 4-5 hours of my day in the hospital doing executive physicals. Each physical exam began with an intake interview to evaluate the patient's current lifestyle. Did they sleep well? What did their nutrition look like? Were they moving their body on a regular basis? Was stress an issue in their life? Were they on any medications? What were their past or present injuries? Most of all, what did they want their future to look like from a health perspective?

After the interview was completed, we moved on to a variety of assessments. These included a stress test on a treadmill, a spirometer test to measure lung function, a flexibility and balance assessment, blood work, and a one-on-one session with the doctor. I learned a great deal about heart rhythms, lung function, and medications, along with listening to how the doctor talked with the patient. What I really enjoyed most about this experience was trying to inspire these people to take that next step to feel and be their best.

The second half of my day was spent speaking with organizations and their people about health and wellness, including how they could improve their blood pressure, type 2 diabetes, cholesterol, weight control, and improve their health. This was my first experience speaking in front of people. In the beginning I was extremely nervous, raw, and most likely not very good at it. But over time I truly enjoyed having fun with the audience and helping people see the light of what was possible!

A few years later, I went to work for a family practice physician, Dr. Barry Saltman. Dr. Saltman was a wonderful man and extremely hard-working. He saw on average up to 40 patients a day. Yes, 40 patients per day! Dr. Saltman wanted to build a small 5,000 square-foot exercise facility in the basement of his practice, and asked me to help him design it, select exercise equipment, and develop nutrition and exercise programs for many of his high-risk patients. This was a wonderful opportunity for me to work with a seasoned physician like Dr. Saltman, but I quickly realized I was in over my head. There were not just a few high-risk patients but hundreds, and most needed one-on-one attention. I had never seen so many unhealthy, highly medicated people in my life.

I kept thinking, "How did all these folks become so unhealthy? Is daily interaction with heavily medicated, high-risk people normal for many doctors in the United States?" Working closely with Dr. Saltman I was given this incredible opportunity to work directly with people who had high blood pressure, chronic obstructive pulmonary disease, type 2 diabetes, severe obesity, and even one man who had a heart replacement. I loved helping this guy get his health and his life back. Dr. Saltman was an incredible doctor, but an even better person, and I learned so much from his teaching and mentorship.

After two years of intense training with Dr. Saltman, I was hired as the Director of Health and Fitness by Carl Porter, the founder and CEO of the Michigan Athletic Club in East Lansing, Michigan. The Michigan Athletic Club at the time was the largest hospital-owned, multi-purpose health club in the world, spanning over 275,000 square feet. My role was to recruit, hire, train, and retain the best and brightest personal trainers and to develop health and fitness programs for the members.

As time went on, we realized many of our personal trainers were not skilled or trained in dealing with the challenging needs of many of our high-risk, highly medicated clients. What we needed was a systematic training program to help teach our personal trainers how to interact with our members and their growing needs. Step-by-step, we looked at body alignment, injuries, nutrition, stress, sleep, breathing, health history, weight loss, medications, motivation, and how to change behaviors. We developed a personal training program that was centered not just on exercise, but the entire person.

Members were seeing wonderful results. Doctors and health professionals started referring more and more of their patients to our program. The word began to spread and within a few short years we were one of the highest revenue-producing, personal training programs in the United States.

For over 17 years I had the privilege to work side by side and learn from some of the best trainers in the world. I have also done a fair amount of one-on-one training, racking up over 20,000 hours.

After watching members struggle with information regarding stress, breathing, sleeping, nutrition, weight loss, cholesterol, blood pressure, medications, fitness, and health, I wanted to help more people, so I began doing live seminars. My first book was titled *Meal Patterning*, based on the eating patterns of the Sumo wrestlers.

In 2006 I went to Colorado to meet with a branding specialist by the name of Dick Bruso. After two days of brain storming, we came up with the name On Target Living, based on my "Food Target."

Attendance slowly grew. I wrote a few more books. Demand increased, and after many years of working on my gigs I decided to take my passion full-time. Today I travel around the world speaking to corporations, organizations, associations, and schools. My mission, our mission at On Target Living is to help improve the health and performance of people from all over the world. . . one person at a time!

Most people want to have great health, more energy, a better night of sleep, look good and feel great. They want to be more energetic and happier, but many are not as healthy and robust as they could be.

What would happen if you knew with 100 percent certainty that something was going to work? No second guessing—no going back—but a true belief that this is your time to shine. When it comes to our health, one of the biggest variables to success is HOPE. When people begin to truly believe, success soon follows. It is the belief that they can do it!

Here is what to expect over the next 34 chapters. You have in your hand a resource guide to help you navigate almost everything you need to know to take care of your greatest asset and that asset is your health!

What makes this book unique is the balanced approach to building your foundational pillars of health—how you **REST**, **EAT** and **MOVE**!

I wanted to write a book that gives you the necessary information to help guide and motivate you to develop a lifestyle that you can learn to love and most importantly sustain. I am so excited for you to take this journey with me as there is nothing more valuable than our health.

I have done the work. I have been in the trenches. I have made the mistakes, and now it is time to share this information with YOU!

Your journey to becoming your best self is about to begin—so buckle up and enjoy the ride!

Here's to a lifetime of Health & Happiness!

SECTION
1

HEALTH BEGINS IN THE MIND

1 The Power of Feeling Your Best

Imagine feeling great, better than you have in a long time—maybe ever. Imagine having lots of energy, getting a restful night of sleep, and feeling strong with greater vitality. Can you remember the last time you felt that good? Have you ever felt that good? Feeling great, or not, is closely related to how you **REST**, **EAT**, and **MOVE**.

The journey to greater health and feeling our best begins in the mind. Before jumping into all the vital information needed to reach that destination, it is imperative to prepare and ready the mind. The rest of the book will cover the important topics of cellular health, pH balance, stress, breathing, sleep, hydration, superfoods, carbohydrates, proteins, fats, fasting, calories, dieting, exercise, motivation, momentum, building support systems, and much, much more.

Information alone is not going to get it done for most people. We all must learn how to use our mind to help us make our lifestyle choices stick.

Changing behaviors is not easy especially when it comes to making lifestyle changes. Over time these new behaviors can become stronger as they move into new habits. If you get stuck at any time throughout the rest of the book, come back to this section again. Because your health truly begins in your mind.

Culture of Health

For most of us, our parents have a huge influence on our lives. I was raised in Michigan in the 1960s and 1970s, with my older brother Nick and my younger sister Paula. We had a great childhood, and our parents were loving and kind. However, they smoked and drank heavily. Fortunately, both of them quit smoking and drinking approximately 25 years prior to their deaths.

My siblings and I sometimes laugh about how we became so focused on health and fitness after growing up in a household that lived on Beefaroni, pot pies, bologna sandwiches with white bread and Miracle Whip, Captain Crunch and Lucky Charms cereals, Little Debbie Oatmeal Pies, Pringles, Hostess Cupcakes, 3 Musketeers and Snickers bars, Kool-Aid, Pepsi, and whole milk. Our favorite diners around town included Kewpee, McDonald's, Jon's Country Burger, Yankee Cone Shop, DeMarco's Pizza, Famous Recipe Chicken, and A & W hot dogs and root beer.

Lessons Learned from My Parents

Our mom was fun, energetic, gritty, tough, loving, and had a heart of gold. She loved her dogs and instilled compassion and kindness in all her kids. Our mom was the "rock" of our family. She was our guiding light.

Mom really turned her life around from a health standpoint starting at the age of 55. Mom began eating better, exercised multiple times per week, and became known in my seminars as the "Bionic Women" due to her multiple surgeries that included ankle fusion and knee and hip replacements. Mom also had high blood pressure and arthritis.

Mom was determined to get her health back and she did. For over 25 years mom was full of life, medication-free, felt great, and enjoyed vibrant health. When mom and I traveled to some of my speaking events, I would just sit back and watch her work the room. Her passion to share her newfound health was extremely contagious.

Mom was a wonderful example that it is never too late to turn your health and life around, and she enjoyed vibrant health during the last years of her life. Mom died a few years ago at the age of 83 due to dementia.

Our dad died over 10 years ago at the age of 78. Dad was my guy. He was funny, curious, engaging, loved to play, was a great listener, was non-judgmental, and loved his kids and grandkids. Dad was not a healthy guy. He skipped breakfast, rarely moved his body, had trouble sleeping at night, and was chronically dehydrated. He always told me his coffee had water in it. Dad ate whatever he wanted whenever he wanted. Dad would ask me on a regular basis, "You feel good, don't you"? He would then say, "I don't think I have ever experienced what it is like to truly feel good." I think dad wanted to feel good, but never got on track with his health.

There are two things I want you to keep in mind as you read through this book. First, don't feel like you must do it all at once. Start slowly and take it one step at a time. This was one big mistake I made with my dad. I overwhelmed him. I wanted dad to feel great and have vibrant health. I would ask him to drink more water, drink less coffee, walk daily, use the foam roller, strength train, eat more fruits, have a big salad, make a healthy smoothie, and work on his breathing. I wanted him to do it all—and it was too much!

Second, I always told dad how much I loved him, but I never told him how much I needed him. Tell people in your world how much you love them, but also tell them how much you need them, and remember how much you are loved and needed.

Here's to Feeling Your Best!

2 Health Our Greatest Asset

I truly believe we are at a crossroads when it comes to our health. Hopefully the pandemic provided an awareness that we all need to take care of our health because it is the greatest asset we own.

There have been many incredible advances in health, fitness, and wellness over the last decade, but are we getting healthier as a society? Some of our latest advances or trends include wearable devices, CBD, intermittent fasting, paleo, keto, collagen protein, CrossFit, Peloton, the Mirror, outdoor fitness, digital fitness, remote personal training, mindfulness, meditation, telehealth, and telemedicine to name just a few. Will some of these new advances become trends that will help us move our society in a healthier direction or will many become fads that will quickly disappear?

Where Has Our Health Gone?

Even with greater advances in medicine, improved technology, more highly trained health professionals, more medications to choose from, wearables that track our stress, breath, sleep, movement, and just about anything that has to do with the health of the mind and body, Americans are doing a poor job when it comes to managing their health.

Obesity has never been higher. Type 2 diabetes has exploded around the world. Digestive health, cancer, heart disease, mental health, and the list of our health challenges continues to grow. The quality of health in the United States and around the globe is moving in the wrong direction.

The United States spends more on healthcare, or as many refer to it as "sickcare," than any other developed nation around the world. Healthcare costs in the United States gobble up 17.5 percent of our GDP to a tune of over $3.5 trillion each year. This equates to over $10,000 per person per year spent on healthcare. Most other countries spend a much lower percentage of their GDP on healthcare, coming in at under 9 percent. Switzerland comes in second to the United States at 12 percent.

If the United States spends the most on healthcare, does that mean that we have the best health? The answer is NO. The United States does not even rank in the top 25 of the healthiest countries in the world. Here is a glimpse at per capita spending on healthcare around the world. Keep in mind these costs continue to rise with no end in sight.

Healthcare Costs Per Capita

- United States: $10,000
- Switzerland: $8,000
- Norway: $6,300
- Germany: $5,700
- Ireland: $5,500
- France: $4,900
- Canada: $4,800
- Australia: $2,500

The Sad State of Health in the United States

- In 1960, 1 in 4,000 people in the United States was diagnosed with type 2 diabetes. Today that number is 1 in 10, trending to 1 in 4.
- Today, one of every three Medicare dollars is spent on type 2 diabetes.
- The United States and New Zealand are the only countries in the world that allow direct-to-consumer drug ads.
- Over 50 percent of the United States population over the age of 65 is on 5 prescription medications.
- Since 1995 the use of anti-depressant medications for teens and adults in the United States has risen over 500 percent.
- Chronic illnesses account for over 85 percent of all money spent on healthcare in the United States.
- Around the world more than $60 billion are spent each year on cholesterol-lowering medications.
- More than 35 percent of women over the age of 50 have thyroid problems or poor bone health.
- In 1970 less than 10 percent of the United States population was considered obese. Today, nearly 3 out of 4 adults are overweight or obese.
- Seventy-two percent of young people between of the ages of 17 and 24 do not qualify for military service because of exceptionally high levels of obesity and poor fitness levels.

The list of everyday problems for many adults continues to grow, including high blood pressure, hormonal imbalances, thyroid issues, atrial fibrillation, type 2 diabetes, obesity, sleep problems, high stress, acid reflux, gout, digestive health issues, allergies, asthma, and arthritis among others.

Medication Free in Her 80s

A few years ago, my mother, 81 at the time, suffered a medical emergency. At the hospital they asked mom what medications she was taking. She replied that she did not take any medications. They then looked at me for confirmation, thinking her memory was failing. I confirmed the fact that my mother knew exactly what she was talking about. They were very surprised and said that they rarely see anyone in their 80s who does not take multiple medications.

Treat the Source Not the Symptom

Unfortunately, most of our healthcare professionals are compensated to fix the symptom not the source of the problem. In many cases our healthcare professionals are incentivized to prescribe a medication or recommend surgery, rather than going after the source of the problem. Why is your blood pressure too high? Why are you having trouble sleeping? Why do you have acid reflux or gout? Why is your knee bothering you? There needs to be a large paradigm shift in the practice of care and how our healthcare professionals get paid for the services they provide.

Bring A New Perspective to Healthcare

Imagine if everyone looked at healthcare from a new perspective. Imagine viewing healthcare as a security blanket. It is there if we need it, but we rarely use it! It is time take back control of our health. Our goal should be having more healthy people, not more healthcare options.

There are multiple reasons why we are moving in the wrong direction when it comes to our health. High levels of stress, lack of sleep, lack of movement, easy access to processed foods and beverages, and poor access to healthcare are just a few of the problems we face that prevent us from living a life in good health.

Looking deeper into our healthcare system in the United States, I think most would agree that we have an incredible trauma care system in place. We are great at putting out fires. If we break a leg or get into a car accident, our healthcare system is the best.

Unfortunately, most of the resources in our current healthcare system are set up to fix people when they are broken. There is little focus on prevention and the quality of a person's health. We have become fixated on the cure and preoccupied with disease rather than prevention.

Our latest cancer research efforts are focused on developing medications that strengthen our immune system. Imagine if we took a different approach and began educating every person on how the immune system works along with simple strategies to rejuvenate it.

During the COVID-19 pandemic, most of our efforts were focused on wearing a mask, washing our hands, social distancing, and most importantly the vaccine. All were necessary components for slowing down the pandemic.

Unfortunately, not much information was given on how to play offense with our health. Little was said about how stress can weaken our immune system and compromise our health. Little was said about promoting strategies on how to balance our nervous system, how to breathe to calm the mind and relax the body, how to get enough sleep and stay hydrated, how to improve gut health, and the importance of moving the body. These are all things that help the mind and body feel and be their best.

The way we currently train most of our healthcare professionals is predicated on a model that the human body heals in isolation. The future psychiatrist needs training in gut health and how the microbiome in the gut affects mental health. The primary care physician needs more training in nutrition to help patients prevent or reverse type 2 diabetes. The physical therapist needs to have a better understanding of stress and rest and how they can impact the recovery process. This is going to take time, but when we start looking at the bigger picture of health and work together, we can achieve a future of greater care.

A Person or a Protocol?

Going in for my annual physical a few years back I had an interesting experience. After taking my vitals and measuring my height and weight, the nurse reviewed my results and informed me that my BMI (Body Mass Index) of 26.0 classified me as borderline obese. Because I have a bit more muscle mass, the BMI calculation classified me as obese. Next, she said that my low resting heart rate of 47 was bradycardic (under 60 beats per minute,) and she was concerned that it was extremely low. Finally, she stated that my resting blood pressure of 106/70 was too low and wanted to know if I was lightheaded on a regular basis.

The point is that she was only looking at numbers and not looking at the patient. The nurse never once asked anything about my lifestyle.

Here is what she could have asked.

Do you have a lot of stress in your life?
Are you a chest or diaphragmatic breather?
How much sleep do you get and is it restful?
What type of downtime activities do you practice?
How much exercise do you get on regular basis?
What type of movement activities do you enjoy?

> *Tell me about your nutritional habits.*
> *How much water do you drink each day?*
> *Do you fast on a regular basis?*
> *How is your energy?*
> *Are your low resting heart and blood pressure numbers typical for you?*
> *Once the doctor came in, he confirmed that the numbers showed something different than my actual condition and that I was out of the norm. However, they had to follow a certain protocol to review the numbers based on my age. I truly believe these healthcare professionals meant well but following a structured protocol without looking at the patient or asking better questions is not the answer.*

Future of Healthcare

Okay enough of the doom and gloom. I wanted to tee up some of the challenges we are all facing to make that point that now is the time for everyone to get in the game of health. Changing our healthcare system for the health of our people can and must be done. There are many incredible minds working tirelessly to improve our current healthcare system. Here are a few strategies that must take place for a healthier world.

Price Transparency in Healthcare Costs

Lack of price transparency is a problem in our current healthcare system. Did you know that the price of a knee replacement surgery ranges between $25,000-$60,000, or the price of a heart bypass surgery ranges between $70,000-$350,000? Why is there such a large disparity in pricing for the same procedures?

We have a pretty good handle on what most of the goods and services we use daily are going to cost. We would never buy a car, go to the movies, get a haircut, buy a pair of shoes, have a massage, or even buy a house without a good idea as to how much it was going to cost. We need to have this same type of price transparency when it comes to our healthcare services. Imagine if there was a menu of procedures, services, and medications with the price tag next to each. Like a menu at your favorite restaurant.

- Colonoscopy: $1,500
- Knee Replacement: $25,000
- Heart Bypass: $80,000
- Childbirth (vaginal delivery): $10,000
- Cholesterol Medication: $200 per month
- Dialysis Treatment: $150 per visit

This type of price transparency is currently being done by many surgical centers around the United States. We need to bring price transparency across all our healthcare systems.

Increased Competition for Healthcare Services

Having competition in any market keeps everyone on top of their game. If there was only one grocery store in town, they could increase prices, and in most cases, not lose a single customer. Why would you pay $30,000 more for the same surgical procedure or $200 more per month for the same medication? What if you had the option to shop around for the best quality of care at a fair market price?

Studies have shown that hospital prices in monopoly markets are 15 percent higher than those with multiple hospitals in the same region. We need to have competition in healthcare to maintain high quality at a fair price.

New Technology

The amount of new and exciting technology coming into the healthcare market has exploded and will continue to expand at a rapid pace. This new technology will drive industry-wide transformation with new diagnostic procedures, healthcare data analytics, artificial intelligence, telemedicine, and security solutions just to name a few. There are many medical advancements currently taking place to improve health outcomes.

There has also been an explosion of personalized fitness tracking wearables. These devices can help measure almost everything we do during the day or night including the amount of stress we have, how much sleep we get, how many breaths we take during the day and night, and how our heart is beating and the variations it goes through every 24 hours. They also track how active we are by tracking steps, body movements, and even how much we sit on a typical day.

Personal Tracking Devices

Many people ask me what I think about all these personalized tracking devices. I think they can be beneficial in creating a sense of awareness of our own health and can also be beneficial when used by many healthcare professionals to learn more about their patients.

Imagine a future doctor's appointment where you breathe or speak into an Artificial Intelligence Box. The information is then transcribed for your health professional to make the necessary recommendations.

Let's Return to the Art of Healthcare

Our healthcare system's focus has been and continues to be placed on treating the symptom rather than the source of the problem. Matching the procedure or pill to the illness is not the answer. The future of healthcare must move in the direction of prevention, on thriving not just surviving, on playing offense versus defense. This is our future.

Our Greatest Asset Essentials

Big Picture

- Health quality around the world continues to decline.
- Healthcare costs in the United States gobble up 17.5 percent of our GDP to a tune of over $3.5 trillion/year.
- The United States spends more on healthcare than any other country in the world.
- Too much time and energy, and too many resources are spent on trying to find cures rather than on prevention.
- The future of healthcare must move in the direction of prevention.
- We are on the verge of a wellness revolution when it comes to health.

Ask Yourself

- Why is the quality of health in the United States declining when we have the latest technology in medicine?
- Did you know that chronic illnesses account for over 85 percent of all money spent on healthcare in the United States?
- Did you know that the average 65-year-old in the United States takes five prescription medications?
- What would result if everyone looked at our healthcare system from a new perspective?

Small Steps

- Take steps to improve your health. This will contribute to the improvement of our entire healthcare system.
- Ask better questions when working with your healthcare professional.
- Change your mindset and take back control of your health.

3 Creating a New Future

The real key to improving our health in the United States and around the globe is to get back to the basics of how we **REST**, **EAT**, and **MOVE**. As I just pointed out, there are many ways to improve our current healthcare system. The greatest movement will come when we focus on prevention.

It is not fair to our healthcare professionals to walk into their office with broken sleep, digestive health problems, high blood pressure, and hormonal imbalances and expect to be fixed in a 15-minute visit.

We all need to take more ownership in our health and work together with our healthcare professionals. The answer is not trying to make our healthcare system more efficient. The answer is getting our people healthier, and everyone must play their part.

Taking Responsibility for Our Own Health

Medical Literacy

We must become smarter when it comes to our health. Medical illiteracy has never been greater than it is today.

Why do we know so little about our medical world? Do you know the cost of a colonoscopy or the cost of medications for type 2 diabetes, blood pressure, or cholesterol? Do you know that homocysteine is a powerful predictor for heart health or that testosterone levels can provide great insight into the aging process for both men and women? Do you know that learning how to use the diaphragm correctly when breathing can quiet the mind and improve blood pressure? Why do we know so little about how to get a good night of sleep or one of the greatest sciences of all, nutrition?

It is this lack of knowledge that keeps many in the dark about taking greater control of their health. Nobody knows your body better than you. We need to learn how to listen to our body, and this needs to be taught at an early age.

Asking Better Questions

Asking better questions comes from knowledge. If we are kept in the dark about our health, it becomes extremely difficult to ask the right questions. Over the next six sections you will learn how to **REST**, how to **EAT**, and how to **MOVE**. You will also learn how to decode your health, improve your numbers, stay motivated, and develop a plan for the rest of your life. As you travel through the rest of this book, your knowledge will grow, giving you the necessary tools to ask better questions. Remember, in the question lies the real answer.

Endless Possibilities

We all have blind spots in our life when it comes to imagining what is truly possible.

A few years ago, my wife Paula and I were in Arizona. At our hotel an astronomer giving hotel guests a peek through the lens of his telescope on one of the largest portable telescopes in the world. This was one big telescope! Guests were raving about this guy. His energy and passion for the planets and stars was extremely contagious. He asked us if we would like to see a second galaxy. My response was, "Are you kidding, you can see a second galaxy through your telescope?"

When I looked through the lens of this incredible telescope, it was like I had stepped into another world with thousands of stars, planets, and a second galaxy. In an instant my world seemed extremely small.

Better Health is a Decision

Are you sitting on the fence? Still wobbling back and forth, thinking about going "all in" and making necessary changes with your health? I understand this is a tough conversation to have with yourself, but it is exactly where you need to be to begin. What do you want? As I write this book, I am 64 years young, and I cannot say that I have this "health thing" all figured out. I have, however, learned and experimented along the way and know what works. It has been a journey and a process, mixed with decisions, patience, mistakes, and perseverance.

Many people are confused when it comes to their health. There is an incredible amount of information to sift through and determine what is correct and what is not. Everyone is going to take a different path or journey. That is why telling a person to eat this and not that or to follow this particular workout will never work. Guidance is good, structure is good, but a rigid plan cannot and will not work long term.

I believe everyone wants to feel good and there are endless ways to make us feel good temporarily. But there is a better, more sustainable way to help you feel and be your best.

It's Never Too Late to Start

Years ago, I received a phone call from one of my longtime colleagues and good friend, Mike Combes. At the time Mike was the Executive Director of three large health clubs in Cincinnati, Ohio. Mike asked, "I know you are coming back to Cincinnati in a few weeks. Would you be willing to meet one of our shining stars, Joan Barber?" He went on to tell me that Joan attended one of my seminars a few years ago and has since lost over 150 pounds. She also went from 16 medications to 3. And get this, Joan began her journey at the age of 65! I was very excited to meet Joan and learn her story.

During our meeting Joan introduced me to her husband Clarence. Then Joan began by telling me about her journey and how she did it. Joan said, "You talked about taking small steps by building one habit at a time, so I stopped drinking soda pop and started drinking only water. I began eating closer to the source with more fruit, vegetables, nuts, salads, and I upgraded what I was eating. Then I started moving my body for 10 minutes every day and eventually began strength training in the pool. Inch by inch, step by step, I built some new healthy habits and the momentum continued to grow."

It was great to learn how Joan did it, but what I really wanted to know from Joan was her "WHY." Why did she do it? What was Joan's driver for this incredible change to take place? In my over 30-plus years in the health and fitness industry, I have never seen anyone take on this type of challenge at the age of 65. Something very powerful must have been pulling on Joan to make this change!

Okay Joan, the big question—WHY? What drove you to make this incredible transformation? Joan said, "It began with my husband Clarence. Clarence and I have been married for over 40 years. Clarence has two loves in his life. His first love is his love for me." She starts to smile, and Clarence starts to smile. "His second love is his love for motorcycles. Due to my size and poor health, Clarence and I had not ridden a motorcycle together in many years. So, I decided it was time to give Clarence back his second love and start riding again."

By creating this powerful emotion around her love for Clarence, Joan created the leverage necessary for her new behaviors. When Joan felt stuck or frustrated, she kept coming back to her powerful emotion of her and Clarence riding a motorcycle together. Joan also shared that over time she started to enjoy the journey she was on. Today Clarence and Joan are in a motorcycle club in Cincinnati and ride together on a regular basis. Joan's story is a great reminder that it is never too late to create a new future!

Are You Living Your Best Life?

What is your vision for your future? Does your health matter? Imagine having greater health, energy, and vitality. How would this impact your future? Are you thriving or just surviving? What new worlds do you want to emerge?

The human body has an incredible ability to heal and self-correct if given the chance. The seeds planted today lead to tomorrow's harvest.

Are You Ready to Change?

When speaking, I like to end each event by asking the audience a few simple questions.

First: Are you ready? Are you ready to make a change? The audience overwhelming puts up their hands and says, YES!

Second: Are you able? Are you able to make a change? Do you have the necessary skills to make a change? Hands again go shooting up and almost everyone again says YES in a loud robust voice.

Now comes the moment of truth. Are you willing? Are you willing to get a little uncomfortable? Are you willing to put in the necessary effort to create sustainable change? Are you willing to take that first step? Unfortunately, not everyone is as fired up as they were just a minute ago. They now realize that to change they must put in the work, and not everyone is ready to put in the work. Willing is a choice!

As we can see from Joan's story, climbing any mountain begins by taking that first step. We all have bridges to cross in our lives and now is the time to cross your bridge. And remember, you do not have to cross your bridge alone.

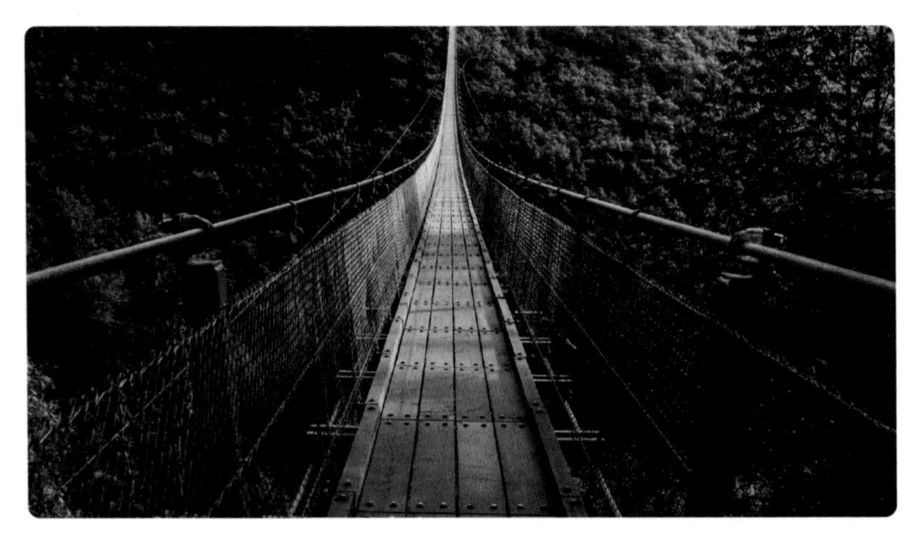

Creating A New Future Essentials

Big Picture

- Your journey for greater health and feeling your best begins in your mind.
- When we open our eyes, heart, and mind, our world becomes full of possibilities.
- Everyone is going to take a different path or journey. The key is to find your own path to follow.
- Joan's story is a great reminder that it is never too late to create a new future.
- Climbing any mountain begins by taking that first step.
- We all have bridges to cross in our lives and now is the time to cross your bridge. Remember, you do not have to cross your bridge alone!

Ask Yourself

- What is your vision for your future?
- Does your health matter to you?
- Are you thriving or just surviving?
- Are you ready to make a change?
- Are you willing to take that first step?
- Are you willing to get a little uncomfortable and understand that you must put in the work.

Small Steps

- Decide today that you can and will develop the future you desire.
- Start planting seeds today for your harvest tomorrow.
- Believe that you have the power to feel your best!

4 The Secret of Change

What is the secret of change? How do we make lifestyle changes stick? That is the challenge that everyone faces. We want to lose weight, have more energy, eat healthier, start working out, become more fit, the list goes on. What holds us back? The secret of change begins with self-awareness and ends when you decide that you are going to make a change.

The Story of Grabwell Grommet

-Art Hoppe, satirist and columnist for the *San Francisco Chronicle*

On the morning of his 42nd birthday, Grabwell Grommet awoke to the sound of ominous thunder. Glancing out the window with bleary eyes, he saw written in fiery letters:

"SOMEONE IS TRYING TO KILL YOU, GRABWELL GROMMET!"

With shaking hands, Grommet lit his first cigarette of the day. He didn't question the message. You don't question messages like that. His only question was, Who?

At breakfast as he salted his fried eggs and buttered his toast, he told his wife Gratia, "Someone is trying to kill me."

"Who?" she asked in horror.

Grabwell slowly stirred the cream and sugar into his coffee and shook his head, "I don't know," he said.

Convinced though he was, Grabwell wasn't going to the police with his story. He decided his only course was to go about his daily routine and hope somehow to outwit his would-be murderer. He tried to think on the drive to the office. But the frustration of making time by beating the lights and switching lanes occupied him wholly. Nor, once behind the desk, could he think a moment what with jangling phones, urgent memos and the problems and decisions piling in as they did each day.

It wasn't until his second martini at lunch that the full terror of his position struck him. It was all he could do to finish his Lasagna Milanese. "I can't panic," he said to himself, lighting his cigar. "I simply must live my life as usual."

He worked until seven as usual. Drove home fast as usual. Studied business reports as usual. And he took his two sleeping pills in order to get his usual six hours of sleep. As days passed, Grabwell fully stuck to his routine. And as months went by, he began to take perverse pleasure in his ability to survive. "Whoever's trying to get me," he'd say proudly to his wife, "hasn't got me yet. I'm too smart for him."

> *"Oh, please be careful," she'd reply, ladling him a second helping of beef stroganoff. The pride grew as he managed to go on living for years. But as it must to all men, death came at last to Grabwell. It came at his desk on a particularly busy day. He was 53. His grief-stricken widow demanded a full autopsy. But it showed only emphysema, arteriosclerosis, ulcers, cirrhosis of the liver, cardiac necrosis, cardiovascular aneurysm, pulmonary edema, obesity, high blood pressure, and a touch of lung cancer.*
>
> *"How glad Grabwell would have been to know," said his widow smiling proudly through her tears, "that he died of natural causes."*

You Can Change!

Developing new lifestyle habits can be challenging for all of us. Change is a true constant in life, but how do we convince ourselves to make a change? This is the challenge we all face in different areas of our life. The diet industry is a great example of how difficult change can be. In 2019 the United States spent over $60 billion in the weight loss industry with more than a 95 percent failure rate. People want to lose weight. They invest their precious resources of time and money, but something is missing.

Five Steps to Sustainable Change

Here are the steps to sustainable behavior change. There is a great deal to unpack here. Take it slow as these points will be discussed throughout the rest of this book. Changing behavior is not easy, but people can and do change.

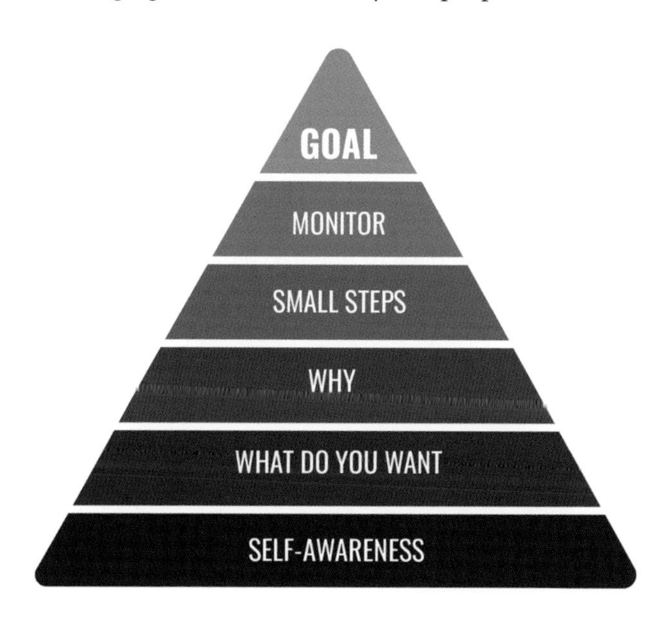

Step 1: Self-Awareness

The story of Grabwell Grommet is a great example of the lack of self-awareness. Grabwell had no idea that his unhealthy lifestyle was slowly killing him. He was ducking, hiding, running away, and trying to elude his killer when in fact he was the killer. Grabwell had many blind spots.

We all have blind spots. How about you? What blind spots do you have?

How many breaths do you take per minute? ________________

What is your resting heart rate? ________________

What is your blood pressure? ________________

How many ounces of water do you drink on average each day? ________

How much time do you spend moving your body on a typical day?

____

Do you consume omega-3 or omega-6 fats on a regular basis? Yes or No

How many hours of sleep do you get per night? ________________

How many hours of screen time do you spend in a typical day? ________

Lack of awareness is a killer for all of us when trying to make a change. If we are not aware, it is impossible to make a change. We all have blind spots in our life, and changing any behavior begins with self-awareness.

Self-awareness is the ability to step outside yourself to make a calculated conscious decision. Once you begin to look around, what do you see? What do you feel? What must change? Are you ready to make a change? On a 1 to 10 scale, are you a 5 or and 8? Maybe you are a 10 and cannot wait to get rolling.

Maybe some of you are thinking, if I am a 3 or 4, then what is necessary to take that first step? Is there something that is holding me back? Some people may feel trapped. Many have tried to make a change before but may have failed. I am here to tell you that everyone can make a change. Having the awareness that you must make a change is step one in your pursuit to feeling and being your best.

How ready are you on a 1-10 scale to make a change? ______________

What has held you back in the past? ______________________________

What blind spots are now coming into view?

____

Step 2: What Do You Want?

Okay, now it is time to develop a clear picture or image in your mind of what you want. Imagine a healthier and fitter you. What does that look like? What does that feel like? Would you like to improve your blood pressure or balance your cholesterol profile? Increase your flexibility and balance? Ski with your grandkids? Walk in the Grand Canyon? Run or walk a 5K? Get stronger? Get off your acid reflux or gout medications? Decrease your back pain? Is your energy and stamina where you would like it to be? How about your sleep? Your body weight? Would you like to balance your hormones? Maybe your health is starting to fade, and your blood work needs to be improved. Or maybe you have begun taking a few medications and do not like where you are heading. Get specific about what you want. If your goal is to lose weight, determine how many pounds, by when, how you will look, how you will feel, how you will move, how it will impact your life. Creating a clear picture in your mind of what you want is very powerful.

Do you have a clear picture of what you want? Yes or No

Are you willing to contemplate your future now? Yes or No

What are the top 3 things you want? Be very specific.

____

____

____

Step 3: Power of WHY

The longer I have been in this space of health and fitness, the more I realize the power of finding our "WHY." Our WHY is the jet fuel for change to take place. It is the emotion that can pull us all out of the mud when we want to give up. When consulting with clients who want to make a healthier lifestyle change, I must help them tap in to their WHY.

When I was speaking in Michigan many years ago, two women approached me and said they had heard me speak multiple times and knew I was all about finding your WHY. They wanted to share their WHY. "Well, the two of us got in a weight loss contest. We both lost over 30 pounds." Here comes their WHY. "The loser had to eat a can of cat food."

When I tell this story, the audience laughs. It is a fun story about how a simple emotion can drive human behavior. The cat food is a small WHY, but a powerful one. Finding a small WHY can be easy and can change like the seasons. Maybe you want to look better for an upcoming wedding or class reunion or increase your flexibility and suppleness so you can work in the yard or play golf again with less back pain. We all need small or short-term WHYs to keep us engaged!

Here comes the challenge. How do you find a "Big WHY?" Going back to Joan's story, over the years Joan had tried to lose weight multiple times with little success. What Joan was missing was the emotional leverage necessary to keep her on track. When Joan's WHY went outside of her, the magic truly began for her. Joan's WHY no longer was just about losing weight. It was much more. Every time she felt like giving up, Joan would think about her husband Clarence and his love for motorcycles. She was driven to give Clarence his second love.

A few years ago, we held an On Target Living Challenge to start the New Year. Over 2,000 people signed up. One of the assignments of the challenge was to come up with your WHY. Reading through all the WHYs, I was pleasantly surprised by the number of people who bared their souls on what was driving them to make a change. One WHY that stood out to our team was from a woman in Seattle. She shared that she needed to get healthier and stronger so she could take care of her disabled son as he grew older. She was his caregiver and his love. She knew if she did not get healthier, she would not be able to care for him. WOW! Reading her story, you could feel the power in her voice. She had enough rocket fuel to go to the moon and back.

Remember, your WHY must always be bigger than your BUT!

What is your small WHY? ______________________________

____

What is your big WHY? ______________________________

____

Step 4: Build a Habit One Step at a Time

Where many people get it wrong is that they try to go too fast. They want results NOW! "I want to lose 30 pounds, so I am going to eat only vegetables, drink only water, and workout and meditate for 60 minutes, 7 days a week." This is a blueprint for failure.

Building sustainable habits takes focus, energy, and time. How can we process everything happening all around us without being completely distracted? It starts in the mind. Our mind has three stages of consciousness that filter our perceptions and thoughts: the conscious mind, subconscious mind, and unconscious mind.

The Conscious Mind

The conscious mind is where our habits begin. It is like working with a piece of clay. It is soft, pliable, and can take on infinite shapes. We can squeeze it and mold it, but all this takes focus, energy, and effort to form the shape we want. Remember when you first learned how to tie your shoes, ride a bike, or drive a car? It took some time and focused energy. Imagine if we had to focus on every little task to start our day: brush our teeth, take a shower, get dressed, put on our shoes, and drive to work. I think we would all be exhausted by 10 a.m. Building a new habit begins in the conscious mind and takes a great deal of focus, energy, and effort.

The Subconscious Mind

The subconscious mind is where most of our habits live. It allows us to process information much faster and with considerably less energy than the conscious mind. Once a habit enters the subconscious mind, it is like going into a vault, locked away but easy to draw upon and execute. Most of our daily habits, like taking a shower, brushing our teeth, getting dressed, having a cup of coffee, looking at our phone, eating breakfast, and driving to work, are on autopilot. It is the subconscious mind that allows our brain to rest a good part of the day.

Unfortunately, when stress is in the mix, our new conscious habits can easily be put on the back burner. We let our guard down, we lose focus, and we lose energy. Most of the time we revert right back to the easy button of our old comfortable habits that live in our subconscious mind. Those conscious habits that we tried to build are hard to resume.

The Unconscious Mind

The unconscious mind is the limitless reservoir of knowledge, creativity, and experiences that make up the largest part of the mind. We have all experienced a time when taking a shower or going for a long walk, some incredible insights pop into our mind. Where did these thoughts and insights come from? They came from the unconscious mind. The unconscious mind holds the answers to many of our questions and challenges.

Because of its infinite capacity, the unconscious mind can be the most powerful part of our mind. To access this information on demand takes training and the ability to quiet the mind. You will learn more about how to quiet the mind and access the unconscious mind in Section 3: Rest, Relaxation, and Rejuvenation.

HUMAN MIND MODEL

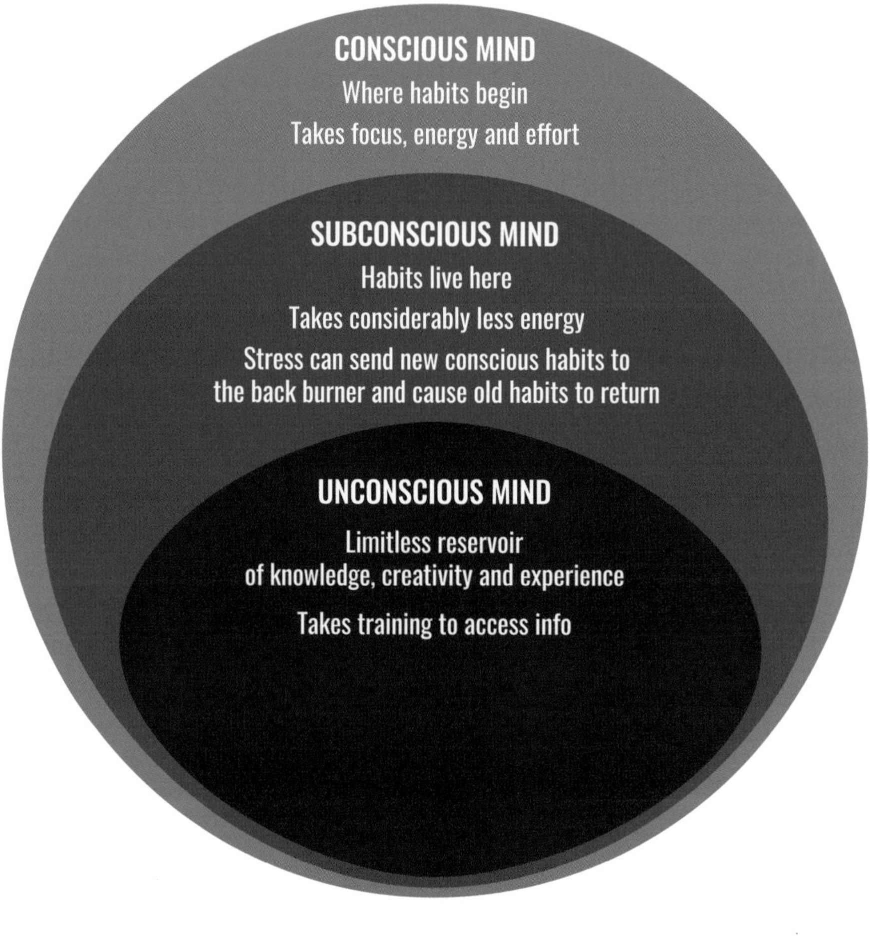

CONSCIOUS MIND

Where habits begin

Takes focus, energy and effort

SUBCONSCIOUS MIND

Habits live here

Takes considerably less energy

Stress can send new conscious habits to the back burner and cause old habits to return

UNCONSCIOUS MIND

Limitless reservoir of knowledge, creativity and experience

Takes training to access info

One Small Step is Better Than No Step at All

A couple of months prior to my presentation to the National Dental Association, I visited my dentist. I asked my hygienist what inside scoop she might have that would help me design my speech to resonate with the crowd. She said, "Why don't you talk about developing the habit of flossing?" She looks at me, I look at her, and we both start to laugh. She knows that I rarely floss. You can't lie to your dental hygienists about flossing. She said, "I am serious. You could build a new habit of flossing and share this with the audience. They would love it." "Okay," I responded. "Please guide me." She advised me to start flossing two times per week. When I asked if that was enough, she replied, "Since you don't currently floss, it is a great start." As I walked out the door I was all fired up about my new flossing plan. In the weeks leading up to the conference I began flossing multiple times per week. I have now become a flossing machine.

When the conference finally arrived, I began my presentation in front of a few thousand dentists and dental hygienists telling my flossing story. The audience was laughing and was super engaged. It was a fantastic opening. Suddenly, a dentist in the front row stated loudly, "Flossing 2-3 times per week is not enough. You need to floss every day." Boom! In an instant the energy in the room evaporated. There was dead silence. After a long pause, I asked the dentist, "How often do you exercise?" He sheepishly answered, "I currently do not exercise." I asked, "If you went for a 10-minute walk a few times a week, do you think that would be good start?"

A few months later I received an email from this same dentist. He said "I want you to know that you inspired me to start taking small steps to improve my health and my life. I walk daily and am now working out with a trainer once each week. I am drinking more water, eating oatmeal with berries and nuts for breakfast, and taking cod liver oil. I have lost 10 pounds and my blood pressure has drastically improved!"

Just like my flossing practice, one small step developed into a lifetime habit.

The key to building a lifestyle that you can love and sustain is learning how to build habits, and you do this by taking **One Step at A Time!**

What is one new habit you would like to build starting today?

____

What is one new habit that you would like to build in the future?

____

Step 5: Feedback

Feedback is the breakfast of champions! We all need regular feedback to measure our new behaviors and habits to see if they are working. We also must have the courage to measure. There are many ways to measure, monitor, and get the feedback necessary to keep us on track. The body is always talking, and we must learn to listen!

Do you monitor your bodyweight? Yes or No

Do you get your blood pressure checked monthly? Yes or No

Do you get your blood work checked on an annual basis? Yes or No

Do you know how many breaths do you take per minute? Yes or No

Do you know your resting heart rate? Yes or No

How many hours of sleep are you getting? ____________

Can you stand with your back against the wall with great posture or get up and off the floor with ease? Yes or No

Success Depends on Feedback

Years ago, I was watching a documentary about the weight loss industry. They were interviewing Eric, a past winner from the TV show, The Biggest Loser. Eric went from 416 pounds to 198 pounds, winning the $250,000 first place prize. He became an overnight success story. Fast forward 18 months, and Eric was being interviewed about his journey. He began by talking about his time on the show, the excitement, the comradery, and how driven he was to win. He said he loved it all except the weekly weigh-ins which were extremely stressful.

Eric then began to talk about what was going on in his life today. He felt as though he had slowly lost his way. The interviewer asked him to elaborate. He said that he started reverting back to many of his old habits of drinking soda pop and eating fast food. He stopped working out. The interviewer asked how much he weighed now. He said that he knew he gained some weight back, but he wasn't sure how much. Then he got on the scale.

This was a live interview, the emotions were real, and you could feel Eric's anxiety as he was about to step on the scale. The scale read 412 pounds. Then there was this long silence. The look on Eric's face was devastating. He had gained all his weight back. Everyone could feel Eric's pain and sadness in that moment. As the interview continued, we learned more about Eric's way of thinking and his beliefs. Eric believed he needed to eat only 1,500 calories and exercise for 2-3 hours every day to keep his weight off. His unrealistic goals, expectations, and beliefs, wrapped with little or no feedback, was a recipe for disaster. We all need some type of feedback to keep us on track and help us pivot when necessary.

How do you plan to monitor your success?

____

Journey of Change

As we begin our journey of change, we can expect to encounter a few roadblocks or challenges along the way.

Stage 1 of our journey begins in the "Honeymoon" stage. The honeymoon stage is a time of bliss. Everything is working great, and we are extremely focused. Our energy and excitement is off the charts, and we are driven.

Stage 2 of our journey is the "Honeymoon is Over" stage. It is during this stage that we may begin to lose some of our motivation. The shiny penny may have lost some of its luster. Our new habits are not yet locked in, and our plan now feels like work. The slope from Stage 2 to Stage 3 is steep and slippery.

Stage 3 is "The Valley of Despair" stage. It is during this stage when most people give up. The journey has become more difficult than expected. We begin to feel stuck and start to believe we cannot do it. We must not give up.

Stage 4, the "Habit" stage, is when habits start taking hold.

Stage 5, the "Ritual" stage, is when habits have turned in to daily rituals.

Stages 4 and 5 take deliberate practice and time to develop. Once habits and rituals are built, success will follow.

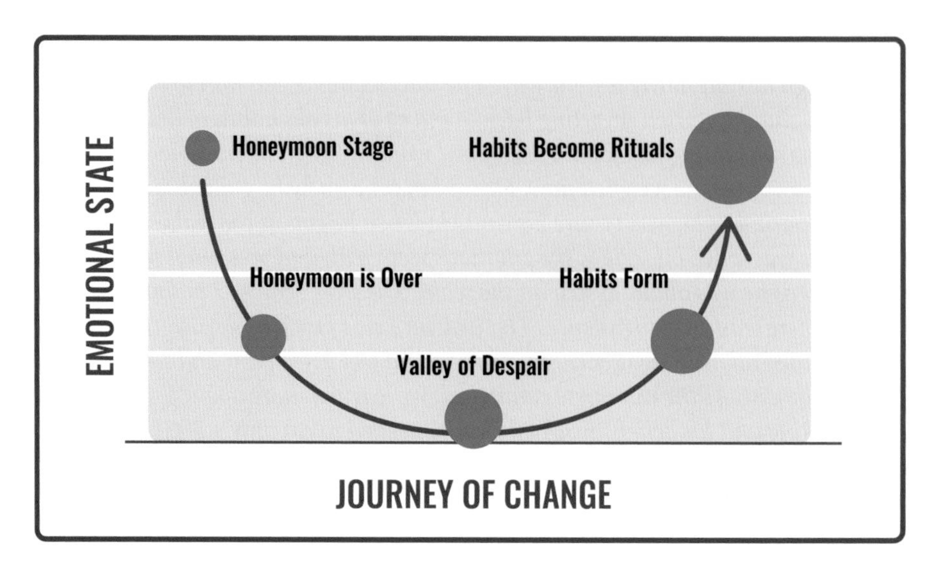

As you continue to work through this book, don't lose hope. Come back and read this chapter repeatedly. You can do this. Visualize a clear picture of what you want. Determine your powerful WHY. What steps can you take? Do not give up; you can do this!

The Secret of Change is to focus all your energy NOT on fighting the old but ***BUILDING the NEW!***

Socrates

The Secret of Change Essentials

Big Picture

- Grabwell was unaware that his unhealthy lifestyle was slowly killing him.
- Developing new lifestyles habits can be challenging for all of us.
- Changing behavior is not easy, but people can and do change.
- The 5 steps to sustainable behavior change include: self-awareness, what you want, power of WHY, one step at a time, and feedback.
- Journey of Change—we all must experience our own journey!

Ask Yourself

- We all have blind spots in our life when it comes to our health. What blind spots do you have?
- Do you have a clear picture of what you want or would like to improve?
- What is driving you to make a change?
- What is one new habit you would like to develop?
- How are you going to monitor your success?

Small Steps

- Take a few minutes now to uncover a possible blind spot.
- Name the top three things that you want.
- Build one new behavior that supports your vision.
- Write down your WHY and post it in clear sight.
- Focus all your energy on what you want and what you are going to do!

5 Beginner's Mind

I was enjoying dinner one evening with my friend and colleague,Dr. Phil Nuernberger, one of the leading experts in the world on stress and how to use the mind. We were discussing the topic of "beginner's mind." Phil asked me an interesting question. If I was speaking to a first-grade class and asked them a question, how many hands did I think would go up? I told him I would expect every hand would go up. He agreed and went on to say that most children have a beginner's mind. They are curious. However, many adults are not. When we lose our curiosity, we lose our ability to solve problems, especially when it comes to our health.

Ask A Better Question

When we ask a better question, the question begins to reveal the answer. Throughout the rest of this book, I want you to stay curious and keep asking better questions. Why is my blood pressure starting to rise or my cholesterol out of balance? Why am I having trouble sleeping? Why have I developed acid reflux or gout? Why is my energy low? If a plant was wilted and I wanted to bring the plant back to life, what would I do? Water, sunlight and soil, simple steps to bring the plant back to life.

Here is a question for you. Does a headache indicate a pain medication deficiency? Of course not. But when most people get a headache, the first thing they reach for is ibuprofen or some type of pain medication. Pain may be a symptom of a headache, but what is the source of a headache? It could be dehydration, not enough omega-3 fats, or a magnesium deficiency. Magnesium is one of the most powerful minerals that keeps our bodies healthy and performing at our best. Magnesium is the mineral of relaxation and helps with many things including blood pressure, sleep, muscles, the heart, and headaches.

When you stay curious and ask better questions, you open up your world to endless possibilities.

Ending Unending Hiccups

Not long ago I received a phone call from a woman in Florida who had attended one of my presentations. She was desperate to find help for her husband who had been afflicted with hiccups for over two years. We set up a call with the three of us to learn more.

He suffered from lack of sleep, low energy, and his body ached all the time. He was really struggling. He had been to multiple doctors and was prescribed medications for acid reflux, muscle tension, sleep, and anxiety, all to help him cope with his hiccups.

We began our conversation with a series of questions.

On a 1-10 scale, how would you rate your current stress level?

Do you breathe with your chest or belly? Fast or slow breaths?

What do you eat? When do you eat? What beverages do you drink?

How often do you exercise? What do you like to do?

What have you and your doctors discussed?

What challenges or roadblocks have been holding you back?

Do you have a WHY that is driving you?

Have you lost hope?

Quickly a few patterns started to emerge. He stated that he felt stressed most the time and his breathing was short and rapid. For the past five years he was on a high protein, moderate fat, and extremely low carbohydrate diet. He had not eaten a fruit, potato, or grain in those years. His morning routine included 2-3 cups of coffee with butter in it, along with eggs and bacon. His lunch and snacks consisted of protein bars and more coffee. Dinner was meat, an occasional small salad, and two glasses of wine. He believed cutting carbohydrates from his diet was the best way to keep his weight down. As you can see, he also liked his coffee, drinking more than a pot a day.

I explained how his stress, his breathing, his poor diet, and his medications all lead to high acid levels, poor gut health, and vitamin and mineral deficiencies. His body was screaming back with chronic hiccups!

We began with the basics, helping him learn how to reframe some of his repetitive negative self-talk, how to relax his vagus nerve, and how to balance his nervous system by changing how he breathed. Nutritionally, we started with drinking more water with orange and lemon slices, hot water with ginger in the evening, and drinking less coffee and wine.

His beliefs around food were challenging at first, but he was desperate and willing to make a change. His new plan included eating more whole foods and less packaged and processed foods. He added healthy carbohydrates including apples, oranges, bananas, oatmeal, potatoes, vegetables, and superfoods, back into his diet. He also began making a smoothie each day for lunch. His smoothie included frozen berries, banana, coconut water, cacao nibs, almond butter, ginger, spinach, hemp, and ground flaxseed. Step by step he began to make more and more changes, and within 90 days his chronic hiccups slowly disappeared.

Beginner's Mind Essentials

Big Picture

- Having a beginner's mind is a powerful tool for future success.
- When you ask a better question, the question reveals the answer.
- When we lose our curiosity, we lose our ability to solve problems, especially when it comes to our health.

Ask Yourself

- Have you remained curious and willing to ask questions and learn?
- If a plant was wilted and you wanted to bring the plant back to life, what would you do?
- Why has your blood pressure begun to creep up?
- Why is your cholesterol out of balance?
- Why are you having trouble sleeping?
- Why have you developed acid reflux or gout?
- Why is your energy low?

Small Steps

- Watch, learn, and listen.
- Learning how to have a beginner's mind is a skill that takes focus and practice.
- Next time you run into a situation or problem, begin by asking a better question.
- Keep digging. When you stay curious and ask better questions, you open up your world to endless possibilities.

6 Box of Beliefs

The average person experiences over 50,000 thoughts each day. Of those 50,000 thoughts, most are repeated over and over, whether they are good, bad, or indifferent. That is an endless loop of repetitive thoughts that need focus and direction.

Our thoughts control how we think, act, and feel. If our goal is to break our patterns of thought, where should we begin? For many, it may begin with self-awareness surrounding our current beliefs. Beliefs may be holding us back from reaching our true potential. It begins with opening our mind to new possibilities. Our life is what our thoughts make it.

Many of us keep our beliefs in a box and nail it shut. We are not open to learning more about opposing views or alternative options. This is what is termed limiting beliefs. We all have them.

What Beliefs Are in Your Box?

Does your belief box keep you from growing and expanding or keep you fearful of the changing world? Maybe it is time to use the box like a stepping-stone to find new ways of thought to expand your knowledge, horizons, and joy.

Recently at one of our On Target Living retreats I asked the group how many of them felt like they did not have enough time or space to move their body on a daily basis. I was shocked when more than half of the group put their hands up. Many truly believed that they did not have the space in their life to fit in daily movement. When they shared all the reasons why they did not have the time to move their body, it revealed that many wanted to keep their box of beliefs nailed shut.

4 Minute Mile

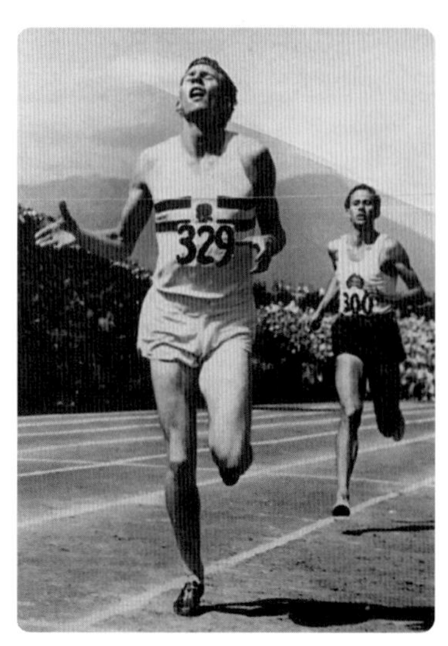

Roger Bannister was the 25-year-old medical student who first cracked track and field's most notorious barrier, the 4-minute mile. Bannister, who was running for the Amateur Athletic Association against his alma mater Oxford University, won that mile race with a time of 3 minutes and 59.4 seconds. He became the first person in the world to break that 4-minute magical barrier!

For years, many athletes had tried and failed to run a mile in less than four minutes. Many believed it to be physically impossible. At the time, the world record for a mile was 4 minutes and 1.3 seconds set by Gunder Hagg of Sweden in 1945. Despite or perhaps because of the psychological mystique surrounding the 4-minute barrier, several runners in the early 1950s dedicated themselves to becoming the first to cross into the 3-minute zone. But it was not until May 6, 1954, that this feat was accomplished by Bannister. Here is the crazy part of the story. Over the next two years, the 4-minute mile barrier was broken 37 times. People now believed it was possible!

Beliefs and Knowledge

Seth Godin, author and former dot com business executive who writes about change, states in his blog that beliefs and knowledge are different. Knowledge changes all the time. When we engage with the world, when we encounter data or new experiences, our knowledge changes. A belief is what we call things that stick around, particularly and especially in the face of changes in knowledge. While more knowledge can change a belief, it usually does not. A belief is a cultural phenomenon, created in conjunction with people around us. The easy way to discern between the two is this question. What would you need to see or learn to change your mind about that?

It is not the lack of knowledge that holds most people back, but their limiting beliefs. Have you ever had a strong belief and at some point realized it was not true?

Commonly Held Limiting Beliefs

- Eating healthy does not taste good.
- Eating healthy is too expensive.
- Eating carbs make you fat.
- A high protein diet makes you lean.
- A high fat diet makes you lean.
- Energy drinks give you better energy.
- Ibuprofen cures headaches.
- The best way to lose weight is to decrease calories.
- You need to exercise more than an hour a day to see results.
- Cardio is the best way to lose weight.
- Exercise is boring.
- You will take more medications as you age.
- High blood pressure or an unbalanced cholesterol is genetic.

Walking on the Moon

On May 25, 1961, President John F. Kennedy announced the dramatic and ambitious goal of sending an American safely to the moon and back before the end of the decade. He, along with many others, believed the United States was falling behind the Soviet Union in the arms race and wanted to change this belief for the entire nation to see. President Kennedy said, "We choose to go to the moon in this decade, not because it will be easy, but because it will be hard. This incredible goal will be extremely hard to accomplish, but if we put our best people, energies and skills in place, anything, including landing on the moon is possible." On July 20, 1969, Neil Armstrong and Edwin "Buzz" Aldrin became the first two men to step on the moon!

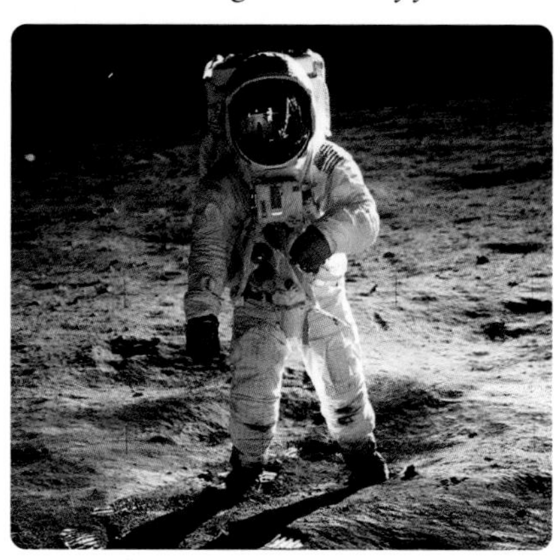

Changing Beliefs

When speaking at live events, I often poll the audience to see how many of them think cod liver oil tastes bad. Most everyone raises their hands. Then I ask them how many believe cod liver tastes bad but have never tried it before. Everyone laughs because they realize they have fallen into the trap of not knowing something but believing it to be true. Then I explain that taking the 1-2 tablespoons of cod liver oil each day provides the health benefits to the brain, heart, and lungs. It improves hormonal balance and reduces inflammation. To ease their fear about the taste, I bring samples for them to try.

When participants try the cod liver oil for the first time, their beliefs change. They are no longer afraid of the taste and have become educated on the benefits. It is a win-win, and an easy step to take in their journey to greater health.

Nailing the Box of Beliefs Shut

Speaking in Colorado a few years ago I was approached by a few guys during our sampling session. This was a large crowd. People were laughing and asking questions. The place was energized. These guys asked me if I would tell their friend my thoughts on eating carrots, potatoes, and bananas. The friend was out in the hallway on his phone during my presentation and had not heard a single word of it.

When I shared my thoughts, their friend jumped in to state that "carrots, potatoes and bananas are poison." He believed that all carbohydrates were damaging to the body. Instantly everyone around the table begins to ask why carrots, potatoes, and bananas are poison. The group was now confused. After I settled the group down, I talked about the source and the benefits of each of these foods. I then asked this guy if he would like to discuss his beliefs after the sampling session was over. He said he did not and walked away. His mind was already made up. His box was nailed shut. Carrots, potatoes, and bananas were poison!

Circle of Success

Here is how the Circle of Success works. First, challenge your current belief. Second, bring in a powerful emotion to help fuel change. Third, recognize your potential. Fourth, take a specific action. Fifth, let the results begin.

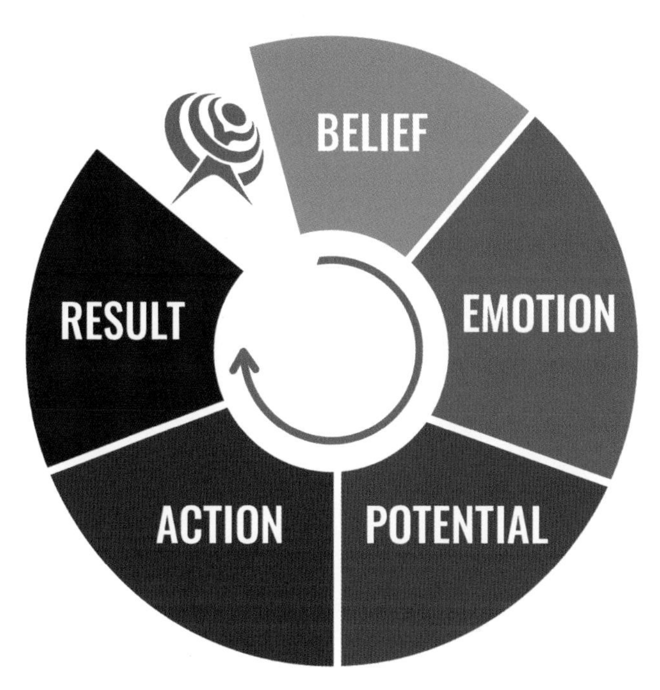

What current beliefs do you have that may be holding you back?

1. ______________________________
2. ______________________________
3. ______________________________
4. ______________________________
5. ______________________________

The Greatest Belief

The greatest belief is the belief that we can do this! No second guessing. No turning back. Follow the plan, stick with the process, and it will work! The one common denominator of success and transformation is the belief that we can succeed. Remember, we are not limited by what we do not know, but by our limiting beliefs.

> ***Believe in Yourself***
>
> *One of my favorite mentors in the world of beliefs was my 6th grade teacher Miss Ellis. Miss Ellis was kind, funny, smart, full of energy, and had an incredible ability to get her students to believe in themselves. I remember her telling me over and over that I was a great student and a fantastic speller.*
>
> *To this day I believe I am a good speller. I think Miss Ellis may have said this to all her students. But you know what? It worked on me. The world needs more of what Miss Ellis was selling—the belief in yourself. Thank you, Miss Ellis, for your love, kindness, and support.*

Box of Beliefs Essentials

Big Picture

- Our thoughts control how we think, act, and feel.
- A belief is what we call things that stick around, particularly and especially in the face of changes in knowledge.
- Many people store their beliefs in a box to try to protect them.
- A belief is a cultural phenomenon, created in conjunction with people around us.
- While more knowledge can change a belief, it usually does not.
- It is not the lack of knowledge that holds most people back, but their limiting beliefs.
- Your greatest belief is the belief that you can do this!

Ask Yourself

- Does your belief box keep you from growing and expanding and keep you fearful of the changing world?
- Why was the 4-minute mile record broken so many times after it was first achieved?
- What belief or beliefs do you need to challenge?

Small Steps

- Take some time to explore your current beliefs.
- Walk yourself through the circle of success.
- Consider what limiting beliefs you may hold.
- Now is the time to act and open your box of beliefs.
- Spread the love of Miss Ellis. Inspire others to believe in themselves!

7 Vibrant Aging

"Wait until you are my age, all those muscles will turn to fat." This is what I was told by one of my parents' friends while at a pool party in the early 1980s. I was in my early 20s, and my parents and their friends were in their mid-40s. Many believed that the muscles I was trying to build would turn to fat as I aged.

We are all aware of aging. We know our chronological age, the age counted from when we were born. Many are us are obsessed with this age and use it as a predicator of health. But why? First, we cannot change our chronological age. Second, chronological age is a poor predicator of health.

We need to shift our focus from our chronological age to our biological age, the age we have control over. Biological age is influenced by our behavior and how we take care of the 50 trillion cells that operate within our body. Over time, our cells age, but we can build, protect, and rejuvenate our cells. It can be possible that our biological age is lower than our chronological age. This is what aging well can look like.

We Have a Say in the Aging Process

We are bombarded with marketing touting the next fountain of youth. Solutions like ancient grains grown in the Himalayas, water coming from the most pristine glaciers, deep freezing the entire body, magical skin creams that make wrinkles disappear, or pills, creams, or pellets to increase our youthful hormones. All promise to slow down the aging process.

I am not a fan of the term, anti-aging. I believe anti-aging sends the wrong message, as if there is something wrong with the aging process itself. What I believe with all my heart is that we have a choice on how we age. Many people, including me, want to live a long and full life. What I truly believe is that most people are interested in the quality of their years, not just the years. What is our potential when it comes to the aging process? Over half of the people born today will live to 100 years old. That is exciting news, and science now tells us that most of us have the potential to live a vibrant, healthy life up to 120 years or more.

The longest human lifespan to date is that of Jeanne Calment of France 1875-1997, who lived to age 122 years and 164 days.

Here is a glimpse of how we have been aging and what we can expect in the future.

Life Expectancy

This chart illustrates the average life expectancy for people living in that era.

Those Alive in:	Live to:
1900	Age 47
1950	Age 68
2000	Age 77
2020	Age 85
2030	Age 90+

As you can see, we are living longer, but what about the quality of our years?

How many people do you know who have died prematurely due to their poor lifestyle choices? Growing up in Michigan I remember so many of my parents' friends who died in their early 50s due to years of neglect of their health with too much smoking, alcohol, processed foods, lack of sleep, and little or no regular exercise. They thought they were living the "good life." Now there is a new statistic that measures early mortality or morbidity. It is called DALY: Disability-Adjusted-Life-Year. DALY measures the years of life lost from both premature death and poor health.

I believe most people want to live a long and healthy life. How vibrant do you want to be at age 70? 80? 90? 100? The lifestyle choices we make in our 30s will show up in our 50s. What we do in our 50s shows up in our 70s. The seeds we plant today will be our harvest tomorrow.

Behavior Matters

What role do genetics play in the aging process? Genetics is the study of heredity and how characteristics are passed down from one generation to the next. Many believe that their genetics determine how long they are going to live and the quality of their years. I believe we have placed too much emphasis on the role our genetics play on our health and how we age. Everyone has a genetic footprint that determines the color of our eyes, our hair, and our height. Our genetics have a powerful influence on who and what we are.

But what about our health? Do genetics have a powerful influence on our health too? Are we doomed if our family history is loaded with type 2 diabetes, high blood pressure, obesity, heart disease, or cancer?

There is a new science in the field of biology called epigenetics. In simple terms, epigenetics refers to how our behavior influences our genes. We now have a science to back up what we have known for decades that our lifestyle has a much greater influence on our genes than our family tree. The amount and quality of our sleep, what and how we eat, physical activity, how we manage stress, and our attitudes all play a large role in the aging process.

In Bruce H. Lipton's book, *The Biology of Belief*, Lipton, a cell biologist, eloquently states, "Twenty years after my mentor Irv Konigsberg's advice to first consider the environment when your cells are ailing, I finally got it. DNA does not control biology, and the nucleus itself is not the brain of the cell. Just like you and me, cells are shaped by where they live. In other words, it is the environment, stupid." What Lipton is saying is that our lifestyle habits create the environment to either thrive or decline.

The movie *Twins* is a fictional comedy based on a genetic experiment of fraternal twins, Arnold Schwarzenegger (Julius) and Danny DeVito (Vincent). The twins are separated at birth and their mother Mary Ann is told both Julius and Vincent are dead. Vincent grows up fending for himself, drinks too much, eats too much, experiences high levels of stress, has little education or love, and ekes out a living in Los Angeles as an unscrupulous street hustler. Julius on the other hand is raised by a scientist and lives in a tropical paradise with access to the healthiest of foods, water, sunlight, daily exercise, high levels of education, and lots of love. Vincent is small, weak, and overweight, while Julius is large, strong, and vibrant. It is a funny movie with a happy ending. The point is our environment plays a very significant role in our health.

Aging Gap

What should we expect as we age? For most people the aging process begins with a slow decline in lung function, followed by decreasing nerve conduction, mobility, flexibility, balance, and strength. From the age of 20 to 100, there is a slow decline in our health even if we maintain a healthy lifestyle.

Here is the bad news. If we have an unhealthy lifestyle, we may begin to see a rapid decline in our health between the ages of 40 and 60, taking us down into the aging gap. The aging gap is space between vibrant health and poor health. Blood pressure begins to creep up. Type 2 diabetes sets in. Joints ache. Body weight increases. Cholesterol is out of whack. Energy is low. Hormones are out of balance. Acid reflux is now a daily problem. Sleep has become broken. We can no longer touch our toes. We get short of breath going to the mailbox and back. The aging process has taken an ugly turn with no relief in sight.

Here is the good news. The human body has an amazing ability to heal and self-correct when given the right environment to heal. If your health is moving in an unhealthy direction, begin by changing one habit at a time. You have the power to move out of the aging gap and bring back the vitality you are looking for.

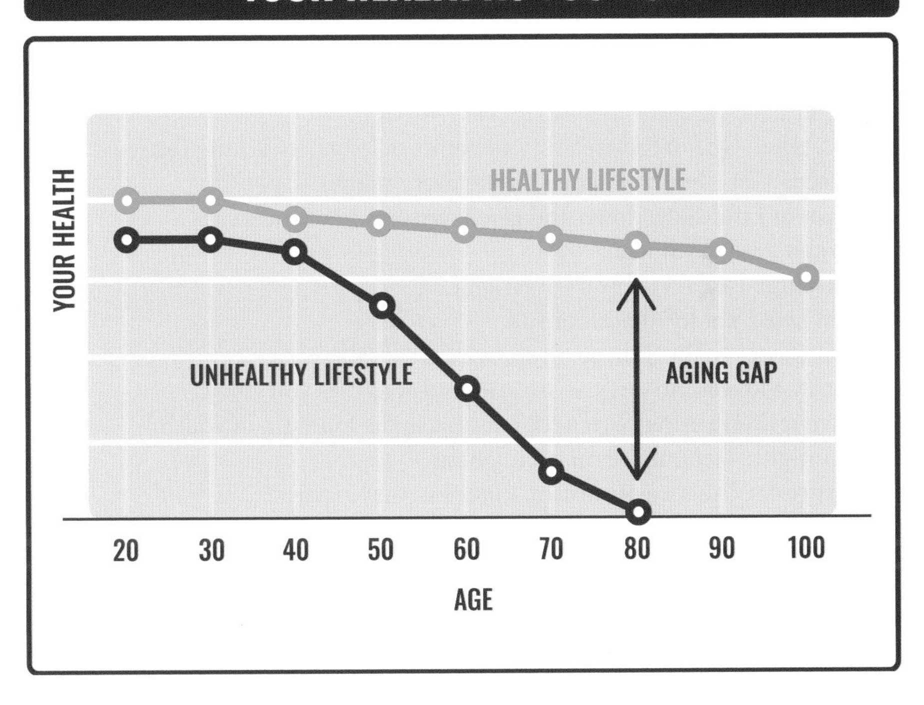

How long do you think you are going to live? ____________________

How long do you want to live? ____________________

Do these two numbers match? Yes or No

What are you willing to change? ____________________

After one of our live events a man asked a question about aging. I answered his question and then asked if he would share with the audience the numbers he wrote down on aging. He said he thought he would live to age 70. The entire audience was a little taken aback by his answer of only 70 years. I asked him how old he was, and he said 63. I then asked him how long he wanted to live, and he said 85. He said that he would love to see his granddaughter get married. I asked him what he was willing to do to make that dream come true. I reminded him that his WHY could drive his future and that now was the time to make a change.

Lifestyle Habits for Vibrant Aging

- **Breathe:** One of the greatest indicators of longevity is lung capacity.
- **Sleep:** Get 8 hours of quality sleep every night.
- **Pace of Life:** Slow down and give yourself some space.
- **Water:** Stay hydrated.
- **Fasting:** Fast 12-14 hours overnight.
- **Eat Less:** Eat to 70 percent full.
- **Eat Closer to the Source:** Improve food quality.
- **Daily Movement:** Stay active and find activities you enjoy.
- **Strength Training**: Strength training is the fountain of youth.
- **Sunlight:** Get outside on a daily basis.
- **Attitude:** Practice optimism, kindness, and gratitude.
- **Laughter:** Laughter is medicine for the soul.
- **Sense of Purpose and Belonging:** You are needed!

Here's to Vibrant Aging!

Vibrant Aging Essentials

Big Picture

- Chronological age is the age when we were born.
- Chronological age is a poor predicator of health.
- Biological age is the age we have control over.
- For people born today, over 50 percent will live to age 100.
- Epigenetics is a new science in the field of biology that states in simple terms that your behavior influences your genes.
- If you have an unhealthy lifestyle you may begin to see a rapid decline in your health between the ages of 40 and 60.
- The human body has an amazing ability to heal and self-correct when given the right environment to heal.

Ask Yourself

- What do you want your aging process to look like?
- How long do you think you are going to live?
- How long do you want to live?
- Do you eat well?
- Do you drink enough water?
- Do you get enough sleep and rest?
- How much time to you spend outside each day?
- Do you move your body on a daily basis?

Small Steps

- To improve your aging process, focus on getting enough rest.
- Get outside on a daily basis.
- Eat more whole foods.
- Move your body on a daily basis.
- Be kind to others.
- Smile more.
- Laugh more.
- Love more.

SECTION

2

THE BEDROCK OF HEALTH

8 On Target Living Health Principles

With the overwhelming amount of information at our fingertips from the internet, media, friends, and family, it can be extremely difficult to understand what is good or bad, healthy or unhealthy.

Years ago, On Target Living developed three principles to help people cut through all the noise. Our three principles, **Cellular Health, pH Balance**, and the **Source**, form the bedrock of our work. Through our live presentations, webinars, consultations, and our ***app*** at ***ontargetliving.com***, we provide the knowledge people need to take greater control of their health.

Principle 1: Cellular Health

Here is a quick science lesson about our cells. There are approximately 50 trillion cells in the human body. One of the most beautiful aspects of the human body is its ability to adapt, self-correct, and heal itself. Each day the cells of the human body go through constant change. In fact, the human body turns over billions of cells each day. Each and every day we have a wonderful opportunity to improve our overall health by improving the health of each and every cell. Improving our cellular health is essential for optimal health.

Cell Membrane

Let's begin with a better understanding of the cell. Every cell has an outer layer called the cell membrane. The main job of the cell membrane is to control what passes in and out of the cell. Think of it as the gatekeeper of the cell. The cell membrane is the brain of the cell, communicating instantly with the mitochondria and nucleus of the cell. Keeping the cell membrane soft and permeable to allow nutrients to be absorbed into the cell is critical to the overall health of the human body throughout our life.

When we eat, blood glucose begins to rise. The hormone insulin is released from the pancreas to stabilize blood glucose and open the cell to receive nutrients. If the cell is hard and brittle due to an unhealthy lifestyle, it may become desensitized to insulin, leading to elevated blood glucose and eventually to type 2 diabetes.

One of the fastest growing medical concerns today is type 2 diabetes. In 1970 the United States had less than 500,000 type 2 diabetics. Today that number has grown to over 30 million. It is very possible that within the next 10 years we could see over 100 million type 2 diabetics in the United States alone.

Type 2 diabetes is not caused by eating a banana or a piece of fruit. It is caused by an unhealthy cell membrane. If the cell membrane becomes healthier, type 2 diabetes can become a disease of the past.

High-quality foods and beverages, hydration, omega-3 fats, foods high in chlorophyll, daily movement, and proper rest all play a role in keeping the cell membrane soft, permeable, and healthy. When we consume too many processed foods, fail to drink enough water, do not move daily, sleep poorly, or experience chronic stress, the cell membrane may become hard and brittle. Think of the cell membrane like an M & M candy, hard on the outside, soft on the inside. That is what can happen to our cells if we do not take care of them.

Mitochondria

Mitochondria are the power packs in the cell. They are equivalent to the engine of a car and relate directly to how the body uses energy. The more active the mitochondria, the more calories the body will use for energy. In each cell there are hundreds to thousands of mitochondria. The number and activity level of each mitochondrion is directly related to lifestyle. Genetics do play a role, but it is small in comparison to a healthier lifestyle.

As we age our metabolism starts to slow down, but we have much more control over it than we might think. The first step to improving the health of the mitochondria is to drink more water and eat more fruits, vegetables, healthy fats, and high-quality forms of chlorophyll—greens. Moving our body daily is also essential for keeping the mitochondria healthy. When we feed our mitochondria the right types of nutrients, we will experience greater energy, increased metabolism, and vibrant health.

If we want to improve our metabolism, we need to take care of our mitochondria.

Nucleus of the Cell

The nucleus of the cell is where our RNA and DNA live. These genetic codes definitely play a large role in who we are. Recent research, however, has shown that they play a much smaller role in our health then we once thought. For years we used to think that the nucleus was the brain of the cell, but we now know that the cell membrane has taken over that role.

Each cell has a genetic makeup that determines everything from the color of our eyes and hair to the length of our bones. Some people are born with better genetics than others, but the good news is that lifestyle choices greatly impact our genetics as well. There may be cancer or heart disease percolating in the nucleus, but healthy choices help us turn on or turn off those good or bad genes. Good lifestyle decisions help our cell membrane have healthier conversations with our nucleus.

Imagine building a house with poor raw materials. Imagine doing the same to your body. If we fail to feed our cells the right raw materials, how can we produce a healthy body?

Feed the Cell High-Quality Nutrients

For years we have been influenced to focus on calories as the most important factor around food. Most people still believe that cutting calories is the most effective way to lose weight. This may be true when starting a diet, but over time calorie restriction can lead to a feeling of deprivation, making the diet extremely difficult to sustain. We need to shift our beliefs away from calories and focus on feeding our cells with higher-quality, nutrient-rich foods.

For many this shift in mindset can be difficult at first. Years ago, one of my personal training clients was not willing to consume a tablespoon of cod liver oil because it contained over 100 calories. Caloric intake depends on many factors, but what matters most is the quality of the calories we are consuming.

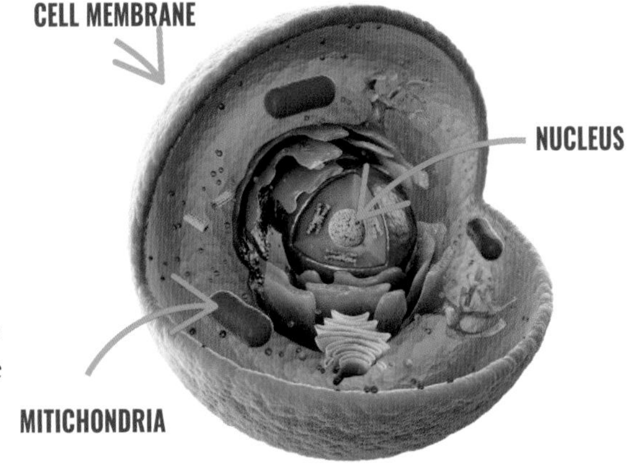

We see more and more people cutting valuable macronutrients like carbohydrates out of their diet in an effort to lose weight. Getting people to focus on feeding the cells high-quality foods in balance can be challenging.

When we begin to understand the importance of cellular health, the way we look at food changes forever. No longer are we afraid to add an extra 100 to 200 calories of healthy fats to our diet or to eat a piece of fruit. Our attention shifts from focusing on calories or cutting valuable macronutrients to feeding the cells higher-quality foods and getting healthier. Skin begins to look better. Hair and nails become stronger. Sleep and energy improve. Clothes fit differently. Inflammation begins to disappear. Cholesterol, blood pressure, and glucose numbers improve. The cells are slowly transforming, and the body is getting healthier.

Everything begins at the cellular level. The way we care for our cells has a huge impact on our overall health and feeling our best.

Principle 2: pH Balance

The second principle we teach at On Target Living is centered on balancing the body's pH.

Acidity and Alkalinity

Here comes a short chemistry lesson. Focus on the concept of having a balanced pH and this will all come together.

Every food, beverage, thought, and emotion impacts the pH level in our blood. It is measured on a scale of 1-14, with 1 being the most acidic and 14 the most alkaline. The pH of stomach acid is 1, energy drinks 2.8, soda pop 3, beer 3.5, coffee 4, and water 7.

> ***"Plop, Plop, Fizz, Fizz, Oh What a Relief It Is!"***
>
> *Alka-Seltzer was the popular over-the-counter medication for acid reflux or stomach discomfort. The magical ingredient in it is sodium bicarbonate, which is extremely alkalizing. Hence the name Alka-Seltzer.*

Food grade baking soda is 12 (similar to Alka-Seltzer). Ideally, the human blood pH should be slightly alkaline, between 7.35 and 7.45. We can monitor our pH on a regular basis by the use of pH strips. These can be purchased online or at a local health food store.

Foods, beverages, thoughts, and emotions are classified as acidic or alkaline depending on the effect they have on the body. An acid-forming food, beverage, thought, or emotion adds hydrogen ions to the body, making it more acidic. An alkalizing food, beverage, thought, or emotion removes hydrogen ions from the body, making it more alkaline.

Foods and beverages are classified as acidic or alkaline based on the effect they have on the body after digestion. For example, lemons and limes are extremely acidic. As we all know, squirt a lemon or lime in your eye and it burns. However, the end product they produce after digestion is extremely alkalizing. A simple way to increase the alkalinity of a glass of water is to add a slice of lemon or lime. This is a simple recipe for those who suffer from acid reflux or gout.

No One Asked the Right Questions

Growing up in Michigan I was a terrible eater. I lived on Beefaroni, bologna sandwiches on white bread with Miracle Whip, Kentucky Fried Chicken, Jon's Country Burger, A & W, Velveeta cheese, Little Debbie's Oatmeal Pies, and frozen pot pies to name a few. My drinks of choice were whole milk, Kool-Aid, and Pepsi. For 15 years, I had severe skin and digestive problems that included psoriasis, dandruff, eczema, and many food allergies.

The doctors recommended Kaopectate for my digestive problems along with prescription oral medications and topical creams for my irritated skin. Nothing seemed to work. The doctors kept telling my parents that I just had "sensitive skin." Never once did they ask about pH balance or anything about my diet.

Once I started asking the right questions and changed my diet, my skin and digestive problems became a thing of the past.

Our bodies are designed to do a wonderful job keeping pH in balance. When the body has to work overtime to maintain a balanced pH, trouble is sure to follow. A pH imbalance is primarily due to the overconsumption of acid-forming foods and beverages, as well as to unhealthy thoughts and emotions. As a society, we consume too much coffee, caffeine, soda pop, energy drinks, beer, alcohol, processed foods, artificial sweeteners, processed protein powders, protein bars, animal proteins, and prescription medications. On top of all our unhealthy food and beverage choices, we live in a world that keeps speeding up, leading to high levels of unhealthy stress.

Causes of Unbalanced pH

High Levels of Stress and Negative Thoughts

There is nothing that moves the body to become acidic faster than excessive stress and negative thoughts. Stress, fear, anxiety, and negative thoughts trigger the hormones adrenaline and cortisol. Adrenaline and cortisol accelerate acid levels throughout the body leading a change in respiration, blood pressure, kidney function, digestion, and mineral depletion.

Food and Beverage Choices

Processed foods, ice cream, fried foods, beef, cow's milk, cottage cheese, artificial sweeteners, sugar, table salt, soft drinks, energy drinks, coffee, and alcohol, along with everything in the red area of the Food Target create high acid levels in the body. More will be said about the Food Target in Section 4: Let Food Be Your Medicine.

Too Much Protein

Proteins are acidic in nature. Consuming more than 25 percent of daily calories from protein may cause the body to become acidic. Plant-based proteins are more alkalizing than animal proteins.

Acid-Forming Diets, Stress, and Health Problems

As you will read throughout this book, the human body has a remarkable ability to heal and self-correct. This is extremely evident with blood pH. If the pH of the blood starts to become unbalanced in either direction by the smallest of margins, the body quickly adjusts to bring it back into balance through several buffering processes. These buffering processes involve the lungs, blood, kidneys, and the use of minerals.

To compensate for high acid levels, the lungs and kidneys have to work harder. The body utilizes many of its precious buffering minerals such as calcium, magnesium, iodine, potassium, and sodium to help reduce high acid levels. These minerals work in the blood, lymph, and extracellular fluids to bind acids, which are then removed through the urine. Over time these minerals become depleted, leading to a vast array of health problems.

It may seem, therefore, that the body has all the checks and balances in place to maintain a balanced blood pH. This may be true in the short term, but when we abuse our bodies with poor food and beverage choices, little or no daily movement, and high levels of unhealthy stress, the body can only do so much before it starts to break down.

Digestive aids are one of the fastest-growing groups of medications in the United States today. More than 75 million people in the United States suffer from chronic acid reflux and other digestive health problems on a daily basis. We currently spend over $20 billion each year on digestive health medications. These digestive health medications may help relieve the discomfort, but they do not fix the problem. In many cases they may lead to even more health challenges. At On Target Living we have witnessed hundreds of people who have completely eliminated their acid reflux or other digestive health medications by changing their diet and managing their stress.

In addition to digestive problems caused by high acid levels and high stress, the depletion of precious minerals in the body has led to many other health challenges. In the United States we have the highest intake of calcium supplements in the world, but still have poor bone health. It is not a lack of calcium causing this. It is that calcium is leached out of the body faster than it is replaced. Atrial fibrillation and an unbalanced thyroid are also common problems today and may be linked to low levels of magnesium and iodine.

It is time to wake up to the power of having a balanced pH.

HEALTH PROBLEMS RELATED TO AN ACID-FORMING DIET AND HIGH LEVELS OF STRESS

- Acid Reflux
- Atrial Fibrillation
- Brittle and Thinning Hair
- Cancer
- Constipation
- Cracked Nails
- Diarrhea
- Fatigue
- Headaches
- Heart Disease
- High Blood Pressure
- Hormonal Imbalances
- Insomnia
- Irritable Bowel Syndrome
- Kidney Stones and Gout
- Muscle Cramps
- Osteoporosis
- Poor Digestive Health
- Premature Aging
- Psoriasis and Eczema
- Thyroid Dysfunction
- Type 2 Diabetes
- Weight Gain

How to Balance pH

Consume Alkalizing Foods

Begin upgrading whatever you eat and drink the most. For example, if you enjoy drinking coffee every morning with a creamer, improve the quality of your coffee and the quality of your creamer. Replace table salt with sea salt. Table salt is very acidic while sea salt is very alkalizing. Fruits, vegetables, ancient grains, and any whole foods are more alkaline than processed foods. The quality of foods, beverages, and even condiments will be stressed throughout this book. Use the pH Target and the Food Target to make healthier selections. Take slow steps to upgrade your food choices.

Women in Japan have wonderful bone health, little atrial fibrillation, and little or no thyroid problems. Their diets are made up of highly alkalizing foods such as fish, leafy greens, tofu, spirulina/chlorella, and sea vegetables. Sea Vegetables! Shushi nori, arame, kelp, dulse, and wakame are all different types of sea vegetables. Because they grow in highly alkaline sea water, they are extremely high in calcium, magnesium, iodine, and many other minerals. It may take some time to acquire a taste for sea vegetables.

Easier ways to improve pH include drinking more water, managing stress, and consuming more fruits, vegetables, ancient grains, spirulina/chlorella, nuts, and seeds to help the body function more on the alkaline side. More on this will be covered in Section 4: Let Food Be Your Medicine.

Consume Alkalizing Beverages

The beverages we consume can have a huge impact on our pH. Water with a lemon is very alkalizing and great for digestive health. When digested, lemons and limes are very alkalizing. Hot water with ginger, green tea, mineral water with a splash of juice, coconut water, and plant-based milks such as coconut, almond, oat, and cashew are all excellent beverage options to keep pH balanced. More on this will be covered in Section 4: Let Food Be Your Medicine.

FOODS HIGH IN CALCIUM, MAGNESIUM AND IODINE

CALCIUM	MAGNESIUM	IODINE
Almonds	Ancient Grains	Ancient Grains
Ancient Grains	Apples	Asparagus
Avocados	Avocados	Blueberries
Bok Choy	Bananas	Coconut
Brazil Nuts	Beans	Eggplant
Brussel Sprouts	Cabbage	Fish
Coconut	Cacao Nibs	Goat's Milk
Figs	Coconut	Leafy Greens
Leafy Greens	Dates	Potatoes
Millet	Figs	Sea Vegetables
Onions	Green Pepper	Seaweed
Sea Vegetables	Leafy Greens	Spirulina/Chlorella
Sesame Seeds	Sea Vegetables	Tomatoes
Spirulina/Chlorella	Sunflower Seeds	Turnips
Wheatgrass	Walnuts	Wheatgrass

Rest and Rejuvenation

Take time for yourself. Focus on breathing, and get more sleep. Walk in nature, and make time for stillness. Take micro breaks during the day and regular vacations. Take Epsom salt baths. Use the foam roller, and get a massage on a regular basis. More on this will be covered in Section 3: Rest, Relaxation, and Rejuvenation.

Taking time to rest and rejuvenate is critical for a balanced pH and to feel your best.

Daily Movement

Moving the body on a daily basis is essential for a healthy mind and body. Motion creates positive emotion. Daily movement along with play can be very alkalizing for the body. Too much exercise or an exercise program that is too intense moves our pH to the acid side, leading to increased inflammation and a breakdown of the body. Incorporating a balanced movement routine is essential for sustainability and balancing pH. Stretching, foam roller, strength training, cardio, and restorative movements along with play are essential for feeling our best and balancing pH. More on this will be covered in Section 5: Movement—The Fountain of Youth.

Balancing your pH is absolutely critical for optimal health performance.

pH Target

To maintain a balance between alkalinity and acidity, aim for 65-75 percent of food, beverages, condiments, thoughts, and emotions from the alkaline portion of the pH Target.

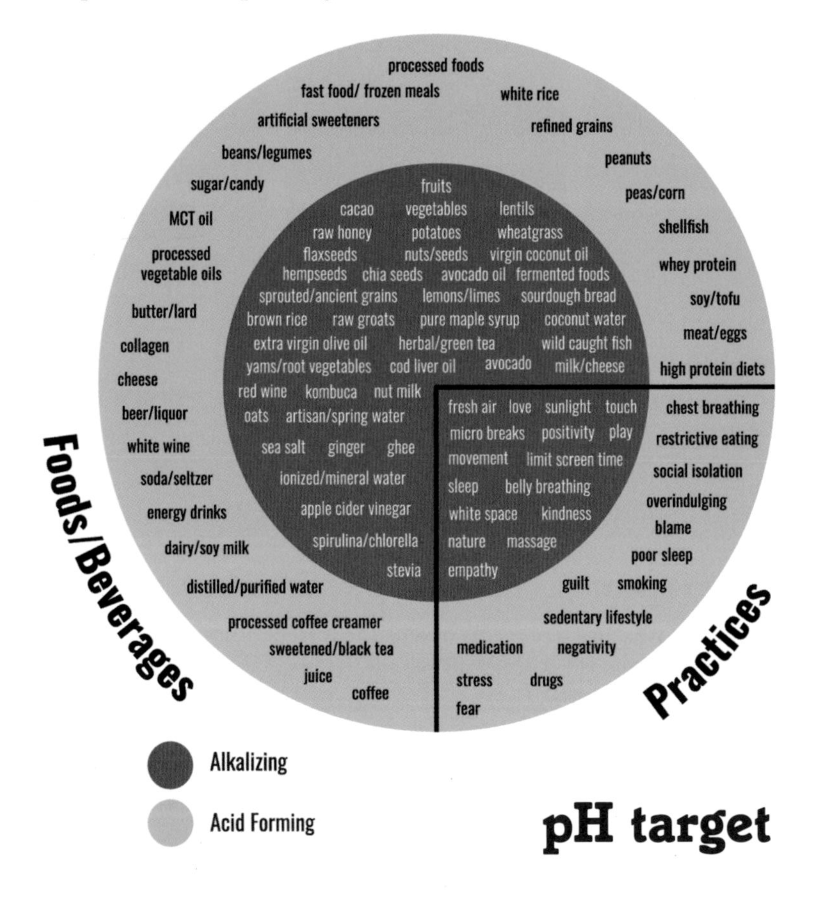

Principle 3: The Source

The third principle is likely the easiest to grasp. There is so much information and confusion on whether a food or beverage is healthy or unhealthy. Organic? Reading labels? How can we make this all simpler to understand? The answer is to get closer to the SOURCE.

A food in its most natural state is the source. It is healthier, easier for the body to break down and absorb, and costs less. Here is a question for you. If a coconut fell from a tree, is the coconut healthy or unhealthy? This coconut is, of course, healthy. This is not the same coconut that grandma put on her German chocolate cake. Coconuts contain a healthy saturated fat and are high in lauric acid. They possess antifungal properties and are great for digestion and brain health. Coconut is one of my go-to superfoods.

Take, for example, an apple. The apple is the source. When an apple is processed into applesauce or into apple juice, both move away from the source. Another example is flaxseeds. Flaxseeds are high in omega-3 fats, fiber, and lignans. They are great for our mind, brain, heart, inflammation, and hormones. And they are very inexpensive. When flaxseeds are converted into flaxseed oil, the fiber and lignans are gone and the price goes up. When converted yet again into flaxseed oil gel tablets, most of the nutrient value has been lost. The price goes up and quality goes down.

To evaluate whether a food, beverage, condiment, household cleaner, or body care product is healthy or unhealthy, check to see how close it is to the **SOURCE.** More will be said about the Source later in Section 4: Let Food Be Your Medicine.

Implementing these three principles form the bedrock to feeling and being our best.

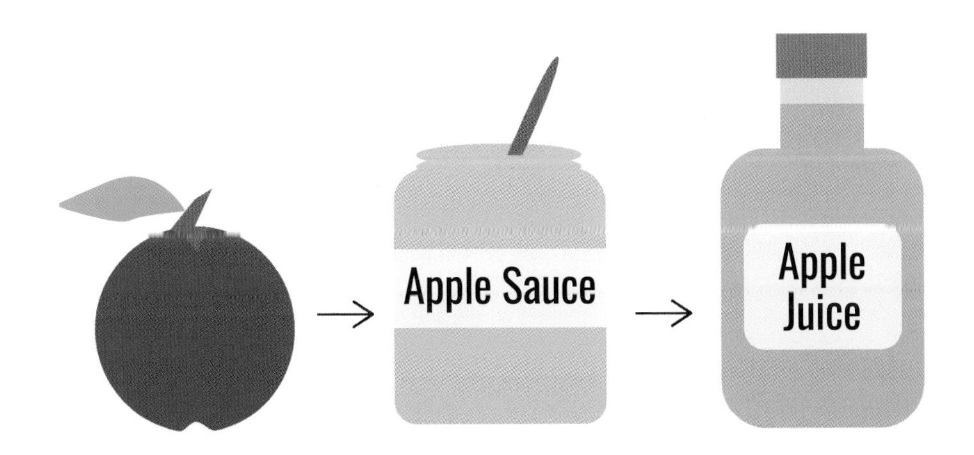

Before selecting a food, beverage, or body care product, can you answer "YES" to all three principles?

Is it good for my cells? Yes or No

Is it balancing my pH? Yes or No

Is it close to the SOURCE? Yes or No

Feeling Alive Again

Thank you On Target Living. Seriously. I feel alive again. Hearing the On Target Living message, and then implementing the principles has improved my attitudes and energies in all aspects of my life. I needed this because I felt dead, but still breathing. It has improved my relationships and my outlook. I don't feel beaten down and I don't stress about things so much. And my kids...my kids have a dad who can run with them and not an old man they come to talk to once in a while.

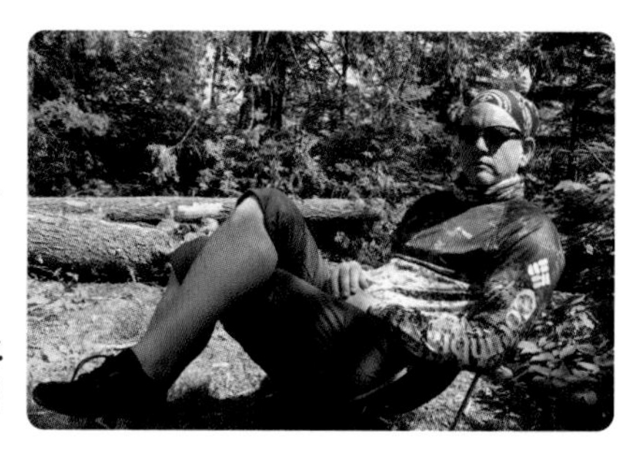

I went to my daughter's elementary school to be a "watchdog dad" for a day at the end of the year. You want a workout? Go play tag at recess (three times in one day) with 20 eight-year-old girls all looking to get you. Being able to run around that playground and keep up with them was worth it all.

I could go on and on about everything, but I want to let you know that I really appreciate all of the insight into "cell health." It is my belief that this was a key component. I now take my pH level seriously and focus on eating closer to the source. If you look at the effort-to-results ratio of my experience, most effort happened at the beginning and most results happened at the end after my efforts became routine. I believe that this is because my body was changing from the inside out.

-Darin Shank

Cell, pH, and Source Essentials

Big Picture

- The three principles of good health are: cellular health, pH balance, and the Source.
- Health begins at the cellular level.
- For optimal health, the cell membrane needs to be soft and permeable.
- Every food, beverage, thought, and emotion impacts your pH level.
- Acid = Inflammation.
- We need to maintain a balanced pH for greater gut health, less inflammation, and improved overall health.
- To maintain a balance between alkalinity and acidity, aim for 65-75 percent of your food, beverages, thoughts, and emotions from the alkaline portion of the pH Target.
- As we age, metabolism starts to slow down, but we have much more control over metabolism than we think.
- Use health and beauty products closer to the Source.
- Consume foods and beverages closer to the Source.

Ask Yourself

- Can you say YES to all three principles: Cellular Health, pH Balance, and the Source?
- Do you feel overly stressed?
- Do you have more positive or more negative self-talk?
- Do you consume too many acid-forming foods and beverages?
- Do you consume alkalizing foods and beverages?

Small Steps

- Choose and implement one or two upgrades in what you eat and drink to improve your pH.
- Consume omega-3 fats and water to help keep your cell membranes soft and permeable.
- Add a slice of lemon or lime to your water to improve gut health.
- Eat 2-3 fruits each day to clean and alkalize the gut.
- Focus on consuming foods and beverages closer to the Source.

9

REST, EAT, and MOVE
The Pillars of Health

Most people want to feel good and have good health. As the saying goes, "When you don't have your health, you don't have anything." What does feeling your best and having vibrant health look like to you? It could be as simple as getting out of bed with fewer or no aches and pains. Is it having more energy and stamina throughout the day? Feeling stronger and more fit? Getting a better night of sleep? Getting off a medication or two? Enjoying clear mental focus and a quiet mind? Or having more pep in your step? Good health leads to feeling your best.

Meeting Basic Needs is Essential to Health

Wouldn't you like to feel your best on a more consistent basis? Abraham Maslow's hierarchy of human needs is a great reminder that there is an order of importance when focusing on our needs and desires.

In his study of monkeys, the American psychologist Abraham H. Maslow observed that some needs were more important than others. If the monkeys were thirsty, water took precedence over food. If food and water needs were not met, the monkeys could not move to the next level of need which is reproduction. They could not move up their hierarchy of needs until the needs below were met.

Maslow then developed these observations into a hierarchy of human needs. At the base of Maslow's pyramid are foundational needs. Breathing, sleeping, hydration, nutrition, posture, and daily movement are our basic physiological needs. The next level is the need to be and feel safe. The third level is a sense of love and belonging. The fourth is esteem. The highest need is self-actualization—finding purpose, the desire to fill potential, to be all we can be.

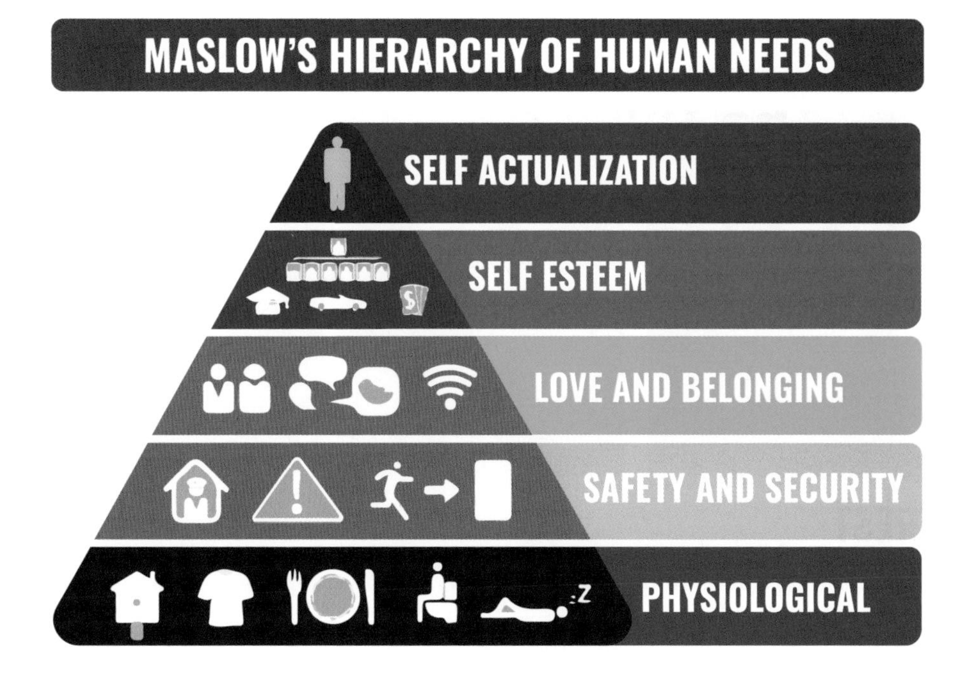

Unlike monkeys, humans like to take shortcuts when chasing their needs. I am always fascinated when I hear people express their needs—working on a new career, making more money, developing personal relationships, or buying a new house or car. In our hurried society some of our most basic needs are often neglected. For many, taking care of their fundamental needs is not even on their radar screen. We seem to have forgotten that it is extremely difficult to feel our best and perform at our best when we do not get enough sleep, are dehydrated, eat poorly, and rarely move our bodies.

Maslow's hierarchy should remind and motivate us to change our perspective and focus on the foundation. Building a stronger foundation is essential for feeling and performing our best.

Build a Healthy Foundation

We all know that building a house does not start with the roof. Think of building a healthy lifestyle as laying the proper foundation. That begins with how we **REST**, how we **EAT**, and how we **MOVE**. These are the three foundational pillars for vibrant health and feeling our best.

The next three sections will drill down into each of these three pillars to help you feel and be your best.

ON TARGET LIVING PILLARS

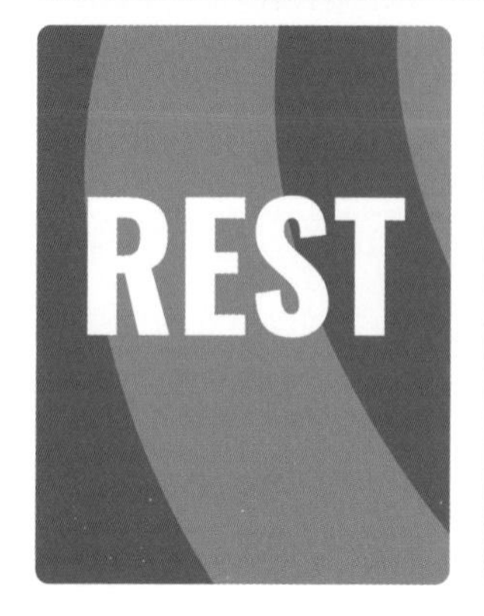

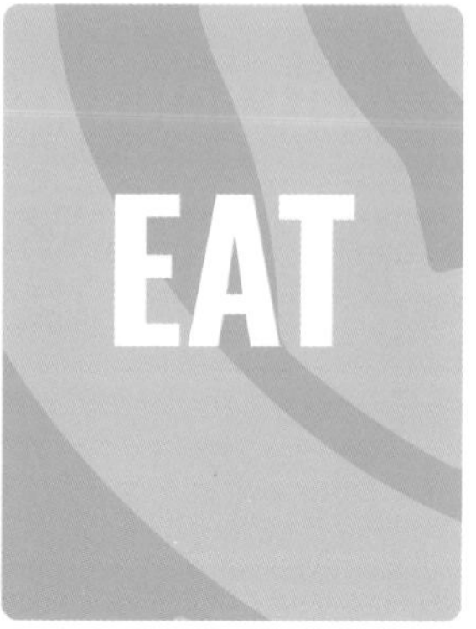

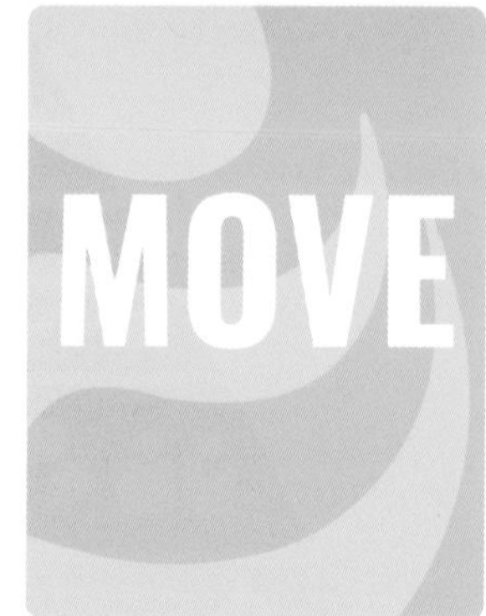

REST

Rest and rejuvenation include the ability to stop and pause to recharge, relax, refresh, and renew. This allows the body to be young again. How we breathe, how we sleep, the amount of space or stillness in our life, and how we handle stress all have a major impact on our health and how we feel.

Whether consulting with individual clients, conducting full immersion trainings at our headquarters, or speaking to large audiences, I always begin with rest and rejuvenation. Rest is the first foundational pillar for feeling our best. Getting enough rest is critical for good health and performing at our best. Have you ever taken a vacation and found within just a few days that your quality of sleep started to improve, you had more energy, and you started feeling like your old self again? We are sleep-deprived in the United States, with a high percentage of our population averaging less than six hours of sleep per night.

Many other countries around the world have rest and rejuvenation strategies plugged into their daily routines. Many countries actually shut down for a few hours every afternoon. It gives people time to eat, rest, and rejuvenate the mind and body. In the United States everything is on 24/7. We need more time to rest and recharge our batteries if our goal is to have greater health and feel our best.

Section 3: Rest, Relaxation and Rejuvenation begins with an important discussion of the science and impact of stress on health. It includes in-depth information on the power of breath and how it can improve blood pressure and gut health and calm the mind. It also illustrates how improving sleep can impact our energy, immune system, waistline, and overall health. Finally, it addresses the essential human need for quality space in life to rejuvenate the mind and body.

EAT

The second foundational pillar for achieving greater health and performance is high-quality nutrition. Food is love and food is social, but food is also medicine for the mind and body. As a society we underestimate the power of food and its impact on our health and well-being. One of the top reasons people end up in the emergency room is due to dehydration. Lack of omega-3 fats can lead to mental health challenges. A healthy gut is essential for having a healthy immune system and getting a better night of sleep. What we eat and drink plays an incredibly powerful role in our health and how we feel.

Section 4: Let Food Be Your Medicine provides information on how the body breaks down nutrients for optimal health and the importance of proper hydration for balanced pH, energy, and brain function. It discusses the power of superfoods and how to slowly upgrade the foods we love. The section also covers the benefits of fasting, the importance of caloric quality over quantity, and how to develop a nutritional plan that is enjoyable and sustainable.

MOVE

The third foundational pillar is movement—the act of physical motion. The human body is designed to move. If movement came in a pill, it would be the most prescribed medication in the world. That is why I call movement the Fountain of Youth. To feel our best and to be our best, we need to move our body on a daily basis. Motion creates positive emotion.

Section 5: Movement—The Fountain of Youth discusses the importance of daily movement. It includes guidance on how to develop a movement mindset, information on how movement can quiet the mind and relax the body, and ways to make movement fun and enjoyable.

The mind and body require a few basic ingredients to stay healthy and help us perform our best. We must be kind to ourselves and focus on the basics so that we can enjoy life to the fullest.

REST EAT MOVE Essentials

Big Picture

- Abraham Maslow's Hierarchy of Human Needs demonstrates how fundamental health is in achieving our other needs.
- **REST**: The ability to stop and pause to recharge, relax, and renew allows the mind and body to be young again.
- **EAT**: The process of being nourished, using food as fuel, growth, and repair.
- **MOVE**: The act of physical motion leading to positive emotion.

Ask Yourself

- What does feeling your best and having vibrant health look like to you?
- How well are you addressing your most basic needs?
- What can you do to get better rest?
- What can you do to start consuming healthier foods and beverages?
- How can you build daily movement into your lifestyle?

Small Steps

- Start building your **REST EAT MOVE** pillars today.
- Starting tonight, add 30-minutes of sleep.
- Drink more water—minimum of 60 ounces per day.
- Eat more whole foods.
- Move your body for 10-15 minutes every day.

SECTION

3

REST RELAXATION AND REJUVENATION

10

Stress and Health Running from The Bear

Adequate rest, relaxation, and rejuvenation practices are among the most powerful tools for optimal health and performance but are also among the most neglected. I tell my clients that if the goal is to build muscle and get in better shape, we can only train as hard as we rest.

Having enough rest is the secret to optimal growth, health, and performance. More than ever people are over-training, over-working, over-breathing, under-sleeping, and under-spacing, all leading to under-resting. Without adequate rest, the human body breaks down very quickly. As our world continues to speed up, it becomes increasingly challenging to balance life's priorities: work, family, friends, and time for rest. Life's demands are in hyperdrive, leaving less time for self-care. As we try to do more, the need for rest increases. To do more, we must do less.

Before jumping into strategies and tactics to bring more rest and rejuvenation into life, the first topic to address is stress. Stress can wreak havoc with our blood pressure, change our metabolism, damage our brain, destroy our gut health, create inadequate sleep, impact our sex life, stimulate under or overeating, and cause our health to go sideways.

Let's begin with a greater understanding of stress.

What is your definition of stress?

____

____

____

When we look around the house, the car, the office, or the grocery store, can we touch stress, grab it, point it out? It is very hard to get our arms around this thing called stress. Everyone has experienced some type of stress in their life, and there is no hiding from it in the future.

One of my good friends and colleagues is Dr. Phil Nuernberger, PhD. He explains common misconceptions about stress.

Stress Myths

Myth: Stress is something that happens to us.
Truth: Stress is our reaction to the things that happen to us.

Myth: There is good stress and bad stress.
Truth: No expert has been able to define the difference between good and bad stress. No one benefits from stress. Stress harms us every time we create this monster.

Myth: To achieve optimal performance, we need stress.
Truth: Stress inhibits performance. Nothing is more powerful than a calm clear mind. We need challenge. We need arousal. We do not need stress!

How Stress Has Changed

Once upon a time most of our stress came from trying to survive predators, find enough food and water, or protect ourselves from the elements. Then our stress progressed into fighting diseases such as scarlet fever, yellow fever, typhus, smallpox, or the bubonic plague.

Today over 80 percent of our medical expenditures can be directly linked to stress. The stress we are now facing can trigger a much deadlier class of diseases that are directly related to prolonged stress. Our nights are filled with worry leading to diseases that create a slow accumulation of damage, such as cancer, heart disease, poor digestive health, autoimmune diseases, and poor mental health.

Occasional acute stress can be extremely beneficial, kicking our bodies into a higher gear and making us more able to ward off imminent threats, like running from a bear. However, prolonged or chronic stress—the kind of stress that can last for days, weeks, months, or even years—is the stress that is killing us.

Life provides many stressors: how to pay the mortgage, pressures from work, relationships, and stressful events that are most often manifested in our heads. These are the types of stress that can suppress our immune system, disrupt our digestive system, destroy our lymphatic system, and much, much, more.

Stress is Physical

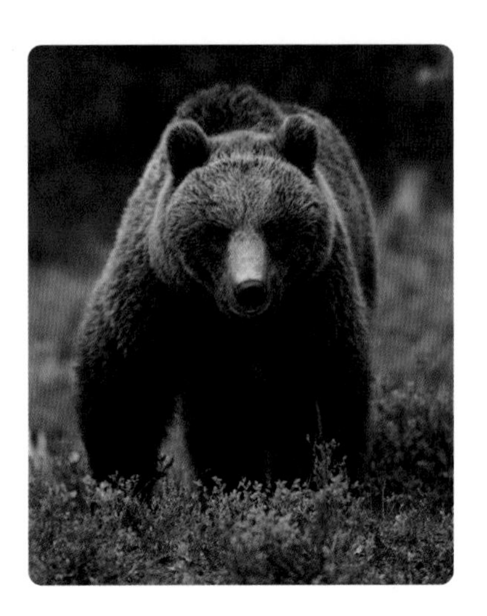

When we feel threatened, the fight-or-flight response immediately kicks in. Breathing becomes short and rapid. Heart rate increases, and blood pressure elevates. Pupils dilate, and hormones are released throughout the entire body. Muscles contract, and digestion shuts down. The immune system becomes compromised. Stress is a physical response to a stressor. Stress has a physiological impact on the mind and body. Too much stress over time takes its toll.

Stressors

A stressor can be defined as anything that moves the body out of balance and into the fight-or-flight stress response. Regardless of the stressor—heat, cold, lack of food, lack of water, an encounter with a bear, worry about paying the mortgage or funding retirement, or a problem with a co-worker—if we feel threatened in any way, the body will elicit the stress response.

The human body is superbly designed to handle acute stress. We are not designed to handle prolonged or chronic stress!

How has stress changed for you over the last year or two?

___

___

___

Most Stress is What We Say to Ourselves

Over 2,000 years ago, the great philosopher Epictetus taught that people are not disturbed by things, but the view they take of them. It is not what happens to us but how we react to it. Pain and suffering come from the stories we tell ourselves about the future. We cannot choose our external circumstances, but we can choose how we respond to them.

Most of our stress today begins in the mind. It is not the stress we experience when we run from a bear, but it is the chronic emotions of worry, frustration, and anxiety that trigger the stress response from these stressors.

These are perceived threats. When we feel threatened, whether it is real or perceived, the body reacts the same way. Have you ever perceived a threat that never came true, but experienced the physical stress that went with it? Most of our stress today comes from what we think might happen, not what actually happens.

The Train of Terror

Years ago, we took our middle school aged kids and a few of their friends to the Cedar Point Amusement Park in Sandusky, Ohio. As we approached this mega roller coaster theme park, we could see the Millennium Force ride from miles away. The Millennium Force stood over 300 feet tall. I called it "The Train of Terror."

My son and his friend quickly announced they were not going on the Millennium Force. My wife added that she was "out." But my daughter and her girlfriend asked me to take them on the ride. I immediately said yes but had no clue what I was getting myself into!

As we approached the Train of Terror, I was becoming extremely anxious. This beast was over 30 stories high! While standing in line, I could barely breathe. My heart was pumping out of my chest, my palms were sweaty, my stomach was in a knot, and my body was trembling. I was a complete mess. The anticipation of getting on this ride was tearing me up physically and emotionally. Mr. Positive was not so positive this time. At this stage of my career, I had little training or the skills necessary to reframe my focus and control my mind.

As we stepped on that Train of Terror, my daughter and her girlfriend were screaming with delight and had no idea how scared I was. The Train of Terror quickly ascended straight up to 300 feet, paused for a second at the top, and then plummeted back to earth at a speed of 93 miles per hour.

After our ride, I was exhausted. I felt like I had been run over by a truck. My hair was a mess, and my shirt was soaked from sweat. I had never experienced this type of anxiety or fear before. It left a mark that was hard for me to understand at the time but has helped me to have a better understanding how powerful the stress response can be, especially if we do not have the proper training to control it.

The human body was not designed to be in fight-or-flight on a daily or regular basis, only during acute stressful situations where the real danger lives. It is not the acute stress that we need to be concerned with. It is the day in, day out prolonged or chronic stress that is breaking us down.

Two Mistakes When It Comes to Stress

First, we overestimate the threat. We worry about having enough money to pay the bills, public speaking, threats at work, threats to family and friends, and threats to our health. These are threats that are easy to overestimate. We need to give ourselves some time to step back and dive deeper into the threat and determine what we can do to feel less threatened. How can we reframe the threat in our mind? What is out of our control? What is in our control? Learning to reframe threats is a skill and takes practice.

Second, we underestimate our ability to handle stress. We can all learn skills, strategies, and practices, such as how to breathe properly, get a better night of sleep, consume foods, and do exercises that help calm the mind and body, and include rest and rejuvenation practices essential to help us recover and become more resilient to stress.

The Science of Stress

It is fascinating how the mind can trigger the fight-or-flight response. Here is a glimpse of what takes place in the body when the stress button is pushed—especially if it is pushed too often.

Autonomic Nervous System

Imagine what it would be like if we had to think about our heart beating or taking a breath while asleep. The human body is truly amazing with all its connected systems and processes. One of the most remarkable is the autonomic nervous system. The autonomic nervous system acts as the control center in the body regulating the heart, digestion, respiration, perspiration, pupil dilation, and sexual arousal as well as many organs and muscles.

The autonomic nervous system is divided into two parts: the sympathetic nervous system and the parasympathetic nervous system. The role of the autonomic nervous system is to synchronize the two systems and maintain balance throughout the body. Our role is to create the self-mastery to control our nervous system.

Sympathetic Nervous System: Fight-or-Flight

The sympathetic nervous system acts as a gas pedal. This is what most people think stress is. When we see or feel a threat, the fire alarm goes off, and the entire body goes into high alert. It is all hands on deck! Stress hormones such as adrenaline and cortisol are immediately pumped into the body to get us ready for fight-or-flight. Our heart rate and blood pressure go up, muscles contract, digestion shuts down, and the immune system is suppressed. When we run from a bear, we do not need to waste energy digesting food.

Remember, it does not matter if the threat is real or perceived. It is all about our reaction to it. Fight-or-flight can be extremely beneficial when we need it, but chronic dominance of the sympathetic nervous system breaks us down physically and mentally. Nerves are overstimulated. Inflammation is increased, and muscles become tight and sore. The mind is easily distracted. Sleep becomes broken. Feelings of chronic agitation make it difficult to relax. Digestion suffers, the immune system breaks down, and our health suffers. The body responds as if it needs to run from the bear.

Running from the Roar

For our 20th wedding anniversary my wife Paula and I took a wonderful, bucket list trip to Tuscany, Italy. Tuscany is an amazing place with beautiful rolling mountains, vineyards, and countless small towns that have not changed in hundreds of years. We stayed at this incredible hamlet where all the food was grown right on property. On our first day there, we decided to explore by taking a hike up into the hills nearby. As we approached the top of the mountain, we stopped to admire the spectacular view of the valley below.

Out of nowhere we were blasted by the loudest roar we have ever heard. We were absolutely petrified, and we instantly experienced the fight-or-flight response like never before! I quickly recognized that whatever made that sound was going to be problem. Paula and I quickly hustled down the mountain and lived to tell the story. We found out later that the powerful roar came from a wild boar. Fortunately, we never encountered it face-to-face, but we will never forget the fear we experienced hearing its roar!

Parasympathetic Nervous System: Rest and Digest

If the sympathetic nervous system is a five-alarm fire, then the parasympathetic nervous system is chilling out in a hammock on a warm summer night. If the sympathetic nervous system is the gas pedal, think of the parasympathetic nervous system as the brake.

The parasympathetic nervous system activates the rest and digest response. Our heart rate and blood pressure drop. Muscles relax, and blood vessels dilate. Brain waves slow down, and pupils constrict. Digestion increases. It helps us calm down and relax for extended periods of time. We all probably need more rest and digest in our lives.

If the parasympathetic nervous system becomes too dominant, we begin to lose muscle tone, and it may become difficult to get out of bed in the morning. We slowly begin to lose our juice, become emotionally flat, and can even experience states of depression. We may begin to lose interest in our passions and feel tired much of the time. Procrastination can become our favorite pastime. Chronic dominance of the parasympathetic nervous system depletes and atrophies the mind and body. This is called the possum response.

Restoring Balance

Some experts suggest we have little control over our stress response. That may be true in cases like running from a bear or avoiding a car accident. Speaking in front of a large crowd, being under the gun for an important work deadline, or having a tough conversation with a colleague can also elicit the stress response.

Most people and organizations believe stress is out of their control. The truth is we actually have more control over stress than we think. It is the perception of threat and the distorted reactions to it that take a toll on us. It does not have to be this way. We can learn how to have greater control over our reactions.

The human body is designed to cope with stress. The sympathetic and parasympathetic nervous systems typically perform opposite functions but work together to create harmony within the body. The sympathetic nervous system is essential in small amounts to provide greater focus, energy, and

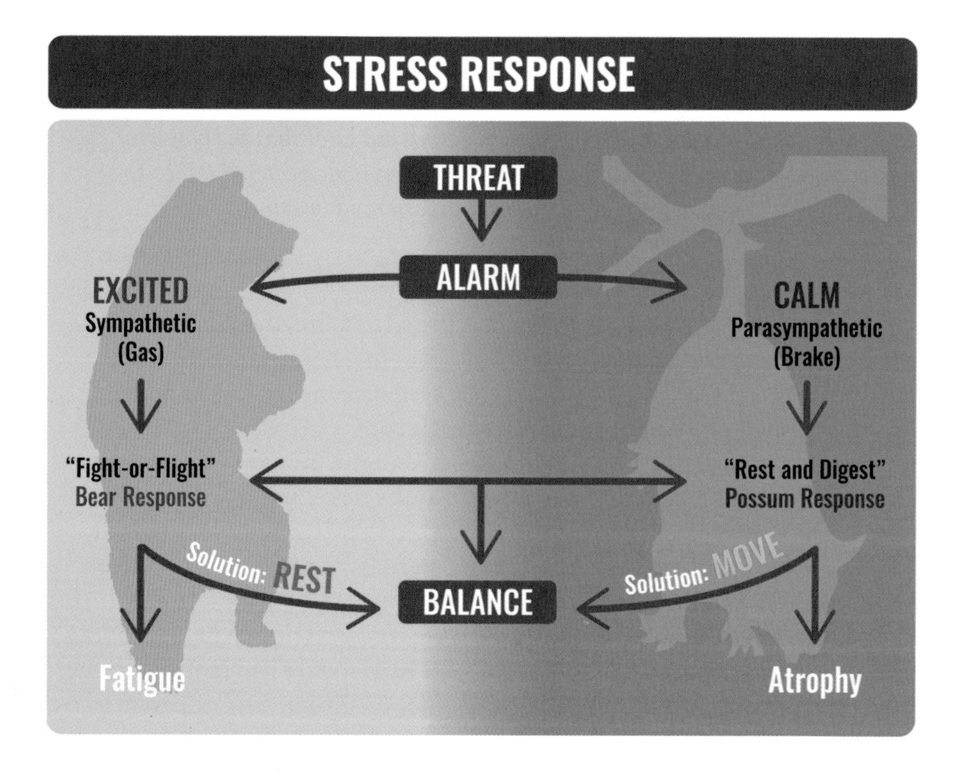

drive. Unfortunately, in our overstimulated world, many of us are forced into unsustainable overdrive.

If we have been running at top speed for a long time, we eventually need the brakes to slow us down. If we have been riding the brakes for a long time, we eventually need to step on the gas to get us moving again. Remember, most stress is what we say to ourselves and how we react to our inner dialogue.

While most actions of the autonomic nervous system are involuntary, many others, such as breathing and heart rate, can be influenced by our conscious mind. Rest and rejuvenation practices are essential to quiet the sympathetic nervous system response and transition to a more parasympathetic response.

Learning how to balance the nervous system is essential for a healthy mind and body. With a little breathing practice, we can lower blood pressure, decrease resting heart rate, improve digestion, improve hormonal balance, relax muscles, and quiet the mind. The Stress Response graphic shows how the body responds based on our stress reactions.

Nasal Breathing Balances the Nervous System

The fastest way to trigger the parasympathetic nervous system is to change how we breathe. For more detailed information on breathing, see chapter 12.

Nasal breathing is one of the most powerful strategies to balance the autonomic nervous system. What is great about this strategy is that we have access to it 24/7. This exercise is one of the fastest methods to quiet the mind, relax the body, and bring balance. Try it now.

Alternating Nostril Breathing Exercise

- Take your right thumb and close your right nostril. Keep your mouth closed and breathe only through the left nostril for one inhalation and one exhalation. (3 seconds in, 3 seconds out)
- Then take your right index finger and close the left nostril and breathe only through the right nostril for one full inhalation and one full exhalation. Repeat this sequence 3-8 times.

Daily Movement Acts as an Anti-Depressant

Another powerful strategy to rebalance the nervous system is daily movement. Movement stimulates the parasympathetic nervous system and is an effective way to get the mind and body back into balance. I will go into more detail about movement in Section 5.

Stress and Hormonal Balance

Hormones are chemical messengers that coordinate physiology and behavior by regulating, integrating, and controlling our bodily functions. Think of the hormonal system as an orchestra made up of many skilled musicians working together to perform beautiful music at Carnegie Hall. All our hormones work hard to bring balance and harmony to the body.

We are bombarded with commercials for problems related to hormone imbalance, including low T, menopause, hot flashes, increased belly fat, low thyroid, poor bone health, and erectile dysfunction. Hormones, like other systems in the human body, are greatly impacted by stress. It is critical to understand how stress affects them. We need to ask a better question. Why do we have such a problem with imbalanced hormones? Let's begin by understanding a bit more about the intricate workings of our hormones.

Hormones affect almost every system in the human body. Here are just a few ways they work their magic. Hormones stimulate and inhibit growth, affect our mood, increase or decrease immune system function, and regulate metabolism. They control our reproductive cycles and prepare the body for new phases of life such as puberty, parenting, and menopause. Hormones also prepare the body for mating, fighting, fleeing, and sexual arousal. They also play a big role in our hunger cravings.

Sleep to Improve Hormonal Balance

A 54-year- old male client asked my opinion about TRT (testosterone replacement therapy). His doctor had recommended it in response to a low testosterone test result. My client was not sure what path to take. I believe good answers are found in asking better questions.

What was he experiencing? He reported low energy, increased belly fat, little or no sex drive, erectile dysfunction, muscle loss, and just not feeling good. His doctor told him that low testosterone causes most of these symptoms and that testosterone levels decline with age.

How well did he sleep? He said that his sleep had been poor for many years, and that he had been taking a sleep medication for two years. We went over the basics of hormonal balance and how stress and lack of rest impact building hormones, including testosterone. During stage 3 deep sleep the body goes into full repair, and hormones, including testosterone, are released. Without adequate sleep, hormones and health can easily get out of balance.

How was his stress level? When asked to rate his stress level on a scale of one to ten, he rated himself an 8.5. He also experienced it on a prolonged basis, working too much, and feeling like he was on a hamster wheel. We discussed the impact of prolonged stress on hormones, especially cortisol and testosterone. If the body is in constant alarm mode, stress hormones such as cortisol dominate and steal from building hormones, including testosterone. Some health professionals refer to this hormone shift as the "cortisol steal." This prevents building hormones from repairing vital body functions.

What medications was he taking? He had been taking acid reflux medications for more than ten years. I explained that most of these medications leach out valuable minerals, including the trace minerals selenium and zinc that are essential to helping the body build testosterone.

He had also taken a cholesterol-lowering medication for four years. We discussed how statin medications block the production of cholesterol, which is the backbone of all building hormones. It also blocks the production of CoQ10, one of the most powerful antioxidants produced in the human body.

Was hormone replacement therapy the best path for him?

We decided that the place to start was a holistic approach to his sleep and stress issues beginning with many of the REST strategies outlined in this section.

To address some of the underlying causes of low testosterone, we also discussed pursuing effective nutritional and exercise strategies to improve hormone balance and overall health. More on this can be found in the EAT and REST sections later in this book.

Stress and Eating

Stress can influence why we eat, what we eat, when we eat, and how we eat. People often talk about being a stress or emotional eater, being addicted to carbs, or eating unhealthy foods when they know they should not. Many people eat not just out of nutritional needs, but out of emotional needs as well.

The duration of stress can have a huge impact on what we eat, when we eat, and the amount we eat. During acute or short-term stress, the body releases corticotrophin-releasing hormone (CRH). One of the main jobs of CRH is to suppress appetite during acute or short-term stress. We do not worry about our next meal while running from the bear.

On the other hand, when the body is stressed for hours, days, weeks, or months, the body secretes another set of hormones called glucocorticoids. Glucocorticoids increase appetite to help us recover from the stress response. For many people, glucocorticoids also increase the storage of that ingested food. When the stress beast is knocking on the door, it does not mean that we have little or no control over our appetite. We actually do. Understanding stress and having strategies to deal with it are essential for optimal health and controlling our appetite.

Stress and Health Essentials

Big Picture

- The human body has an amazing ability to heal and self-correct if given the right resources.
- Over 80 percent of medical expenditures are linked directly to stress.
- Stress is physical. It affects our heart rate, blood pressure, brain waves, hormones, and most importantly, our health.
- The sympathetic nervous system is our fight-or-flight response.
- The parasympathetic nervous system is our rest and digest response.
- It is the imbalance of the sympathetic and parasympathetic nervous systems that leads to poor health.
- A healthy and vibrant immune system requires a balanced nervous system.
- We are superbly designed to handle acute stress, but we are not designed to handle prolonged or chronic stress.

Ask Yourself

- How do you define stress?
- Do you sometimes overestimate the threat?
- Do you have tools or strategies to manage your stress response?

Small Steps

- Review your answers about stress in this chapter.
- Recognize the physical signs of stress.
- When you feel stressed, stop, evaluate the threat, and reframe it.
- Get enough sleep.
- Practice the nasal breathing exercise.
- Move your body daily.

11 The Source and Solution to Your Stress is You

As Viktor Frankl once said, "Everything can be taken from a man but one thing: the last of the human freedoms—to choose one's attitude in any given set of circumstances, to choose one's own way."

Reframing Stressors

The logical place to begin with managing stress is with the stressor. Stressors come in all shapes and sizes with varying degrees of intensity. Can you identify some of the stressors that bother you? Can these stressors be eliminated or looked upon from a different light? Reframing is a coping strategy to help take greater control of the stressors in life.

Step 1: Take a few minutes now to recognize your top stressors.

What are the stressors that keep you awake at night?

____

____

____

A New Way to Look at Things

One of my goals was to write a book. I wanted to share my thoughts with others, and I knew it was essential for future growth. However, the process seemed too overwhelming. When I began my first book, I dreaded the thought of writing. I would do almost anything to avoid sitting down to write. I would read the newspaper, vacuum, do the dishes, or look for something to eat. I would do almost anything but write. Writing a book was a giant stressor to me!

I was telling my mentor Al Arens, an author of accounting textbooks, about this during one of our regular meetings. Al said, "You are looking at this all wrong. You need to enjoy the process of writing." I asked him if he really enjoyed the writing process, wondering to myself how anyone could enjoy writing textbooks on accounting. But his answer was, "Absolutely."

So, I began to reframe my writing process from a negative to a positive. I blocked out uninterrupted time in my schedule and created a warm writing environment of Baroque music and aromatherapy and looked at writing as an adventure in growth and learning. Today, I truly enjoy the writing process.

Step 2: Identify the stressors that can be eliminated.

If you walk by your neighbor's house each day and their dog is not friendly, is there a different route? How do you feel every time you walk by the closet and all you see is clutter, or when you look at your desk and all you see are heaps of books and piles of paper? Does it feel like there are too many things to do and not enough time to do them? I think we all feel like this now and again.

Imagine tackling projects in small blocks of time. Are there some relationships that can or should be avoided? Or is it possible to repair some of these relationships whether they involve work, family, or friends? Are you spending too much time focusing on the future and not enough time in the moment? Are your nights filled with worry? Are you opening the bottle of wine before its time?

What stressors can you easily eliminate from your day, week, or month?

____

____

____

Step 3: Look at those stressors in a different light and reframe them.

I travel around the world on a regular basis and sometimes get frustrated with travel. Don't get me wrong, I love what do, but travel can beat us up both mentally and physically. If I have to take a long flight, I have to look at it differently. What can I do to enjoy the travel process? How can I engage with people more? Smile more? Can I enjoy the solitude and stillness of the flight?

When trying to lose weight, many people focus too much on the outcome and not on the process. Imagine reframing the process of losing weight into something enjoyable. What if we start to focus on what we are achieving versus what we are giving up? Could this make the process of losing weight more enjoyable?

Many people do not exercise or move their body on a regular basis because they find it unpleasant, or it just adds to the list of things that they should do each day. Imagine exercise or movement as something we look forward to and enjoy. Can we find 10 minutes each day to move our body? Is it possible to reevaluate our current strategy and try another movement activity?

What stressors can you reframe?

____

____

____

Learning how to recognize, eliminate, and reframe our stressors can be extremely powerful coping strategies in the quest to manage stress!

Stress Sources and Solutions Essentials

Big Picture

- You have the power to manage your stress.
- As Viktor Frankl once said, "Everything can be taken from a man but one thing: the last of the human freedoms—to choose one's attitude in any given set of circumstances, to choose one's own way."
- Reframing is a coping strategy to help take control of the stressors in life.

Ask Yourself

- What stressors keep you up at night?
- Are there specific stressors you can eliminate?
- How can you reframe a few of your stressors and place them in a different light?

Small Steps

- Take time to identify your top stressors and write them down.
- Identify one stressor you can eliminate and create a plan to do it.
- Identify one stressor to reframe and develop your new narrative.

12 The Lost Art of Breathing

The REST Pyramid takes the mystery out of rest and rejuvenation strategies to help build a solid REST plan that can be easily followed. The REST Pyramid consists of three solid rest building blocks: Breathing, Sleep, and Space. The first building block is Breathing.

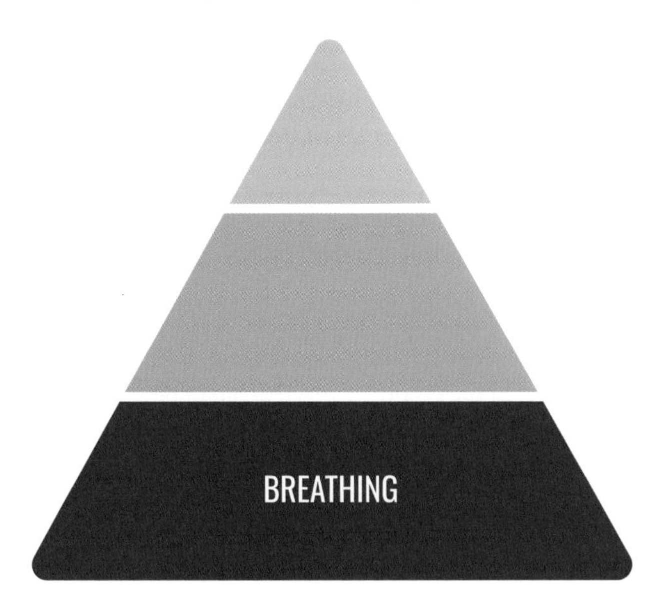

The Power of Breath

One of the most powerful and effective methods to bring greater balance, energy, and health back into our lives is learning how to breathe correctly. Breathing has incredible power to influence the mind. This power has been used for over 1,000 years. Imagine having the skill to calm the mind, improve blood pressure, lower resting heart rate, improve digestion, decrease anxiety, improve hormonal balance, strengthen the immune system, get a better night of sleep, improve posture, develop healthier teeth and gums, increase lung capacity, and improve overall health. Believe it or not there is such a thing, and it is free. It is called breathing.

Breathing Techniques Lower Blood Pressure

Recently a great friend of mine and I we were discussing of all things—health. He told me his blood pressure had been slowly creeping up over the past few years and his doctor wanted to put him on a blood pressure medication. He wanted to know if I had any ideas on how to lower his blood pressure. I suggested he eat some celery and foods rich in magnesium, and take Epsom salt baths, which also provide magnesium.

There was a better question. How did he breathe? The fastest and most powerful way to improve blood pressure is to practice breathing through the nose, taking slow breaths using the diaphragm. We went over the power of the diaphragm and how it activates the vagus nerve, which leads to an increase in the parasympathetic nervous system. Once activated, this system quiets the mind, improves digestion, relaxes muscles, lowers heart rate, and lowers blood pressure. I suggested practicing diaphragmatic breathing once in the morning, sometime during the day, and before he falls asleep. Just a few short weeks later, he called me to share the exciting news that his blood pressure had improved almost overnight by changing how he breathed. He wanted to share his new diaphragmatic breathing skills with everyone he knew. One of our greatest gifts is sharing simple but important information with others.

Breathing is more than just the biomechanical or physical act to move air in to feed hungry cells and move air out to remove waste. How we breathe influences every internal organ in our body by telling them when to turn on or turn off. These organs affect our heart rate, blood pressure, digestion, mood, attitude, hormones, and so much more. How we breathe influences everything that goes on in the mind and body.

Unfortunately, we have become a society of unhealthy breathers. We breathe too much through the mouth, breathe too much with the chest, and breathe too fast. All these ways of breathing lead to an array of physical and emotional health problems. How we breathe is a vital to health and is a skill we can all learn.

How We Breathe Matters

Breathe through the Nose

The ancient Chinese called the breath inhaled through the mouth "Ni Chi" or adverse breath. We all experience breathing through the mouth when talking, eating, drinking, climbing a few flights of stairs, working out, or when we have a cold and a stuffed-up nose.

Habitual mouth breathing is extremely unhealthy and may lead to an array of health problems ranging from high anxiety levels, snoring, sleep apnea, broken sleep, high blood pressure, heart disease, asthma, dehydration, poor memory, bad breath, periodontal disease, and increased inflammation in many adults. In children it may also be linked to ADHD, allergies, asthma, crooked teeth, and bed wetting. Have you looked around your local pharmacy or grocery store recently and seen the explosion of nasal sprays and decongestants?

Why is breathing through the nose or nasal breathing so important to our overall health and well-being? It is our most intimate connection to our surroundings.

Smell is life's oldest sense. This incredible organ—our nose— has over 400 scent receptors and can identify over a trillion smells, from freshly brewed coffee in the morning to the smell of a spring rain or a bouquet of flowers. Women have a greater sense of smell than most men, but don't lose hope fellas. We can improve our smeller with use. The nose can also detect fear, rotten food, bad breath, body odor, and so much more. The nose is a work of art.

The nose also plays many intricate roles in our overall health, acting as a gatekeeper to the body by filtering out harmful bacteria before it enters the body. The nose also warms and moistens air before it reaches the lungs, improving gas exchange along with keeping the lungs and other parts of the respiratory system from drying out. Breathing through the nose stimulates our limbic system, the system that controls emotions, memory, and arousal. Nasal breathing puts less stress on the heart and lungs, improves digestion, balances hormones, strengthens the immune system, and helps to quiet the mind and relax the body for a better night of sleep. Breathing through the nose is essential for feeling and being our best.

For most of my life I thought the nasal passages were just two exhaust pipes helping air to flow in and out of the body. The fact is our nasal passages act as a switchboard to the autonomic nervous system. Inhaling through the right nostril controls the sympathetic nervous system. When activated, this gas pedal to the fight-or-flight response speeds up circulation, raises blood pressure and heart rate, releases cortisol, and increases body temperature. Inhaling through the left nostril controls the parasympathetic nervous system. This system acts as a brake and activates the rest and digest response, which has the opposite effect on the body by lowering blood pressure, heart rate, body temperature, and anxiety.

It is important to be aware of how much of the day and night we breathe through the nose. To increase nasal breathing, focus on doing this for a few minutes, and gradually build up more time. If you are going for a walk, or doing some light exercise, try to breathe only through your nose. Continue building up the amount of time you breathe through your nose. With time and practice, I am now able to breathe only through my nose, even during my workouts.

Remember, the nose is like a muscle and needs to be exercised. Keeping the nose constantly in use trains the tissues inside the nasal cavity and throat to stay open. This helps those who snore or have asthma or sleep apnea. The more we use the nose the stronger it will become and so will our health. Breathing through the nose is a skill we can all learn and is one of the great secrets of longevity. Today is the day to stop mouth breathing and begin to breathe through the nose all day and all night.

Diaphragmatic Breathing

One of the most powerful and effective ways to bring more balance, rest, rejuvenation, and health back into life is to learn how to breathe using the diaphragm.

There are basically two types of breathing: chest breathing and diaphragmatic or belly breathing. As babies we are all belly breathers, but as we age, many people slowly become chest breathers.

When was the last time you tried to blow up a balloon or blow out the candles on a birthday cake? Was it easy or difficult? Imagine having the strength in your lungs, diaphragm, and core muscles to blow up a hot water bottle. Really, a hot water bottle! In the early 1970s, Franco Columbu, the Sardian Strongman and two-time Mr. Olympia, stood 5'5", weighed in at 185 pounds, and was known as one of the strongest bodybuilders of all time. He blew up a hot water bottle until it popped in only 55 seconds! How did he do it? It was the power of the diaphragm that gave him the force to deliver this amazing feat of strength.

The diaphragm is the dome-shaped muscle located at the base of the lungs and one of the most important muscles in the human body. Abdominal muscles help move the diaphragm, which provides the power to empty our lungs.

Diaphragmatic breathing decreases the workload on the heart and lungs by over 50 percent. It also balances the autonomic nervous system, lowers heart rate and blood pressure, relaxes the mind, lowers inflammation, helps keep pH in balance, and improves digestion, memory, and sleep. Chronic chest breathers put themselves in a chronic fight-or-flight arousal state, which may lead to more stress on the heart and lungs, increased inflammation, inability to quiet the mind, tight muscles, broken sleep, high blood pressure, inability to digest food properly, and a weakened immune system.

As we age, we all slowly lose strength, mobility, flexibility, and balance. But what most of us lose the fastest is lung capacity, our capacity to breathe. It is not about getting air in. It is that we cannot get the air out. We lose the ability to exhale fully. If we seldom use the diaphragm to breathe, it, like all muscles, gets weak. By age 70, most people who have not used the diaphragm for breathing have lost over 30 percent of their lung capacity. The greatest indicator of health and longevity, you guessed it, is lung capacity. Here is the good news. We all can learn how to maintain and improve our lung capacity simply by learning how to use the diaphragm as we breathe.

Using the diaphragm not only expands lung capacity, it also plays an important role in the balancing of the autonomic nervous system and its two branches: the sympathetic and parasympathetic systems. As we saw in chapter 10, the autonomic nervous system is a vast network that acts largely unconsciously or automatically. How we breathe can influence it. Breathing through the nose greatly influences the autonomic nervous system. So does breathing with the diaphragm, but in a different pathway.

The human body has a power switch that can influence the autonomic nervous system. This power switch is called the vagus nerve. This seems almost magical due to its ability to calm the mind and relax the body especially in times of stress. The vagus nerve, the longest cranial nerve in the human body, attaches to the base of the diaphragm and travels up into the brain, signaling the parasympathetic nervous system to turn on. When the parasympathetic nervous system is turned on, it stimulates relaxation and restoration.

When the parasympathetic nervous system is turned on, it also turns off the sympathetic nervous system, giving the mind and body a nice relaxation break. Isn't the human body amazing? Whenever we take a slow breath using the diaphragm, the vagus nerve is stimulated. Our heart rate slows down, blood pressure drops, digestion improves, energy increases, brain waves slow down, and emotions become balanced. The only time chest breathing is useful is during exercise. The rest of the time should be spent breathing with the diaphragm.

Is it possible to learn how to become a diaphragmatic breather? Absolutely. At the end of this chapter, there are several diaphragmatic breathing exercises. Diaphragmatic breathing is extremely therapeutic for the mind and body. With regular practice it can become your standard way of breathing.

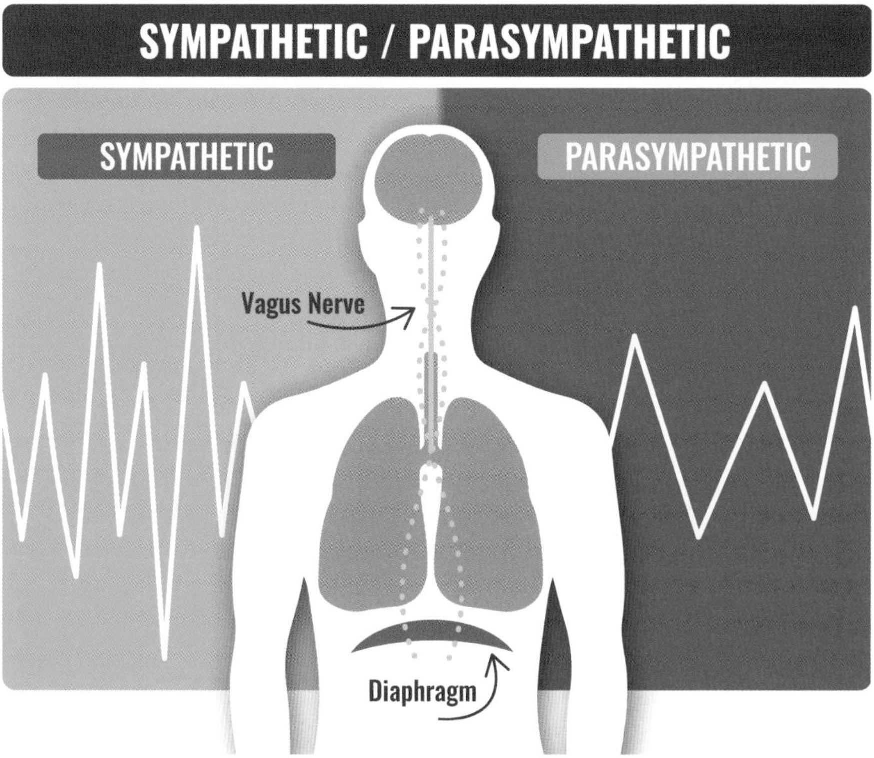

SYMPATHETIC / PARASYMPATHETIC

SYMPATHETIC
PARASYMPATHETIC
Vagus Nerve
Diaphragm

Slow Breathing

We have become a society of overbreathers (or hyperventilators), averaging up to 18 breaths per minute—equating to over 25,000 breaths per day. That is a lot of inhalations and exhalations each day. Overbreathing puts an enormous amount of physical stress on the entire body, especially the heart and lungs. Slow diaphragmatic breaths through the nose create efficiency and balance throughout the entire body. Imagine taking 10 breaths or less per minute, equating to 9,000 to 14,000 breaths per day. Would this change affect your health, energy, and mind? I think your mind and body would love the new you.

When breathing at a normal rate, our lungs can absorb about a quarter of the available oxygen we breathe from the outside air. The majority of that oxygen is exhaled right back out. By taking longer slower breaths, we allow the lungs to soak up more oxygen in fewer breaths. When we slow down our breathing, we train the lungs to be more efficient. Fewer breaths actually increase oxygen due to greater absorption.

Learning how to slow down the breath is easy to learn and just takes some regular practice. Practice! Practice! Practice!

Facing a Colonoscopy with Calm

Recently I went to get my third colonoscopy. I highly recommend everyone over the age of 50 get this easy diagnostic exam every 5-8 years. It can save your life! Anyway, back to my exam.

As I lay on the table getting ready for my exam, I was hooked up to a monitor to check my resting heart rate and blood pressure. The nurse came in and asked if it was normal for me to have such a low resting heart rate. My resting heart rate was fluctuating between 46-48 beats per minute, and I told her that was normal for me. As I waited to be taken in for the procedure, I closed my eyes, breathed only through my nose, and began taking slow, rhythmic diaphragmatic breaths with the intention of calming my mind and body.

When the nurse came back, my resting heart rate was hovering between 39-40 beats per minute. She asked what I had been doing to get my heart rate so low. I explained that I had been working on my breathing, taking slow, rhythmic, diaphragmatic breaths. I think the nurse wondered how this guy lowered his resting heart rate and blood pressure just prior to getting a colonoscopy.

Holding the Breath and Overbreathing

Breathing is an autonomic function we can consciously control. While we cannot simply decide to slow or speed up our heart rate, lower blood pressure, or improve digestion, we can choose how and when we breathe.

We have all tried to consciously hold our breath at some time in our life, whether it was learning to swim or plugging your nose to see who could hold their breath underwater the longest.

Overbreathing to Hold My Breath Longer

When my kids were young, we had a pool in our backyard. We often challenged each other to see who could swim the farthest under water. I would stand at one end of the pool, rapidly overbreathe (hyperventilate) for 30-60 seconds, then hold my breath and dive under water. My goal was to swim under water for at least four lengths of our pool. On a rare occasion I reached five and sometimes six. Now that I think about it, our pool was not very big! My kids were always amazed at how long dad could hold his breath.

I am not recommending hyperventilating and then holding your breath to swim under water. But if you ever get into a life and death situation, this technique may save your life!

Most people can hold their breath comfortably for 1-2 minutes. Holding our breath gives our cells more time to absorb oxygen and produce carbon dioxide, creating a training effect for the lungs. It also strengthens the diaphragm and increases lung capacity.

Intentional fast and heavy breathing (overbreathing) is a more advanced form of breathing that takes time to learn and develop. Here is a quick look into what takes place during intentional overbreathing.

Under normal circumstances, we maintain a breathing pattern that allows sufficient diffusion of oxygen into the blood and carbon dioxide out of the blood. When exercising or moving our body more intensely, our rate of breathing increases because our cells consume more oxygen and produce more carbon dioxide. When breathing matches the increased demand by the body, it is called hyperpnea.

In overbreathing or hyperventilation, a person moves more air in and out of the lungs than is needed. The major effect of hyperventilation is decreased concentration of carbon dioxide in the blood. The imbalance of oxygen and carbon dioxide informs our nervous system to increase or decrease the rate and depth of our breathing.

Breathing also affects our pH levels. When carbon dioxide concentration levels in the blood become too high, our blood becomes more acid than normal. This signals the nervous system to increase the rate and depth of breathing. When carbon dioxide is too low, our blood becomes more alkaline than normal, signaling a decrease in the rate and depth of breathing. This is why hyperventilation prior to holding our breath results in being able to hold our breath longer.

Breathing slowly stimulates the vagus nerve. This moves us into a parasympathetic state and provides a chill pill for the mind and body. Breathing fast and heavy (overbreathing) flips the vagal response in the other direction, pushing us into a sympathetic or stressed state.

The ability to control the autonomic nervous system can help calm the mind and relax the body. It may also train the body to handle extremes of hot and cold, to speed up metabolism, or to possibly get out of a funk. It creates a powerful reset when the body is out of balance. Intentional overbreathing may be beneficial in more advanced breath work.

How we breathe has the power to affect every cell in the human body!

Do you breathe through your mouth or through your nose? __________

Do you breathe from your chest or your diaphragm? ________________

How many breaths do you take per minute? _______________________

Do you hold your breath during the day or night? Yes or No

Do you snore or have sleep apnea? Yes or No

Have you ever been trained on the art of breathing? Yes or No

Breath Work

Now is the time to put our knowledge of how to breathe into practice. Here are a few steps to begin intentional breath work. This is a skill that takes regular practice. Taking just a few minutes each day can change your life!

Breath Awareness – Nasal Breathing

- Lay flat on your back, close your eyes, and breathe only through the nose. Relax and count the number of breaths you take in one minute (inhalation and exhalation = one breath). This gives you a beginning baseline and an awareness of how fast you are breathing.
- How many breaths did you take in one minute? _________________
- How long can you hold your breath? ___________________________

Diaphragmatic Breathing

Here are a few easy tips to follow to become a regular diaphragmatic breather.

- Lie on a flat surface, foam roller, or bed with your legs straight out or if it is more comfortable for your back, bend your knees. If your knees are bent, place a pillow under them. Put one hand on your belly and the other hand on your chest. Close your eyes and mouth.
- Breathe in slowly through your nose so that your belly moves up against your hand, as if you are blowing up a balloon. Your chest should not move. As you take a breath, your belly expands or rises. As you exhale, your belly comes back down.
- Feel the coolness of the breath through the nose (breath awareness). By focusing on your breath, your mind will become clear and your body will relax.

- Practice this exercise daily for 1-5 minutes.
- If you want to practice diaphragmatic breathing while standing or sitting, follow the same principles along with maintaining good posture.

Slow Breathing

- Assess how many breaths you currently take per minute. Lay on you back, close your eyes, and count how many breaths you take in a minute (full inhalation, full exhalation = one breath). What is that number?________________________________
- Go with the flow. Lay on your back. Close your eyes, and breathe only through your nose. Put one hand on your belly, and just breathe. Feel the slight coolness during the inhalation and a touch of warmth during the exhalation (breath awareness). No counting. No holding. No stress. Just breathe.
- Now begin to experiment with your breath work. There are many different breathing techniques. Here are a few of my favorites.
- Start with a 3-second inhalation and a 3-second exhalation. Repeat this sequence for 1-2 minutes. This will get you to 10 breaths or less per minute. This is a great place to start!
- 4 x 4: Inhale for 4 seconds, exhale for 4 seconds. Repeat for 2-5 minutes (7.5 breaths per minute). Simple micro breathing breaks calm the mind and relax the body.
- 5 x 5: Inhale for 5 seconds, exhale for 5 seconds. Repeat for 2-5 minutes (6 breaths per minute). The Perfect Breath!
- 4 x 8: Inhale for 4 seconds, exhale for 8 seconds. Repeat for 2-5 minutes (5 breaths per minute). This is a very effective exercise at bedtime to create an optimal state of relaxation.
- 4 x 4 x 4 x 4 "Box Breathing": Inhale for 4 seconds, hold for 4 seconds, exhale for 4 seconds, hold for 4 seconds. Repeat for 2-5 minutes (5 breaths per minute).
- 4 x 7 x 8: Inhale for 4 seconds, hold for 7 seconds, exhale for 8 seconds. Repeat for 2-5 minutes (3 breaths per minute). A little more advanced, but extremely restoring.

Breathing Essentials

Big Picture

- How you breathe can change your life.
- One of the most powerful and effective methods to bring greater balance, energy, and health back into our lives is learning how to breathe correctly.
- Our breath is our greatest connection to the outside world.
- Learning how to breathe correctly can calm the mind, improve blood pressure, lower resting heart rate, improve digestion, decrease anxiety, improve hormonal balance, strengthen the immune system, get a better night of sleep, improve posture, develop healthier teeth and gums, increase lung capacity, and improve overall health.

Ask Yourself

- Are you breathing through your mouth or nose?
- Are you breathing using your chest or diaphragm?
- How many breaths per minute do you take?
- Is your breathing rhythmic or are you holding your breath unintentionally?
- Do you snore or hold your breath while sleeping?

Small Steps

- Breathe through your nose 24/7.
- Intentionally use your diaphragm to breathe.
- Slow down your breath.
- Practice! Practice! Practice!

There is nothing more essential to our health and well-being than learning how to breathe properly. Here's to a life of nasal, diaphragmatic, and slow breaths!

13

Sleep
Nature's Elixir of Life

The second building block of our REST Pyramid is Sleep. Every night, if we are lucky, we take part in one of the great mysteries of biology called sleep. Sleep is a natural state of rest for the mind and body. Sleep is anabolic, repairing and building the mind and body.

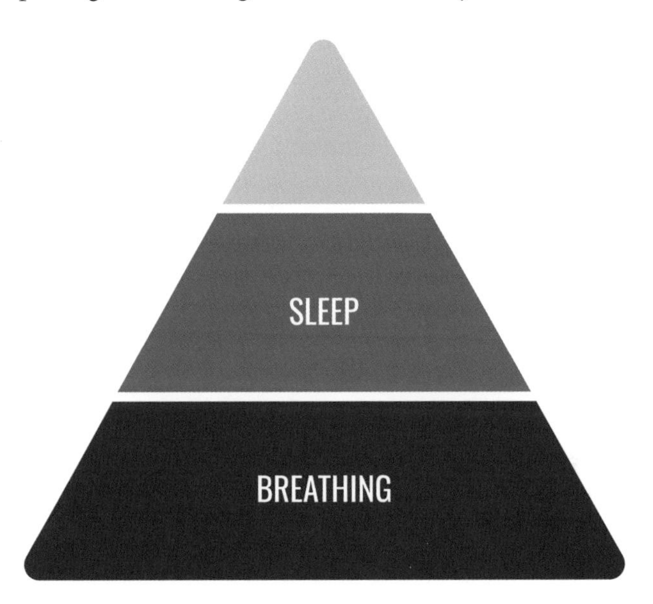

A Growing Understanding of Sleep

Until the early 1950s, most people thought of sleep as a passive, dormant part of our lives. Today we now know that our brains and many parts of the body are very active during sleep. It is as if elves come out at night to repair and make new again.

When we sleep the body collapses and the brain tunes out to most sights and sounds. Muscles become somewhat paralyzed, and hormones come out to play/ The digestive system begins the process of cleaning itself, and the brain takes out the trash.

Although scientists are still trying to learn exactly why humans need sleep, we know for certain that sleep is necessary for every cell in the human body. Without sleep we cannot survive!

Learning about Sleep Loss the Hard Way

The year was 1982. The alarm went off. The time 2:30 a.m. I climbed out of bed, walked into the shower with my eyes glued shut, dried off, dressed quickly, grabbed my lunch box, and off to work I went. One of my first jobs out of college was driving a bread truck for Butternut Bread. Yes, it is true, I was driving a bread truck selling white bread along with Dolly Madison cakes and cupcakes.

Each day looked the same. I would wake up at 2:30 a.m. and return home around 6 p.m. after 15 straight hours of non-stop movement. I was in the prime of my physical life, fit, strong, and energetic. But within just a few short months my body started to break down. I lost weight and lost my desire to exercise and play. I was totally exhausted and had lost my juice. Unfortunately, finding another job at this time was tough and my work schedule from hell continued for over a year. This job really beat me up—so much so that after I left Butternut Bread, it took the next six months to get my sleep and my life back to normal. Out of the 20 drivers I worked with, many are gone today. If you asked what killed most of these men, there is no doubt in my mind that it was the lack of recovery and most importantly, lack of sleep!

The Importance of Sleep

Nervous System

Sleep is essential for our nervous system to work properly. Too little sleep leaves us drowsy and impairs concentration, memory, and physical performance. If sleep deprivation continues, hallucinations and mood swings develop. Most sleep experts believe sleep gives our neurons a chance to shut down and repair. Without sleep, neurons become so depleted in energy and built up with toxins that they begin to malfunction.

The Boy Who Stayed Awake for Eleven Days

In 1963, San Diego high school students Randy Gardner and Bruce McAllister decided to break the world record for staying awake as a science fair project. The record at the time was held by a DJ who had managed to stay awake for 260 hours, or just under 11 days. Gardner and McAllister quickly realized that only one of them should try to stay awake while the other would help them stay awake. So, they flipped a coin and Gardner was the lucky one selected to go without sleep! As time went on, they brought in another friend, Joe Marciano, to help keep Gardner awake. Sleep researcher William Dement from Stanford also joined in to report his findings. After 11 days and 25 minutes Gardner broke the world record. Afterward, Gardner slept for 14 hours and woke up feeling fine, so he thought. Going without sleep for over 264 hours had not done him any harm. Or had it?

A psychiatrist who examined and monitored Gardner reported otherwise. By day two Gardner had trouble with his eyes. By day four Gardner started hallucinating and became paranoid. His memory was fragmented, and his speech slurred. Gardner recovered afterward, but while it lasted, this experiment had seriously affected his brain. The Guinness Book of World Records no longer accepts sleep deprivation records, thank goodness! Obviously, this is an extreme example of sleep deprivation, but we now know that lack of sleep destroys the mind and body.

Brain Health

Sleep is also necessary for a healthy brain. It is during stage 4 REM (Rapid Eye Movement) sleep that the brain has time to repair and take out the trash. As the day goes on amyloid plaque begins to build up in the brain. This may lead to an array of neurodegenerative diseases. Getting enough REM sleep allows the brain enough time for the glymphatic system to clean and remove amyloid plaque. We have to ask questions. Why are Alzheimer's, Parkinson's, and many forms of dementia rising so quickly around the world? Are researchers asking the right questions? Are they focusing on the role of sleep in these diseases?

Growth and Repair

Sleep is essential for growth and repair. It is during stage 3 deep sleep that our building hormones come out to play. These building hormones are essential for cellular growth and repair, making the body young again. Unfortunately, high levels of stress and the lack of sleep are leading to an epidemic of hormonal problems. If we want a balance of healthy hormones, we must value our sleep.

Immune System

Sleep has a huge impact on the immune system, which protects the body from outside invaders. Neurons that control sleep interact closely with the immune system. As anyone who has had the flu knows, infectious diseases make us feel sleepy. Cytokines, the chemicals our immune system produces while fighting an infection, are powerful sleep-inducing chemicals. Sleep helps the body conserve energy and other resources to help the immune system do its job.

Another way sleep impacts the immune system is through the gut. Did you know that approximately 80-90 percent of the immune system lives in the gut? The intestines are home to a large concentration of microorganisms that make up what is known as the "microbiome." The microbial world within us plays an important role in digestion and the health of our immune system. The microbiome is in constant communication with the brain and our central nervous system, helping regulate hormone production, appetite, digestion, metabolism, mood, stress response, and immune system function.

The microbiome produces and releases many of the sleep-influencing neurotransmitters such as dopamine, GABA, serotonin, and melatonin, which are also produced by the brain. Our microbiome is regulated by our circadian rhythm, our body clock. When circadian rhythms are disrupted, the health and functioning of the microbiome suffers.

Weight Control

The amount and quality of sleep plays an important role in weight control. The body produces two opposing hormones that help control energy balance. Leptin and ghrelin are directly influenced by sleep or the lack of it. When the body gets enough quality sleep it releases leptin, which create a feeling of satiety. On the other hand, when the body is deprived of sleep, it releases ghrelin, which initiates a feeling of hunger triggering the desire to eat, and in many cases, to overeat!

Overnight Therapy

What can we do about a problem that is bothering us? "Sleep on it" has always been great advice.

Sleep is one of nature's greatest gifts, releasing the burden of some of life's greatest challenges. I think we have all experienced taking that magical elevator into sleep. We wake up the next morning and our troubles from the day before do not seem as bad. Sleep makes everything better! Sleep is extremely powerful in keeping us feeling and being our best!

Rhythm of Sleep

For an activity that we all participate in every 24 hours, most of us know very little about sleep. Let's take a deeper dive into how we sleep.

Circadian Rhythm and Melatonin

Circadian rhythms are the body's internal clock, determining wakefulness and sleep. It is our circadian rhythm that controls body temperature, heart rate, and hormonal regulation.

Creating a consistent sleep pattern is critical for maintaining a healthy circadian rhythm. If we constantly change the time we go to bed or get up, it is very difficult for the body to find its rhythm and release melatonin at the right time. This is one reason we feel jet lag when changing times zones or exhaustion on Monday mornings after staying up too late over the weekend.

Melatonin is known as the hormone of darkness, and it is darkness that cues us to go to sleep. I never have to tell my dog Floyd when to go to sleep. When the sun goes down, Floyd winds down. Melatonin plays an important role in regulating our circadian rhythm. It winds the body down to a more lethargic and sleep-ready state. Without melatonin, it would be impossible to achieve a relaxed and restful night of sleep. Some melatonin is produced in the pineal gland of the brain and comes out at night. To stimulate melatonin, we need to turn off the lights. Melatonin loves the dark. This is one reason why we should avoid electronics prior to bed. Electronics, blue light, or anything that gets the mind racing may stimulate the stress hormone cortisol, which shuts down melatonin production.

Melatonin is also produced in the gut. This is a big reason why people who have an unhealthy diet may have trouble sleeping. They may not be producing enough melatonin. Taking a synthetic melatonin is not the answer to get us to sleep. Most commercial melatonin products are offered at dosages much higher than are naturally produced in the body. Taking a typical dose (1-3 mg) may elevate blood melatonin levels 1 to 20 times normal. To improve melatonin production, turn off the lights and clean up our diet.

Sleep Pressure

Sleep Pressure also determines wakefulness and sleep. Sleep pressure is created by the sleep-promoting chemical adenosine. Adenosine is a key mediator of sleep homeostasis. Adenosine continues to build up in the brain every minute of the day that we are awake. The longer we are awake, the more adenosine accumulates in the brain, creating pressure to go to sleep. Unfortunately, in today's fast-paced frenetic world, our circadian rhythms, melatonin production, and sleep pressure can be compromised or destroyed. We mask or block our body's desire to sleep with too much light, too much work, too much caffeine, and too many electronics. All lead to broken or little sleep.

Sleep Cycles

During sleep, the human body travels through four stages of sleep. These stages progress from falling asleep to stage 4 Rapid Eye Movement (REM) sleep, and then they start all over again. Each sleep cycle takes approximately 90-110 minutes to complete. A great night of sleep includes 4-5 cycles. Broken sleep may only include 2-3 cycles, with very little REM sleep.

Stage 1: Falling Asleep

Stage 1 is a transition to sleep. We have all experienced the feeling of falling or twitching while sitting in a meeting, flying on an airplane, or even in a movie theater. This is when we are on the edge of sleep. We drift into stage 1 of sleep within 5-10 minutes. Heart rate and breathing begin to slow down. Awareness of where we are gradually fades, and the body may begin to twitch now and then.

Stage 2: Light Sleep

As the body slowly moves into stage 2, the twitching slows down, and heart rate and breathing slow even more. Body temperature drops and brain waves

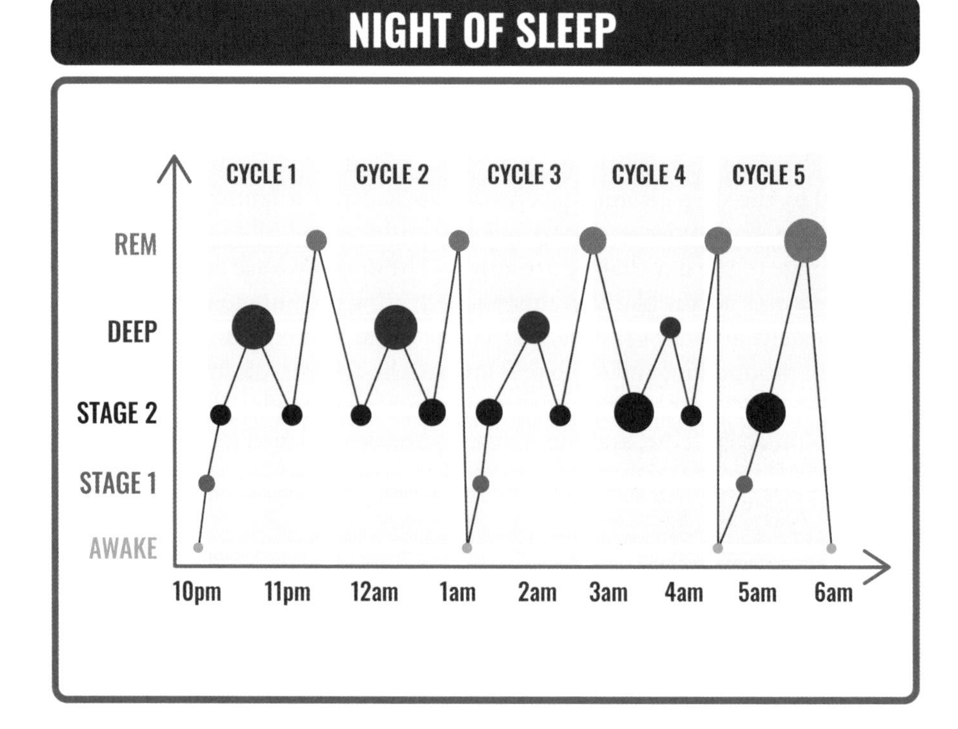

begin to change. Stage 2 takes up to half of our sleep time each night. Stages 1 and 2 very quickly set us up for stage 3, our state of hibernation or deep sleep.

Stage 3: Deep Sleep

In deep sleep, extremely slow brain waves begin to appear. There is no rapid eye movement or muscle activity. It is very difficult to wake someone during deep sleep.

Deep sleep is when the body goes into full swing to build, heal, and repair itself. Our building and sex hormones all become very busy building and repairing the damage done by the rigors of the day.

Stage 4: REM (Rapid Eye Movement) Sleep

As we move into REM sleep, our breathing becomes rapid, irregular, and shallow. Our eyes jerk rapidly in all directions, and the muscles of our limbs are temporarily paralyzed. Heart rate increases, blood pressure rises, and males develop erections. It is during REM sleep that we dream.

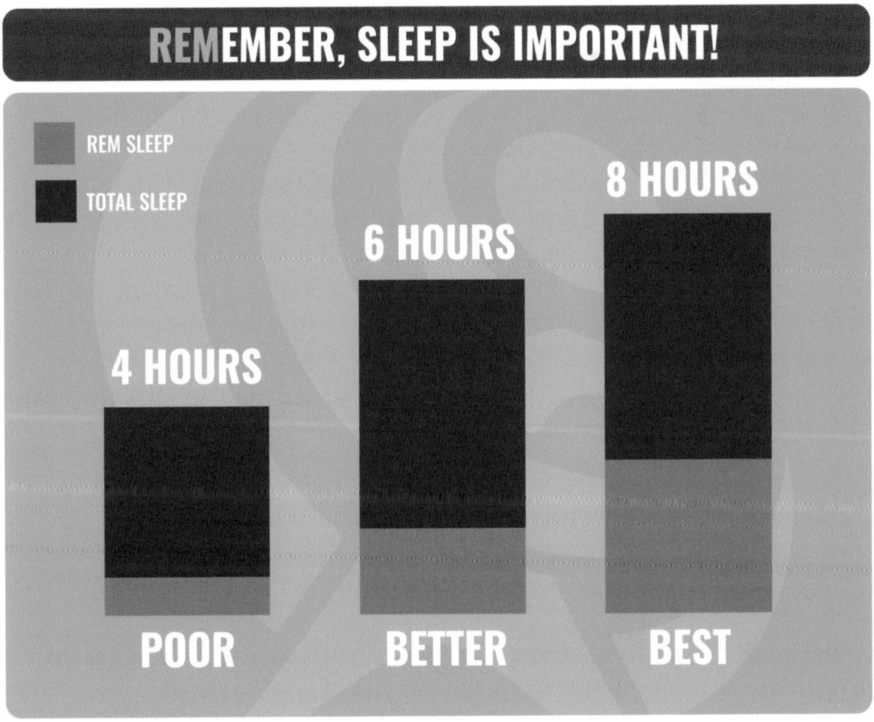

Our first REM sleep stage usually occurs about 70-90 minutes after we fall asleep. The first cycle of sleep contains very little REM sleep and long periods of deep sleep. As the night progresses, REM sleep periods get longer, and deep sleep periods get shorter. By the morning hours, people spend nearly all their sleep time in stages 1, 2, and REM sleep.

During REM sleep the brain is in full repair and cleaning mode, allowing the glymphatic system to heal, build, and take out the trash that has built up throughout the day.

If we sleep 4, 5, or even 6 hours a night, we limit the amount of time we spend in REM sleep. If we normally get up around 6 a.m., but decide to interrupt our normal REM sleep by getting up at 4 a.m. to work out or to prepare for an important meeting, we have not only lost two hours or 25 percent of our sleep time, we have also lost 60-85 percent of our REM sleep. Ouch!

The brain needs this necessary time to clean, build and repair. One reason why it is so important to get 7.5 to 8.5 hours of sleep is to be sure we get enough REM sleep. By sleeping 8 hours every night, we may double the amount of REM sleep that is so essential to a healthy and happy brain!

Sleep Needs as We Age

Sleep is really necessary for optimal health, growth, and performance as we age. How much do we need?

- Infants: 14-17 hours
- Babies: 12-16 hours
- Toddlers: 11-14 hours
- Children: 10-13 hours
- Teenagers: 8-12 hours
- Adults and Seniors: 7-9 hours

During our developmental years we need much more sleep. Our infants and babies sleep a lot, and they should. Toddlers, children, and teenagers also need a great deal of sleep, sometimes up to 14 hours a night. Adults and seniors need their sleep too. I know how good I feel when I get in my 8 hours of sleep. The thought that older adults simply need less sleep as they age is a myth. There are many scientific findings that support the fact that older adults need just as much sleep as they did in midlife. Unfortunately, in many cases they are simply less able to create that sleep.

How many hours of sleep do you get on a typical night? ____________

Is your sleep restful or broken? ______________________________

For adults, including seniors, the greatest performance enhancement drug in the world is not just sleep, but 8 hours of *quality* sleep!

Fun Facts!

Sleep is crucial for humans, but sleep is also important to the entire animal kingdom. Every animal from whales to sloths and even insects exhibit sleeplike behavior. Giraffes sleep very little, sometimes less than 30 minutes a day. Elephants sleep 4 hours a day, sloths 10 hours, lions and tigers 15 hours, and the brown bat more than 20 hours a day. That brown bat must have a grueling schedule the other 4 hours of the day! The length of sleep varies widely from creature to creature, but they all need their sleep.

When to Sleep

One of the keys to getting a better night of sleep is to go to bed and wake up at the same time on a consistent basis. Each person must find his or her own circadian rhythm. I remember as kids my older brother Nick would sleep until noon on the weekends, and I was up with the birds. Nick would go to bed after midnight, and I was in bed when the sun went down. If Nick had to get up early in the morning, he was a grouch. If I stayed up too late, I would turn into a pumpkin. What was behind these completely different sleep schedules?

It was our chronotypes. A chronotype is a person's circadian rhythm defined by differences in activity and alertness in the morning and evening. Are you a morning person or are you a night owl or something in between? Knowing our chronotype may help us to understand how our body clock works, and how we can synchronize our sleep patterns to line up with our activities for greater productivity.

There are four different chronotypes: Larks, Bears, Owls, and Dolphins.

Lark Chronotype

Larks like to rise early in the morning. Larks may easily wake up before dawn and are their best up until noon. Typically, Larks like to wind down in the early evening and fall asleep between 9 p.m. and 10 p.m.

Bear Chronotype

Most people fall into the Bear category. That would be me. Bears sleep and wake according to the sun. Bears wake easily and fall asleep with no problem. Bears are most productive until 2 p.m.

Owl Chronotype

The Owl chronotype often has trouble waking up in the morning. This would be my brother Nick. Owls dread activities in the morning. Owls like to go to bed after midnight and prefer to awake late morning. They are their most productive from noon to 4 p.m. and again after 6 p.m. While most people are winding down from the day, the Owl may be getting his or her second wind.

Dolphin Chronotype

If you have trouble following any sleep schedule, then you may be a Dolphin. Sleep is difficult for Dolphins. They often do not get enough sleep due to their sensitivity to disturbing factors like light and noise. Dolphins may also get stuck into a cycle of worrying about not getting enough sleep, which causes them to stay awake. If you find your mind racing at night, put a notebook and pencil on your nightstand to write down your worries so you can get back to sleep.

Identifying your chronotype can provide greater insight into your sleep and wake cycles, as well as peak productivity time.

What chronotype are you? ______________________________

How Sleep Has Changed

Within the space of a mere hundred years, human beings have abandoned their biological need for adequate sleep, a need that evolution has spent millions of years perfecting. As a result, lack of sleep is having a catastrophic impact on our health, our performance, and our life expectancy.

Sleep and Light

Thomas Edison's invention of the electric light bulb in 1879 has been called the most important invention since man-made fire. The light bulb helped establish social order after sundown, extended the workday, and allowed us to navigate and travel safely in the dark. Without the light bulb, there would be no nightlife. Prior to the invention of the light bulb, people slept an average of 10 hours per night. Today that number has shrunk to less than 6.5 hours per night. Ouch! I am tired just thinking about this.

When our activities were no longer limited by the day's natural light, our sleep habits began to change, and change they did. Satellite photos of the earth taken at night show that every major city around the world is lit up by artificial light. Our cities never get the chance to sleep. I do not think any of us wants to live in the dark, but maybe we can learn something from history and learn to respect sleep once again.

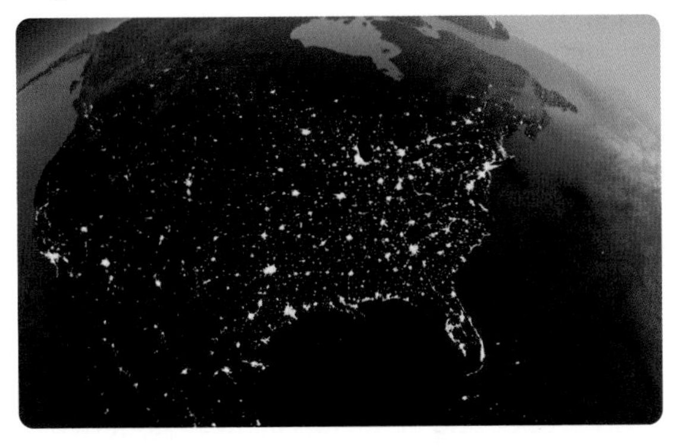

Today, the sleep industry has become big business, not only in the United States but also around the world. The use of prescription and over-the-counter sleep medications continues to skyrocket. Pillows, mattresses, sheets, blackout shades, sound machines, temperature-controlled mattress pads, and sleep apps are all being gobbled up in our quest to get a better night of sleep. But is it working?

I think most of us have experienced what a good night of sleep feels like and its impact on how we performed the following day. We all have nights when we do not sleep well, especially as we age. Life can be challenging. Maybe there are too many demands on our time, and we cannot get to bed early enough. Maybe we cannot shake off some of our troubled thoughts. Whatever it is, our quality of sleep can suffer now and then. An occasional night of poor sleep is not the problem. What I see in my profession is an epidemic of chronic sleep issues.

A Night of Sleep Medications

We have a serious problem in the United States when it comes to our sleep, evidenced by the explosion of prescription sleep medications. Many years ago, while staying at a hotel in Denver, Colorado, a fire alarm went off at 3 a.m. As I left my room, I could see that many people on my floor could hardly walk. They looked like a bunch of zombies! This situation was serious, so I quickly grabbed a few people and carried them down the stairs to an outside door. Thank goodness our hotel was only three stories high.

I began to notice that many of these people were drugged up from sleep medications. It was not just a few people, but many of them. Everyone got out safely, but I never realized how many people feel the need to take a sleep medication to fall asleep and stay asleep.

The Power of Sleep

In my work, I ask people about their sleep. I seldom hear that they get a solid 8 hours of quality sleep each night. Most often people report getting 5-6 hours of sleep. The list of reasons why they do not sleep never ends. They have to get up early to exercise, to get ready for work, and to get the kids off to school. When I ask what time they go to bed, they often report 11 p.m. or midnight, because they have work to do, need time to unwind, want to watch TV, or get on their phone or electronics. Many say they do fine on 5 hours of sleep. Most believe that in order to get ahead in life, they need to steal some time. And the only place to find this time is to cut back on sleep.

In an 1889 interview with *Scientific American*, Thomas Edison claimed he slept no more than 4 hours a day, and he apparently enforced the same practice among his employees. Jack Dorsey, the founder of both Square and Twitter, once said he spends up to 10 hours a day at each company. If so, I wonder what he does with the other 4 hours. This type of thinking continues to grow in our work culture. How does someone who sleeps 3-4 hours a night compete with someone who sleeps 8 hours a night? They don't!

If the goal is to increase performance in all aspects of our life, including work, getting enough quality sleep is foundational to sustainable performance and health.

Stealing time from sleep destroys the mind and body. Lack of sleep is one of the fastest ways to age the human body. Poor sleep can lead to many health-related problems, such as heart disease, cancer, hormonal imbalances, obesity, headaches, high blood pressure, dementia, erectile dysfunction, inflammation, joint pain, back pain, and poor energy. The answer to our sleep problems lies within all of us. With a little planning and practice, we can all learn how to sleep better!

The shorter your sleep, the shorter your life!

Sleep Better

Unlike learning how to breathe better, eat better, and move better, we cannot just generate sleep. We cannot rush sleep. We have to let sleep unfold naturally. We must give sleep time. Sleep is a dance we all participate in each and every night. It cannot be rushed or compromised.

Now is the time to get the valuable sleep we all need and deserve! Here are some important steps to help you sleep better.

Step 1: Value Sleep

Not long ago I consulted with a 63-year-old man with a variety of health challenges, including low energy, high blood pressure, acid reflux, an imbalanced cholesterol profile, low testosterone, obesity, and joint pain. When I asked him how important sleep was to him, he gave sleep a value of 4. A 4 out of 10! After a long discussion he admitted that he never realized what an important role sleep plays in our health.

Many people do not respect the power of sleep. They may view sleep as an indulgence, or that it gets in the way of things they want to do, such as work, exercise, play, socialize, and even binge-watch shows. Surely, they think, it does not hurt to cut back on sleep to live a fuller life. It does hurt. Sleep is essential for the health of our mind and our body. Sleep improves performance in almost all aspects of life, whether it is on the playing field or in the board room. Sleep is extremely important if we want to feel and be our best!

For many, sleep loss is a badge of honor, a sign that they do not require the 8-hour biological reset that most of us do. Others feel that keeping up with their peers or competitors requires a sacrifice of sleep to gain more time. This type of thinking is a fast track to aging and a decline in overall health and performance.

Commit to sleep!

On a 1-10 scale, 10 being the top, what value do you place on sleep? ____

Step 2: Plan Your Sleep

It is very interesting that people plan many things in life, but sleep is not one of them.

All new parents understand the power of developing a sleep schedule for infants. If we want our new baby to sleep, we have to develop a plan for bedtime, naps, eating, and changing diapers. If we want to sleep better, we have to develop a consistent process around sleep.

Do you keep a regular sleep schedule? Yes or No

What time do you normally go to bed? ______________________________

When do you normally get up? ______________________________

Do you give yourself enough time to get 8 hours of sleep? Yes or No

What is your sleep chronotype? ______________________________

Keeping a regular schedule is critical to maintaining a synchronized circadian rhythm and conditioning the body to expect specific sleep and wake-up times.

Getting to bed at the right time is a big part of a healthy daily lifestyle routine. Timing is critical for consistent release of our sleep-inducing hormone, melatonin, and for our waking hormone, cortisol. Sunlight in the morning boosts natural cortisol levels to wake us up.

Set up a consistent sleep schedule and do the best you can to follow your plan.

Step 3: Sunlight and Cod Liver Oil

Get more sunlight during the day. Make a point to get outside each day. Morning is especially beneficial. Facing the sun for just a few minutes each day is critical to produce the melatonin necessary to keep your circadian rhythm in sync. Sunlight exposure along with the daily consumption of cod liver oil (see chapter 17) helps to increase vitamin D levels. Low levels of vitamin D have been directly associated with many sleep disorders.

Step 4: Closing the Door on Stress

Stress can break us down in so many ways. One of the biggest is how it impacts our sleep. Most of the time it starts slowly, but over time it can be a real killer. If our stress hormones are always on, the adrenals get worn down, which may lead to chronic sleep problems. Remember, if the sympathetic nervous system is on prior to bed, it will most likely keep us up.

Before moving forward with more strategies on how to get a better night of sleep, the big task at hand for many is shutting the brain off at night. When we leave work for the day, we shut the door. But how do we shut the door in our mind? I think we have all experienced some form of rumination—when our thoughts continue to swirl around in our mind. Round and round they go with no end in sight. It is no wonder we cannot get back to sleep.

We all need to define when the day ends. We need to stop checking emails or looking at the phone. We need to protect ourselves from rumination. A great way to shut the door in our mind is to ritualize the transition to the end of our day. This can be done by doing a few simple things:

- Change clothes
- Drink a glass of mineral water with lemon
- Listen to music
- Change the lighting
- Move your body
- Walk outside

- Change how you breathe
- Practice stillness (see chapter 14)

We all need to put up guardrails to define when the day ends.

Step 5: Daily Movement

When I was a kid growing up in Michigan, we played outside from morning to night, only coming in the house to eat dinner. Within an hour or two, I was in bed with no prompting, no begging. Nobody ever had to tell me to go to bed. My body was telling me to go to bed.

Regular movement has a way of burning up the stress hormones, allowing a calming effect post movement or exercise. We can go for a walk, get outside, breathe the fresh air, go for a swim, or ride a bike. Get moving for a better night of sleep. Avoid intense exercise in the evening as it may keep you awake. Improving our lifestyle can help us sleep better. Getting a good night of sleep does not have to a be a thing of the past.

Step 6: Hydration, Caffeine, and Alcohol

Staying properly hydrated has a powerful impact on our overall health and our sleep. Dehydration causes the body to become acidic, thus increasing inflammation, constricting blood vessels, and depleting valuable minerals. If you are a coffee or other caffeinated beverage drinker, give yourself a caffeine curfew at 1 p.m. Consuming any type of stimulant after 1 p.m. may interfere with your sleep. I do not want to be the alcohol police, but it is important to understand that alcohol inhibits REM sleep. Having a nightcap or alcoholic beverage before sleep may help you relax, but heavy alcohol use robs us of REM sleep.

Step 7: Magnesium—the Mineral of Relaxation

Maintaining a balanced pH is important for overall health and good sleep. When blood levels are too acidic, the body depletes valuable buffering minerals such as magnesium. Magnesium, known as the relaxation mineral, helps calm the mind and body, and help us stay asleep. Green foods are rich in magnesium along with dates, figs, raisins, bananas, cacao nibs, oatmeal, and chia seeds.

One of the greatest ways to get a better night of sleep is to take an Epsom salt bath prior to bed. Dissolve two cups of Epsom salt in a warm bath, and soak for 10-15 minutes before bed. Epsom salt is high in magnesium and is great for muscles as well.

Step 8: Naps

More and more organizations are recognizing the value of taking short recovery breaks during the day. These include naps. Okay, just to let the cat out of the bag, the Johnson Family comes from a long line of nappers. And why not? Taking a short 5 to 15-minute nap can do wonders for the mind and body. In the United States, a land inhabited by insomniacs, nappers may be looked upon with suspicion. In Latin countries, it is the opposite. People who do not nap are considered odd. In Italy, Spain, and the south of France, napping is a sacred, post lunch, digestive ritual observed by all, except tourists. I do not recommend napping late in the afternoon if it interferes with sleep. If you feel drowsy during the day, take a short nap, and leave the guilt in the garbage!

Step 9: Sleep Environment

One of the keys to getting better sleep at home or on the road is creating a great sleep environment. Start by making your room completely dark. If this is challenging, buy some eyeshades or blackout shades. Exposure to excessive light at night, including the use of electronics, can disrupt your sleep or exacerbate sleep disorders especially in children and adolescents. Any light at night can be disruptive and suppress our sleep hormone melatonin.

Second, make your sleep environment quiet. For many people, some type of relaxing sound or white noise can be extremely helpful in drowning out noise.

Third, make your sleep environment cool. Cool temperatures play a huge role in stimulating the parasympathetic nervous system, making the body slow down and relax. Decrease the temperature in the bedroom to 65 degrees or less. I personally use a cooling mattress pad, which allows me to control the temperature without having to turn my bedroom into an igloo.

Lastly, put several important things on your nightstand: water to keep you hydrated, a small notebook and a pen to write down anything that is keeping you up, and books to read to help you relax and quiet your mind. Lastly put the phone away. Creating an ideal sleep environment can have a huge impact on the quality of your sleep.

Step 10: Breathing and Progressive Muscle Relaxation

Often the reason why we cannot fall asleep, sleep peacefully, or sleep soundly through the night is mental or physical tension. If we can completely relax mentally and physically before falling asleep, we will always have restful sleep.

Coupling breathing exercises with Progressive Muscle Relaxation Therapy joins two powerful practices to quiet the mind and relax the body.

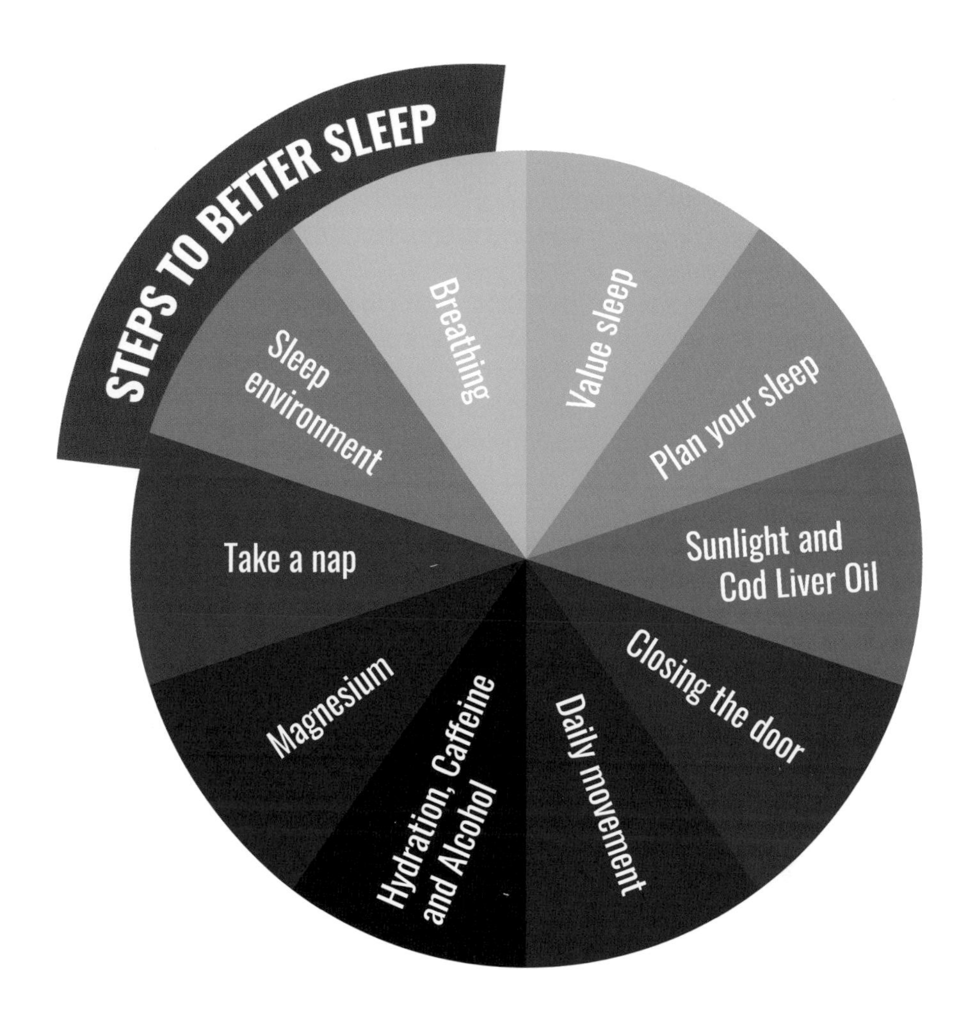

Sleep Exercises

Breathing is a key element in relaxation. Sleep exercises take advantage of the breathing process to help you get to sleep and also help you sleep more restfully. This exercise should be done with diaphragmatic breathing, not chest breathing. Follow the directions closely, but focus on the breath, not the counting. Very few people are able to finish this exercise because they fall asleep. Practice this exercise every night until you have trained yourself to fall asleep within five breaths.

Breathe Yourself to Sleep Exercise

This exercise is based on exhaling for twice as long as you inhale.

- Use a comfortable breath count of 6:3 or 8:4. You are not trying to empty or fill the lungs completely. The breathing ratio of 2:1 should be effortless.
- Pay close attention to your breath. There should be no stops, pauses, or shakiness during either the inhalation or the exhalation. Minimize the pause between inhalation and exhalation.
- Begin with 8 breaths (2:1) lying on your back.
- Then take 16 breaths (2:1) lying on your right side.
- Finish with 32 breaths (2:1) lying on your left side.
- There are times when the mind is still too preoccupied to sleep peacefully. If you are still awake, repeat the exercise once more. Then focus on smooth 2:1 breathing until you fall asleep.

Progressive Muscle Relaxation

The purpose of this exercise is to allow the sympathetic nervous system to relax.

- Lay on your back.
- Start with the muscles in your toes. Contract these muscles for 15 seconds and then release them.
- Then move up to your ankles, contracting them for 15 seconds and releasing them.
- Continue moving up the body – to the calves, hamstrings, quads, buttocks, back, arms, hands, fingers, and face, contracting and releasing the muscles as you go.
- Contract the muscles of each area of the body for 15 seconds. You will get the hang of this with practice.
- Repeat if necessary.
- Breath work and PMR are extremely helpful for better sleep!

Sleep Essentials

Big Picture

- You have the power to get a better night of sleep.
- Sleep is essential for life.
- Sleep is a natural state of rest for the mind and body.
- Sleep is anabolic, repairing and building the mind and body.
- Prior to the invention of the light bulb people slept an average of 10 hours per night. Today that number has shrunk to less than 6.5 hours per night.
- The greatest performance enhancement gift to your mind and body is 8 hours of restful sleep.

Ask Yourself

- How many hours of sleep do you average per night?
- Is your sleep restful or broken?
- How much value do you place on your sleep?
- What is your chronotype?
- How does knowing this change your thinking about sleep?

Small Steps

- Value your sleep.
- Develop a plan to get 8 hours of sleep per night.
- Get a daily dose of sunlight, vitamin D, and cod liver oil.
- Have a rigid end to your day to close the door on stress.
- Move your body daily.
- Stay hydrated throughout the day, and limit alcohol and caffeine.
- Take an Epsom salt bath.
- Take a nap if needed.
- Turn the thermostat in the bedroom down to 60-65 degrees.
- Practice diaphragmatic breathing and muscle relaxation strategies.

14 Give Me Some Space

Our third building block of the REST Pyramid and one of my favorites is Space. Space caps off the REST pyramid.

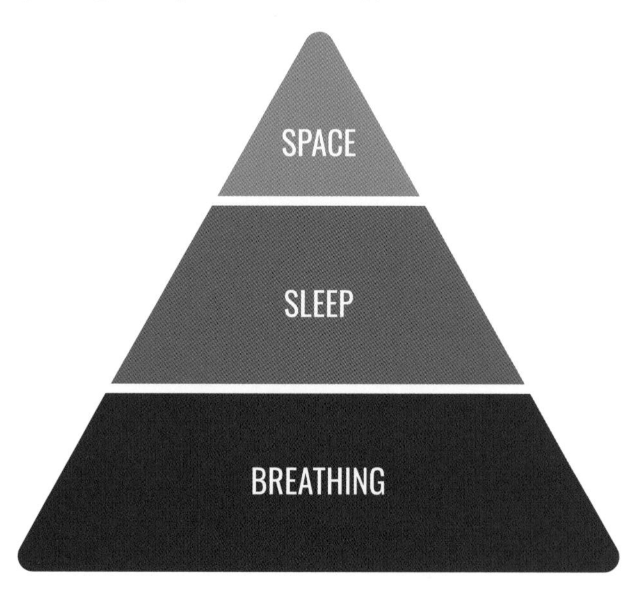

Space is Where Our Memories Are Made

We all need Space in our lives for the special and the meaningful. Important people, occasions, and memories make life magical. These are the things we will remember and value at the end of our lives. How we choose to spend our time reveals who we are as unique individuals.

Unfortunately, our space seems to be shrinking. Over the last 15 years, it is estimated that the average person has lost over 3 hours of space per day. Is your life like your sock drawer? Filled to the brim with no room for even one more pair of socks? This is happening to many people. It leads to increased stress, increased speed, and a decrease in stillness, calmness, and serenity.

Imagine a more confident, calm, and serene life. How would this impact your life and those around you? Is it possible to learn how to slow down, quiet the mind, and relax the body? Is it possible to learn how to bring more calmness, serenity, and tranquility into life?

Rejuvenation—To Make Young Again

I love the word rejuvenation—to make young again, to restore to a youthful vigor, make fresh again, like a springtime rain in the forest where all the plants and animals come out to play. We can feel and smell the energy in the air. The forest is alive and rejuvenated.

As our lives continue to speed up with work, deadlines, obligations, family, friends, community, and technology, we are tugged in so many directions that time may feel like it is shrinking. We are running out of space to move our bodies, space to eat the right types of foods rather than go to the drive-through, or space to get enough sleep because there are only 24 hours in the day. We do not take the time to step back and recharge our batteries. We are running out of space to enjoy our lives.

When was the last time you went for a walk in the woods, had a massage, paid attention to your breath, took a nap, sat at the dinner table, or had a vacation that did not include work?

Do you feel like you have enough space in your life? Yes or No

Do you have enough space to:
- **Sleep 8 hours per night?** Yes or No
- **Work on your breath?** Yes or No
- **Go for a walk in the woods?** Yes or No
- **Get a massage?** Yes or No
- **Read a good book?** Yes or No
- **Take a few breaks during your day?** Yes or No
- **Move your body for 10-30 minutes each day?** Yes or No
- **Prepare healthy meals and snacks?** Yes or No
- **Provide for self-care?** Yes or No
- **Have lunch with a friend?** Yes or No

Creating Space

Bringing more rejuvenation into life begins by creating space—essential space—the space and time needed for rejuvenation to take place.

How do you feel when you look at your calendar and see that you have very little scheduled or planned for your day? Or your weekend? I think we all agree that having more space in our lives is a great feeling.

If your life is so tightly scheduled that you have little time for sleep, exercise, eating right, fun, or relaxation, you may have to step back and

SPACE

SLEEP | WORK + COMMUTE | SURVIVAL | SCREEN TIME | SPACE

	SLEEP	WORK + COMMUTE	SURVIVAL	SCREEN TIME	SPACE
1940	8 HOURS	8 HOURS	3 HOURS		5 HOURS
2008	7 HOURS	9 HOURS	3 HOURS	2 HRS	3 HOURS
TODAY	6.5 HOURS	9.5 HOURS	2 HRS	5 HOURS	1 HR

consider making some changes to allow for more space. We are trending in the wrong direction when it comes to preserving our space.

I ask clients how much time they take to recharge their batteries, and if they plan regular rest and rejuvenation breaks. Most say they take a vacation now and then, but that is it. Bringing more calmness, more serenity, and more tranquility into our lives can be extremely challenging for almost everyone. We know we need to slow down, but do not know how. We know we should try to relax more, but feel like there is too much to do. How do we quiet the mind and stay in the moment? How do we bring more mindfulness and stillness into each and every day?

Silence is Golden

A few years ago, Dr. Phil Nuernberger and I were discussing the silent retreat he holds every summer in Montana. I asked him what he did on this retreat for an entire week. He reported that people hike, meditate, and experience an entire week of stillness. And oh, by the way, there is no talking on a silent retreat! Seriously, no talking? It sounded to me like an entire week of doing nothing. It made me think of a Seinfeld episode—a show about nothing.

I asked Phil if he thought his retreat was something I should attend. He recommended I start a little bit slower, by trying to go for an entire day or two without talking to see how I did. He suggested that my next trip on the road by myself offered a good opportunity. He told me to go without talking for an entire day and only speak when spoken to. I took his advice and did not talk for an entire day. I would have never thought that staying silent for an entire day would have such a powerful impact. I started to look at my surroundings differently. I felt a calmness around me, and the entire world seemed to slow down. I now follow this practice regularly when I travel.

Space has a purpose—a powerful purpose. It allows us the necessary space and time to bring more stillness into our lives. One of my favorite sayings is: **The time we love to waste is not wasted time!**

Time pressures exist for all of us. To create space, it is necessary to take time to step back, reflect, and find ways to bring more planned recovery into our days, weeks, months, and years.

Begin by creating a plan that allows the necessary time to recharge by developing micro, medium, and macro breaks into your life.

Animal Wisdom

The Calm Donkey

Many years ago, trekking up the North Rim of the Grand Canyon, I was astonished to see four donkeys and their riders ascending the North Rim. The North Rim is a spectacular sight to see, with incredible rock formations and beautiful pine trees. The vistas inside the Grand Canyon are breathtaking. The North Rim is extremely steep with tight switchbacks. Danger can be found around every corner.

As I was hiking up the North Rim, I wondered who in their right mind would be riding a donkey on this steep terrain. One false move and you could fall thousands of feet. My stomach was in knots just watching the donkeys and their riders. What if the donkey slipped or became spooked? Death would be imminent!

The next day I asked a few park rangers about the donkeys. They all said the same thing. Donkeys are remarkable animals. They are stronger and more adaptable than horses. They have great endurance, and their senses are extremely acute. It is their confidence, calmness, serenity, and gentle soul that set the donkeys apart. I no longer look at donkeys in the same light.

The Smart Sloth

Another animal that I find intriguing and believe we can all learn from is the sloth, nature's slowest mammal. Everything a sloth does is slow. They move slow, eat slow, and digest their food slow. They are the energy-saving icons of our world. The sloth has only one speed—SLOW! And nothing is going to speed up the sloth.

Learning how to intentionally slow down and quiet the mind are skills that can be learned. I am now beginning to understand the power of the donkey and sloth. I no longer look at them in the same light.

Micro Breaks

When life is busy, it is easy to say no to a big break, but it is nearly impossible to say no to a micro break. There are hundreds of ways to bring more rest and rejuvenation into daily life. Taking a micro break is simple.

- Take a stillness break. Close your eyes and breathe slowly for 60-120 seconds.
- Take a hot and cold shower. It is a great way to rejuvenate and build your immune system. Start with hot water and then slowly change to cold. Go back and forth with the temperatures, ending with cold.
- Listen to Baroque or spa music. Music calms the mind.
- Walk in nature. Look and listen to all the beauty surrounding you.
- Do some restorative stretches: wall extension, standing up dog, and down dog.
- Use your foam roller. This is great for posture and muscle tension. See Section 5.
- Do some diaphragmatic breathing, taking slow rhythmic breaths.
- Have a healthy snack, such as an apple, a banana, or a few nuts.
- Drink some water or have a hot cup of herbal tea. This is very hydrating and improves energy.
- Take a nap. A 5 to 20-minute nap can do wonders for your mind and body.
- Stare at the moon or clouds. Lay on your back and look up into the sky.
- Take an hour out of the office. Just step away from the action.
- Schedule a massage 1-2 times each month.
- Meditate. It is a powerful way to clear the mind, creating peace and serenity.

Medium Breaks

Each and every week plan a longer rest and rejuvenation break. When I see a medium break on my calendar it makes me smile. Get creative and give yourself the necessary space to recharge your batteries.

- Go to the movies.
- Read a book.
- Play a board game or put a puzzle together.
- Work in the yard or garden.
- Move your body with stretching, strength training, or cardio. This washes the brain.
- Walk along the beach.
- Play. Find activities you love.
- Take a hike in the woods. Bring some stillness back into your life.

- Take Wednesday mornings off. It is so nice to see this in the calendar.
- Take a peaceful drive in the country. I used to do this with my grandpa.
- Spend a few hours at the spa, get a massage, use the jacuzzi, or take a hot and cold shower.

Macro Breaks

- Take a 12-hour electronic break. Give your brain a needed break.
- Take a 24-hour work vacation. No work for 24 hours.
- Take a 3-day weekend away. Get a change of scenery.
- Experience complete silence for one or multiple days.
- Go on a silent retreat.
- Take a 10-day vacation. See how you feel after day 8.
- Plan a 3-month sabbatical. It could be life changing. I may need to look into this for myself!

Stillness

Practicing stillness is essential to bring calmness, serenity, and tranquility into our world. Learn how to quiet the mind to create a sense of stillness. We often hear parents ask their children to "be still." We may ask them to be still, but do we teach them how to be still?

The structure of our mind is a vast and energetic field. Every thought we have is a movement of energy—energy of the mind. In a world where it is easy to become distracted, people quickly move from thing to thing to thing. Some call it a "monkey mind." Like a monkey that continually jumps from limb to limb to limb, the mind of a very distracted individual never slows down to focus on one thing.

Learning how to quiet the mind builds a pathway to our inner wisdom and strength. Learning how to build access to the mind begins with stillness. Learning how to be still is a skill that takes practice. It can begin with some simple breath awareness exercises and then move into deeper forms of stillness such as meditation, prayer, or contemplation.

Have you ever had some amazing insights while lying in bed, taking a shower, driving down the highway, or going for a long walk? What was it that allowed your mind to open up? The answer is stillness.

Meditation

Meditation is a chosen or conscious relaxation exercise with the goal of quieting and clearing the mind, bringing stillness, creating peace and serenity, and opening ourselves up to greater insights. It is a state of thoughtless awareness. True meditation is a state of peace that occurs when the mind is calm and silent, yet completely alert.

Meditation is a skill. When practiced on a regular basis, it can help control stress, improve sleep and health, lower inflammation, and improve focus. This state of calmness and serenity helps us find the answers to our questions. The challenge is how to achieve this state.

There is a whole lot more to meditation than simply sitting still with your legs crossed and your eyes closed, but it does not have to be difficult. At the most basic level, meditation is simply thinking thoughts and then letting go of them. It is about learning to distinguish thoughts that may help and thoughts that do not.

Techniques for Effective Meditation

- Block out time. Start with just 5 minutes a day. The key is just to begin.
- Make an appointment for meditation in your day. Start slowly.
- Find a quiet place where you will not be interrupted.
- Posture is important. Sit up straight, hands resting on your thighs. I have found sitting propped up with a pillow against the back of a chair or wall can work great. Get comfortable.
- Close your eyes and mouth. Breathe only through your nose. Think of nothing except the coolness of your breath. This will quiet your mind and relax your body. If thoughts keep popping in and out, no problem. Just keep coming back to your breath.
- Some days are better than others. Some days may be more difficult than others. It is okay. Let your thoughts come and go and keep coming back to your breath.
- Candle Gazing. As you continue your meditation practice, an easy way to enhance your stillness and training is candle gazing. Do this exercise in a dark, quiet room. Get in a comfortable seated position. Place a small candle on a plate and light it. Stare at the light. Try not to blink. Once you blink start the exercise over again. Focus your attention on the flame, ignoring all other thoughts, sensations and feeling. Keep your gaze steady and unblinking. Continue to focus on your breath and stare at the candle. This is a great focus exercise and can be extremely powerful in your journey to create stillness in your mind. Start candle gazing for 2-3 minutes prior to your meditation practice.

Give mediation a try. The benefits can be life changing! Meditation is an extremely powerful practice that consciously brings stillness leading to greater calmness, serenity, and tranquility into our daily life.

Practice meditation exercises using our ***app*** which can be found at ***ontargetliving.com.***

Laugh, Smile, Cry, and Practice Gratitude

Learning to become more intentional about spreading greater love and kindness in our world can be extremely powerful. It is a mindset that requires awareness.

How do you feel when you have a good belly laugh, sing a song, experience a touching moment that makes you cry, or get a warm smile from a stranger?

I love the saying, "Act your way into right thinking." We all have days when we just do not feel like exercising or being nice to a family member, friend, or coworker. When we focus on the task at hand, we begin to develop the muscle to act our way into right thinking. This practice can help us all achieve what we want. If we wait to eat right, exercise, be kind, or meditate when we feel like it, right thinking may never happen.

Act your way into an attitude of gratitude. Smile more and be kind to others. There is no greater wisdom than kindness.

Practice Kindness

Take this challenge for an entire week. Smile or say hello to everyone you walk by. It is the simple things in life that touch our hearts and those around us. Let's all spread more love and kindness in our world!

Practice Gratitude

First thing every morning, identify three things you are grateful for. It is almost impossible to feel bad when we focus on gratitude. Give it a try right now!

1. ______________________________
2. ______________________________
3. ______________________________

Rest, Relaxation and Rejuvenation

The first goal of this section is to deepen our understanding of stress and how detrimental it can be to the mind and body. The second is to provide some solid rest, recovery, and rejuvenation strategies that we can build into our lifestyle to help us feel and be our best.

Use our Rest Target as a guide to help you slowly upgrade and build a few new rest and rejuvenation habits into your life.

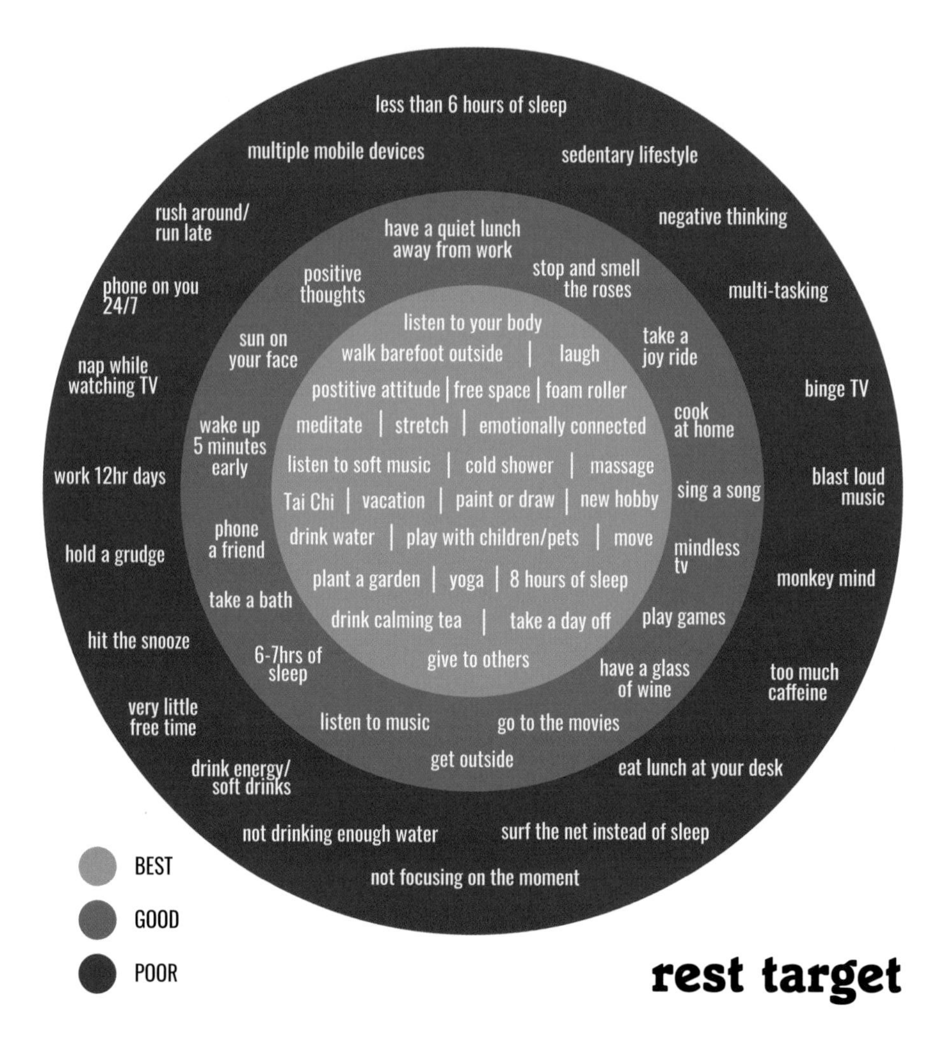

Space Essentials

Big Picture

- We all need space in our lives to rejuvenate the mind and body.
- Space in our lives is shrinking faster than ever before.
- We sleep less.
- We work more.
- Stillness is a skill that needs to be practiced.
- Having enough space is imperative to feel and be your best!

Ask Yourself

- What can you learn from the donkey and the sloth?
- Are you satisfied with the amount of space you currently have in your life?
- What can you do to expand and protect your space?
- How do you feel when you have an open calendar for the day?
- Do you take time to unplug and recharge your batteries on a regular basis?
- How do you feel when you get a good night of sleep or return from a restful vacation?

Small Steps

- Be still each day for 90 seconds.
- Read a book.
- Play a board game or do a puzzle.
- Act your way into right thinking.
- Laugh and cry more. Smile and be kind more. Show gratitude and love more.
- Move your body daily.
- Take a walk on the beach or in the woods.
- Get a massage.
- Play more.
- Take the morning off from work.

SECTION

4

LET FOOD BE YOUR MEDICINE

15 The Power of Food

In Section 3 we discussed the first foundational pillar of health, **REST**, and the importance of having enough rest, recovery, and rejuvenation to feel and be our best. The second pillar is **EAT**. What we eat and drink can change our lives. It sure has changed mine and has for so many others.

Food is love; food is social; and food is taste. Food is energy, and food is health. Much of life is centered around food. Before we jump into a deep discussion of calories, vitamins, minerals, carbohydrates, proteins, fats, superfoods, hydration, meal patterning, fasting, weight loss, shopping, meal planning, recipes, and dining out, let's start with a brief understanding of the science of food.

The Greek physician Hippocrates, born in 460 BC, is considered the father of medicine and was the first to believe that the human body was not a collection of isolated parts. He argued that the human body functions as one unified organism and must be treated both in health and in disease as an integrated whole. Hippocrates was the first to say, "Let food be thy medicine and medicine be thy food."

In the late twentieth century, food finally began to be recognized in the West as an important healing force. Holistic practitioners have always seen marked improvements when individuals make appropriate dietary changes. What we eat and drink can impact our lives with more energy, greater health, expanded capacity, and increased vitality.

Mindset of Food

People have a huge interest in food and nutrition. We see it in social media, television, radio, print, movies, and on the internet. The talk of food is big business. Yet, we know so little about the science of nutrition.

Growing up in Michigan, I learned how to spell, read, and write. I studied math and history. Not once was I introduced to the subject of nutrition, a science that impacts our energy, our welfare, our health, and plays such an important role in our existence.

In my first year of college at Western Michigan University, I took the basics: psychology, geography, math, creative writing, and biology. The subject of nutrition was not included in any of my choices. It was offered only as an elective if you were majoring in dietetics or another similar discipline. Even my graduate degree in Exercise Physiology from Michigan State University only required two classes on nutrition. Just two. Both of those nutritional classes had little practical application. Even today, most medical or nursing schools provide very little training on the subject of nutrition. I still do not fully understand why a science that is so powerful in keeping the human body healthy is not in greater demand in our educational system.

Why is it that 90 percent of our cancer research dollars today are spent trying to develop medications that enhance and improve our immune systems rather than researching how our lifestyle and the food we eat can rejuvenate and build our immune systems?

Why is so much money and energy spent on trying to find the cure? Doesn't it make more sense to go after the source of the problem instead of trying to fix the problem down the line? It is so much easier to keep the car running smoothly with regular checkups than trying to fix the car when the engine light comes on.

My son Matt asked me, "If you could change one thing related to the health of our planet, what would it be?" Without hesitation I answered, "Our educational system, as it pertains to our health." From an early age, we have to teach people self-care. We need to learn how to take care of our own health from grade school all the way up through higher learning. The magic is right in front of us, and our educational system needs to change. Prevention needs to be front and center. We also need to place more of our resources into prevention and compensate our healthcare professionals for driving prevention. These are big issues with even greater possibilities.

I am a strong believer in the power of food. We have been trained as a society to reach for a pill when our blood pressure is too high or when our cholesterol is out of balance. Imagine if we changed our thinking to the power of food, choosing food as our medicine and experiencing the miraculous way the body can heal itself if given the right ingredients.

Dr. Jeffrey Bland, the father of Functional Medicine, says it best. Food is information for the human body. Food speaks to our genes. Food turns our genes on, and food turns our genes off. There are millions of molecules of information in every bite of food that get translated by our genes into cellular instructions. These instructions control our health.

We all need to get on board with moving our mindset towards prevention. We have a wonderful healthcare system when it comes to trauma care. However, if our goal is to stay healthy and prevent most illnesses, we need to take advantage of the power that is in our own hands and not rely on the healthcare system to take care of us in that way.

Prevention is our future!

Nutrition 101

Think of nutrition as the process of being nourished and giving the mind and body nutrients to grow, heal, and self-correct. When we eat or drink nutrients, the human body breaks down these nutrients, and uses them for fuel, growth, and repair.

In 1970 the average person in the United States consumed approximately 2,200 calories per day. Today we consume a whopping 4,100 calories per day. Even with those extra calories, many of us are deficient in the necessary nutrients that keep the mind and body healthy.

There are two types of nutritional deficiencies.

- A **primary** nutrient deficiency occurs when the body lacks a specific nutrient like omega-3 fats, vitamin C, calcium, magnesium, or B vitamins.
- A **secondary** nutrient deficiency occurs when the body fails to absorb or utilize the food or beverage that has been consumed. We may be eating the necessary foods, but the body is not absorbing the nutrients.

How Nutritional Deficiencies Progress in the Body

- **First Level:** Nutrient reserves begin to deplete.
- **Second Level:** The body starts stealing nutrients from tissues.
- **Third Level:** Lab findings start to change (low vitamin D, elevated homocysteine, elevated highly sensitive C-reactive protein, low testosterone, low GFR).
- **Fourth Level:** The body begins talking to us (colds, flu, allergies, acid reflux, kidney stones, broken sleep, high blood pressure).
- **Fifth Level:** Anatomical changes appear (shrinkage of bone, muscles, and tendons, and stressed adrenal glands). Symptoms become anatomical.

The human body has an incredible ability to heal and self-correct if given the proper nutrients.

Nutrition begins with the quality of foods and beverages that we ingest. It is what we ingest and assimilate that fuels the body. This process is called digestion. During digestion, the entire body works to not only break down the foods or beverages that have been consumed, but it also helps these nutrients absorb into the body. After the digestion process is complete, the body moves into the elimination phase. Elimination is the process of excreting what is not needed during the digestive process.

If the body does not use or absorb the foods or beverages that were ingested or does not effectively eliminate the waste, it can lead to toxicity. It is this toxicity that causes many of our problems to begin.

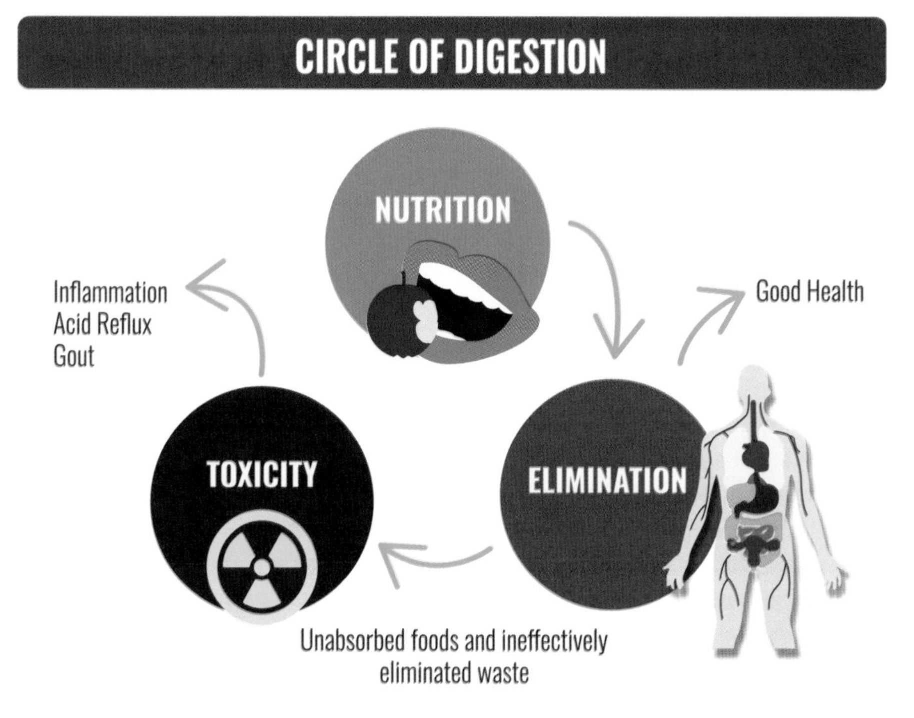

Gut Health and The Immune System

What takes place in the digestive system over the next 24-72 hours after a meal? Think of the digestive system as a 30-foot-long drainpipe from the mouth to the anus. Acids and enzymes melt food particles into sludge while tiny microbes convert food into energy to power your brain, muscles, and immune system. Subtle changes in gut health can have a powerful impact on digestion. Research has linked an imbalance of gut bacteria to a weakened immune system which leads to more than 70 chronic diseases.

The Immune System and How It Works

The immune system protects the body from outside invaders. It is like a suit of armor. The stronger the armor, the more difficult it is for invaders to penetrate the body. The immune system learns from the past. From the time we were young playing in the dirt or going to school for the first time, our bodies were subjected to outside invaders. The body slowly built up the immune system, creating a bank of protection.

Upwards of 80 percent of our immune system lives in the gut. If our gut is not healthy, then we are not going to be healthy. We have seen an explosion in the amount of digestive health problems in the United States and around the world for acid reflux, irritable bowel, Crohn's disease, constipation, diarrhea, gluten intolerances, food allergies, bloating, skin problems, asthma, cancer, headaches, low energy, inflammation, type 2 diabetes, poor immune function, and liver and kidney stress, just to name a few. The digestive aid aisle in most grocery stores and pharmacies continues to expand.

A person who does not digest food properly cannot obtain the optimum amount of nutrients to help build, repair, and regenerate the body.

Digestive Issues on the Rise

First, we eat and drink too much low-quality food. Processed foods, fast food, soda pop, energy drinks, alcohol, artificial sweeteners, and dairy all lead to poor gut health.

Second, we consume too many medications, especially antibiotics and anti-inflammatory medications. While antibiotics have saved many lives and cured many infections, they are not without side effects. The same is true for anti-inflammatory medications. If we have a toothache or a bee sting and need some relief, it is not a problem to take an occasional anti-inflammatory. The problem lies in taking these medications too often or habitually. Over time gut bacteria begins to change leading to an increase of pathogens.

Third, air and water pollution along with an increase of pesticides can have adverse effects on the microbiome, leading to inflammatory diseases, compromised gut lining, and increased pathogenic bacteria. Using some form of water filtration for drinking water and consuming pesticide-free foods are great ways to help improve gut health.

Building Your Garden

Think of the gut as a garden. In the spring we till the dirt and get the soil ready for planting the seeds. If the soil in our garden is dry and depleted of nutrients, nothing grows except weeds. Now imagine a garden that contains a healthy colony of good bacteria and other microorganisms. Foods that help promote beneficial bacteria create an environment where organisms can flourish.

Prebiotics are foods and beverages that develop the soil in the gut to get ready for planting. These are fibrous foods that feed the good bacteria.

Probiotics are the seeds. They are live beneficial bacteria found in food.

Synbiotics are foods that contain both prebiotics and probiotics. That is why I tell people to start eating real foods before taking a prebiotic or probiotic in supplement form. Adding some of these pre-, pro-, and synbiotic foods and beverages into our diet builds a healthy garden in the gut.

Our health begins in the gut and now is the time to build our garden.

Real Food Bacteria

We are dependent on certain bacteria to help digest our food, release energy, produce certain vitamins, regulate our immune system, and keep us healthy by protecting against disease. Improving the quality of bacteria in our gut can also improve overall brain health, mood, memory, and mental health issues like anxiety and depression.

GUT BIOTICS

PREBIOTICS ARE FIBROUS FOODS THAT FEED BACTERIA

PROBIOTICS ARE LIVE BENEFICIAL BACTERIA FOUND IN FOOD

SYNBIOTICS ARE FOODS THAT CONTAIN BOTH PRE AND PROBIOTICS

PREBIOTICS

- Ancient Grains
- Apples
- Artichokes
- Asparagus
- Bananas
- Barley
- Beans
- Berries
- Chia seeds
- Flaxseeds
- Garlic
- Ginger
- Greens
- Jicamas
- Leeks
- Legumes
- Nuts
- Oats
- Onions
- Oranges
- Potatoes
- Quinoa
- Root Vegetables
- Seaweed
- Seeds
- Sweet Potatoes

PROBIOTICS

- Cheese
- Kefir
- Kimchi
- Kombucha
- Lemons
- Miso
- Pickles
- Raw Unfiltered Apple Cider Vinegar
- Sauerkraut
- Yogurt

SYNBIOTICS

- Apples
- Cacao
- Coconut
- Raw Honey
- Seaweed
- Sourdough Bread
- Spirulina/Chlorella (Algae)
- Unpasturized Wheatgrass

How to Improve Gut Health

Here are a few additional tips for improving gut health and creating a healthy and vibrant immune system.

Step 1: Balance Your Nervous System

We need a balanced nervous system to have a healthy gut. If our stress button is chronically on, digestion shuts down making it extremely difficult to have a healthy gut and healthy immune system. Breathe, sleep, and create some space.

Step 2: Eliminate Low-Quality Foods

Consuming a lot of processed foods and beverages will make the body cry "uncle."

Step 3: Chew Food Slowly

The digestive process begins in the mouth. The mouth is full of digestive enzymes that help break down and absorb nutrients. Slow down and chew your food.

Step 4: Maintain Hydration

It is impossible to have a healthy gut and immune system if we are chronically dehydrated. Water increases energy and detoxifies the body.

Step 5: Consume Super Greens

Foods high in chlorophyll clean and detoxify as well as strengthen the gut, leading to a healthier immune system.

Step 6: Balance Your pH

Consuming more alkaline-based foods and beverages together with daily movement and managing stress is essential for optimal gut health.

Step 7: Add Prebiotic, Probiotic, and Synbiotic Foods

Adding in friendly bacteria from foods and beverages is like having a healthy garden. Your garden begins in the gut.

Step 8: Eat Foods Closer to the Source

Eating more live foods increases the amount of fiber, antioxidants, vitamins, minerals, and necessary digestive enzymes needed for a healthy gut.

Step 9: Get Sunshine

Get a daily dose of sunshine. Sunshine is essential for so many aspects of our health, including gut health.

Step 10: Move Daily

Motion creates positive emotion. The human body thrives on daily movement which is essential for a healthy gut and immune system.

Gut health is critical for optimal health, and it is the key for building a healthy, vibrant immune system! Eat more prebiotic, probiotic, and synbiotic foods.

Gut-Brain Connection

I think we have all "gone with our gut" to make an important decision or felt "butterflies in our stomach" when we were nervous. Where do these sensations come from? Hidden in the walls of the digestive system (the gut) is our "second brain." The concept of the "second brain" is revolutionizing medicine's understanding of the links between digestion, mood, health, and even the way we think.

Scientists call this second brain the Enteric Nervous System (ENS). The ENS is one of the main divisions of the autonomic nervous system and consists of two thin layers of more than 100 million nerve cells lining our gastrointestinal tract from our esophagus to our rectum. Unlike the big brain in our skull, the ENS cannot balance a budget or solve a puzzle. The main role of ENS is controlling digestion from the moment we chew our food to the moment we eliminate it.

Our two brains work beautifully together and play a key role in certain diseases in our bodies and overall health. Unfortunately, Western medicine really struggles with this mind-body connection. Our medical system is designed on isolation and specialization, so it is no wonder we lack research and education on this connection.

There are hundreds of examples of how our two brains communicate and work together. When a person feels danger, the fight-or-flight response is triggered. At the same time, the ENS slows down or stops digestion. This is done so that more of the body's energy can be diverted to dealing with the threat. There is no need to digest food when running from a bear.

This connection goes both ways. Bad gut health leads to poor mental health, and poor mental health leads to bad gut health. Our two brains are constantly talking to each other, so treating one without the other makes little sense. Think about this. Thirty to forty percent of our population has functional bowel or gastrointestinal (gut) disorders, such as constipation, diarrhea, bloating, acid reflux, gout, IBS, celiac, and other pH imbalances, not to mention asthma, allergies, sensitivities, and ADHD.

Antibiotics, oral contraceptives, acid blockers, NSAIDS, cholesterol-lowering medications, antidepressants, and many other medications negatively affect the gut. For example, anxiety and stress may be a psychological concern, but we now know that gastrointestinal problems can create anxiety and stress, and that anxiety and stress can create gastrointestinal problems.

When suffering from digestive problems, we need to begin with a greater understanding of stress and learn how to develop strategies to quiet the mind and relax the body (see Section 3: Rest, Relaxation, and Rejuvenation). A great place to start to address stress, anxiety, depression, broken sleep, a compromised immune system, and poor digestion is gut health.

The 5 Superhighways of Elimination: BULLS

A key component in the health of the human body is the ability to eliminate on a regular basis. The old adage "out with the bad and in with the good" fits when maintaining great health. The human body is designed to eliminate unwanted intruders and toxins. Without regular elimination processes, the body can become extremely toxic leading to many health problems. During our seminars and trainings, I find that most people do not know how often they should eliminate. I also find that this subject is considered private and seldom discussed.

If our goal is to lose weight, improve energy, rejuvenate the immune system, improve gut health, decrease disease, and enjoy amazing health, then, we need to learn more about elimination.

The five superhighways of elimination are the bowel, urine, lungs, lymphatic system, and skin (BULLS).

Bowel

How often should we have a bowel movement? Once a day, after every meal, every other day? The correct answer is 1-2 times per day. That is an important goal that everyone should strive for. Imagine if your dog did not have a bowel movement on a daily basis. You would probably take a ride to the vet.

Humans should have 1-2 bowel movements per day. The shape of the stool depends on how long it has been in the colon, with 72 hours being ideal. It should look like a soft banana. If it is not soft, then we are most likely constipated. If we eliminate more than three times per day and it is still

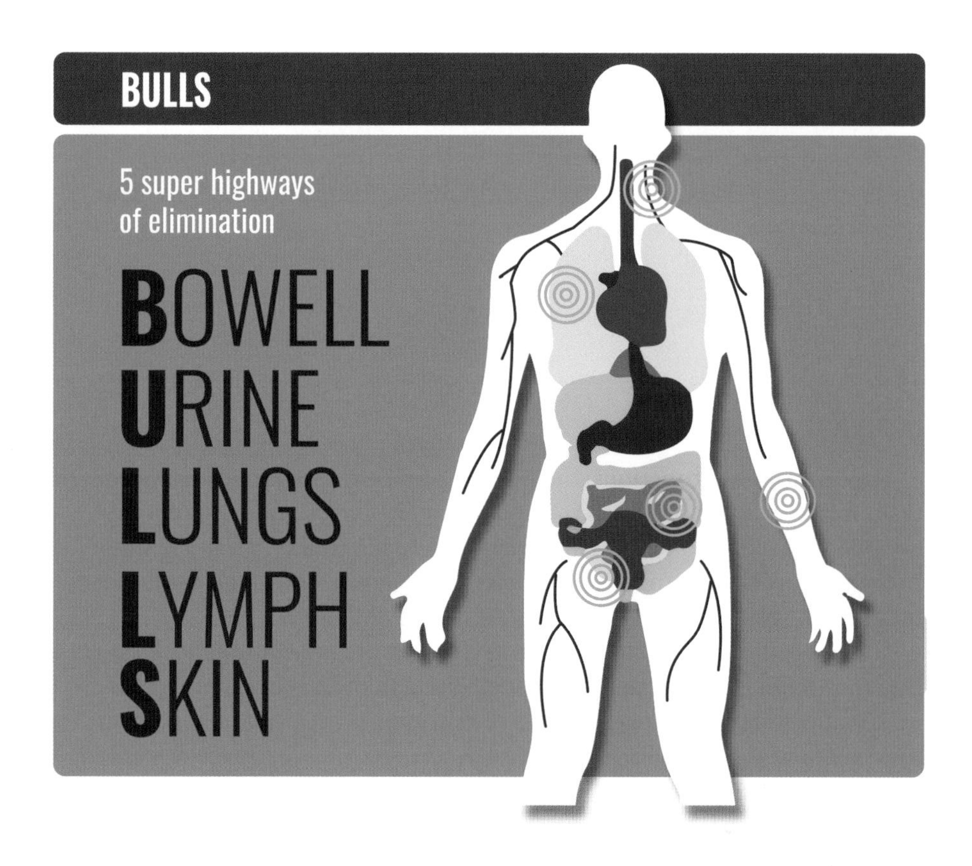

shaped like a soft banana, we are most likely eating too much. If we suffer from loose stools, it indicates inflammation or illness.

How often do you have a bowel movement each day? ________________

Urine

Another way the body eliminates is through the kidneys and urine. Urine should take on the color of Chardonnay, not too dark and not too light. This is one of the major reasons why being hydrated plays such an important role in your health and keeping the body clean. If urine is too dark, it may be due to dehydration. If your urine is too clear, it could mean too much hydration.

What color is your urine? ________________________________

Lungs

We eliminate through our lungs when we breathe. This is one reason why having good posture and regular exercise or movement is essential for the lungs to expel toxins. Breathing with the diaphragm is also extremely beneficial to the elimination process.

Do you breathe with the diaphragm regularly? Yes or No

Lymphatic System

Among its other functions, the lymphatic system acts as a sewer system for the human body. It helps keep the body clean by filtering out and carrying away carcinogens and toxins from every cell, tissue, and organ in the body. Lymph nodes located under the armpits, in the groin, and along the neck and inner thighs play a large role in the elimination of toxins.

Using deodorants or antiperspirants that contain aluminum block the lymph nodes under the arm, thus blocking the elimination process of perspiration. Parabens are chemicals widely used as artificial preservatives in cosmetic and body care products. They are also found in propylene glycol used in anti-freeze or artificial fragrances. All can add toxins to the body and compromise the elimination process. Avoid skin products such as creams, lotions, shampoos, soaps, shaving gels, moisturizers, and cosmetics that contain parabens.

Unlike the heart, the lymphatic system needs a pump. We are that pump. To optimize the lymphatic system, we need to be part of the solution.

How to Stimulate the Lymphatic System

- Move daily, especially using the arms and upper body. I am also a huge fan of using a mini trampoline to stimulate the lymphatic system.
- Maintain proper hydration.
- Take hot and cold showers.
- Get a massage.
- Use a foam roller.
- Practice deep breathing.
- Make good food choices: leafy greens, spirulina/chlorella, wheatgrass, garlic, flaxseeds, chia seeds, almonds, avocados, beets, and apples.

What daily practices are you doing to help your lymphatic system do its job? ____

____

____

Skin

Skin is the largest organ in the human body and tells us when our digestion in not working correctly.

I had skin problems for more than 15 years of my life. Doctors gave me oral medications and topical creams, but nothing seemed to work. The doctors told my parents that I just had sensitive skin. The truth was that I did not have sensitive skin, I was just a poor eater. Due to my unhealthy eating habits, I developed an unhealthy gut and a weak immune system. When I cleaned up my diet and improved my gut health, my skin improved almost overnight.

Regular movement or the occasional use of an infrared sauna can also help the body eliminate. What we put on our skin, such as lotions, oils, soaps, shampoo, perfume, colognes, and even dry-cleaning chemicals, can all affect the level of toxins the body is exposed to. More will be discussed on body care in Section 6: Your Health Keeps Score.

What are a few of your daily practices to take care of your skin?

____

____

____

The Power of Food Essentials

Big Picture

- Harness the Power of Food!
- Food is love and food is social. Food is medicine and food is information.
- In 1970 the average person in the United States consumed 2,200 calories per day. Today that number has grown to 4,100 calories per day.
- There are two primary nutritional deficiencies: what are we missing and what we are not absorbing.
- Your health begins in your gut.
- The enteric nervous system (ENS)—sometimes called your "second brain"—is the gut/brain connection.
- There are 5 superhighways of elimination— the BULLS: Bowel, Urine, Lungs, Lymph, and Skin.
- Building a nutritional plan is a process that takes time.

Ask Yourself

- Do you believe in the power of food to heal and self-correct the body?
- What nutrients may you be missing?
- How can you take more ownership of your health?
- What can you do to rejuvenate and build your immune system?
- How can you make your gut healthier?
- Are your superhighways of elimination—BULLS—running smoothly?

Small Steps

- Stay hydrated.
- Move your body daily.
- Practice diaphragmatic breathing 1-2 minutes per day.
- Use the foam roller.

16 Hydration

Now that we have you have a better understanding of nutrition, let's get cracking on the fun part—the how. To help navigate the world of nutrition, we developed the EAT Pyramid as a guide to building a solid nutritional plan that can be easily followed.

The EAT Pyramid consists of six nutritional building blocks: **Hydration—Superfoods—Quality—Meal Patterning—Quantity—80/20 Rule.** We will cover each of these in subsequent chapters. The goal is to build healthy and sustainable nutritional habits.

Our first EAT Pyramid building block is Hydration. Over the past 50 years the variety of foods available and the consumption of certain foods has drastically changed. The same is true with the types and quantity of beverages that we drink. Many of the popular beverages being consumed these days are causing as many health problems as the poor-quality foods we are eating.

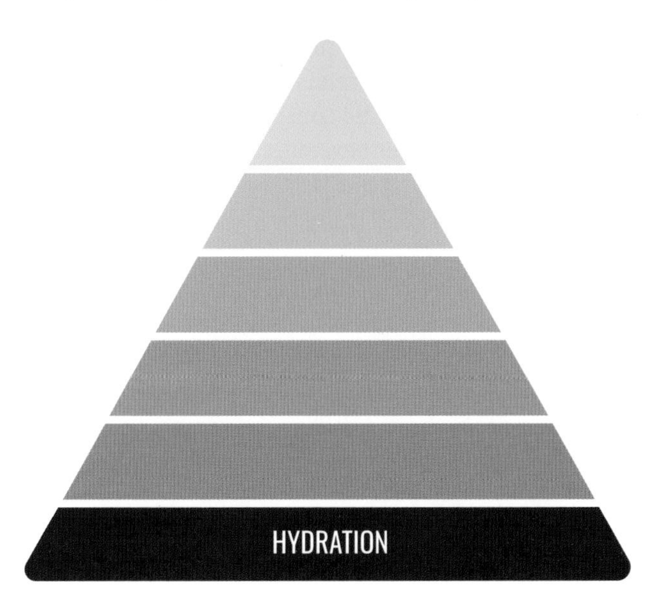

Beverages

Soda Pop

Soda pop is the number one beverage consumed in the United States outside of water. ***Number One!*** The average American drinks 1.6 cans of soda pop every day. That might not sound like much, but it adds up to 597 cans of soda pop per year. This number continues to grow, especially among our children and teenagers.

Mexico has now taken the lead as the number one consumer of soda pop per person in the world. It is no coincidence that Mexico now ranks number two in type 2 diabetes in the world, just behind the United States. This is not a statistic to be proud of.

An occasional soda pop now and then is not so bad, but it is important to understand that soda pop is extremely acidic. It can leach out minerals such as calcium and magnesium, which leads to weak brittle bones, increased inflammation, and poor digestive health.

Soda pop, even diet soda, can also increase the probability of gaining weight. One of the many buffering minerals it leaches out is iodine. Iodine is a powerful mineral that helps support the thyroid gland that plays key role in body metabolism. Years ago, I was consulting with a very obese women and asked her about the beverages she consumed. Her first answer was water. When asked if she drank any other beverages, she reported consuming 6 to 8 diet sodas each day. She believed that because there were no calories in diet soda, she was actually doing a good thing by avoiding sugar. I explained to her about pH balance and how her body was working against her, not with her.

As I said, don't worry about an occasional soda pop. If soda pop is consumed as a primary beverage several times a day, it is time to make a change to achieve greater energy and better health. A better alternative would be to drink mineral water with a splash of fruit juice. Mineral water is very alkalizing and is naturally carbonated. The juice adds a little sweetness and is very refreshing.

Energy Drinks

This is a product line that I have become very passionate about and not in a positive way. Do people truly believe that having an energy shot from a can is a good thing?

Let's start with the facts and just the facts. When I began an internet search for "healthiest beverages to consume," I expected water to be number one. I was shocked to see that an all-natural energy drink came up first. Seriously, who believes that an all-natural energy drink is healthy? I am here to let you know that there is no such thing as a healthy energy drink!

Today energy drinks have exploded into the marketplace and are the fastest growing group of beverages around the world. The first energy drink introduced in the United States was Red Bull back in 1997. The energy drink industry has grown into big business today with powerful marketing and advertising that targets our kids, our teens, our young adults, and now adults. Look out seniors! Are they coming for us next?

We currently spend over $70 billion each year globally on energy drinks with over 100 different types of energy shots and drink options on the market today.

> ***Can We Buy Energy?***
>
> *One day I took a trip to one of the big box grocery stores in my community to check out the energy drink aisle. I could not believe the overwhelming number of energy drink options. The section was over 50-feet long and included Red Bull, 5-Hour Energy, Monster, Full Throttle, Red Thunder, Redline, Hyde, Spike, Bang, Cocaine, Outlaw, and External. These were just a few of the many options available. Then I began wondering who comes up with these names? You could buy the 2-5-ounce energy shot or up to a large 32-ounce energy drink that came in a gigantic can. Can you imagine what your gut would say to the brain when downing these 32 ounces of TNT?*
>
> *Believe it or not, I even spotted a 16-hour energy drink. I had to buy this rocket fuel to see what it looked and smelled like. It was a light blue color and smelled like cough syrup, the same cough syrup I was given as a kid. That smell is still etched into my brain. Imagine trying to get a good night of sleep after drinking this volcanic concoction.*
>
> *I can only imagine what the conversation in the lab may have sounded like. "You know George, there are so many energy drink options on the market offering 5, 8, 10, and 12 hours of energy. How do we stand apart from the rest? I have it—let's make a 16-hour energy drink." What's next? A 24-hour energy drink?*

Three Important Questions to Contemplate Regarding Energy Drinks

First, why are so many people looking for more energy and why would a somewhat healthy person be unable to make it through their day without an injection of one of these powerful stimulants?

Second, where do people think we get our energy from? Energy comes from the food we eat, how we breathe, how we sleep, and daily movement. I get that life can beat us up, but do we truly believe that getting energy from a shot or a can is healthy for the mind and body? Can it be sustainable?

Third, what is in these rocket fuel beverages that makes them so unhealthy?

Most of these high-octane drinks are loaded with thermogenic compounds such as taurine, choline, inositol, L-carnitine, tyrosine, yerba mate, and ginseng. Thermogenic compounds produce heat and can overstimulate your adrenal glands leading to many serious health problems. In addition to the thermogenic compounds, many energy drinks have extremely high levels of caffeine, synthetic B vitamins, niacin, sugar, and artificial ingredients.

Some of the common side effects from energy drinks include dehydration, energy and mood swings, mineral depletion, adrenal fatigue, anxiety, sleeplessness, inflammation, irritability, increased urination, decreased bone health, acid reflux, increased heart rate, increased blood pressure, heart arrythmias, and even death.

The answer to chronic fatigue and loss of energy does not come from any type of energy drink. I recommend avoiding all energy drinks and want you to help educate our next generation on the potential hazards lurking in these powerful drink stimulants.

Coffee

Americans love their coffee, consuming over 450 million cups per day. Coffee shops are everywhere. Ordering a cup of coffee has a language all of its own. People enjoy the taste, the aroma, the warmth, and the quick pick-me-up that coffee provides. For many drinking a cup of coffee is a big part of their morning ritual.

A few years ago, my sister Paula told me she was having a hard time giving up her coffee habit. When I asked her why she wanted to give it up, she said she knew it was not good for her. I did not ask for a scientific breakdown, but she gave it to me anyway. Coffee is acidic, places stress on the adrenal glands, leaches out valuable minerals, and inhibits the absorption of iron, magnesium, zinc, and some B vitamins. I told her that I knew all that. The bottom line was she loved her coffee – the taste, the smell, everything about it. She drank only one cup in the morning. I told her to stop feeling guilty about her coffee habit. In fact, I suggested she upgrade the quality of coffee, and continue to enjoy one cup a day.

Whenever possible buy organic coffee. Coffee and tea are two crops with high pesticide levels. Also, if you like to use a creamer in your coffee, avoid creamers with trans fats, artificial sweeteners, and chemicals. Get a creamer with fewer ingredients that are closer to the source.

Tea

Tea is the most widely consumed beverage in the world, second only to water. For years, followers of alternative medicine have touted the health benefits of drinking tea. There are many different types of tea to choose from, including white tea, Oolong tea, black tea, green tea, and herbal tea. I am a big fan of herbal teas such as peppermint, cinnamon, licorice root, and my favorite—ginger. I like the taste and smell, and it is great for gut health and digestion. Make your own infusion. Ginger root can be found in most grocery stores. Peel and shave it, and then add it to hot water. When choosing your favorite tea, buy organic whenever possible.

Milk

In the United States, we drink over 25 gallons of milk per person per year. Of the milk we drink, over 90 percent is cow's milk. It is touted as a great source of calcium.

Why then, when we drink so much cow's milk do we still have such poor bone health? Cow's milk is not a great source of calcium to begin with and is also highly acidic. It also has a very large protein molecule making it extremely difficult to break down and absorb, causing digestive challenges, skin rashes, psoriasis, allergies, and asthma. Not ready to give up cow's milk? Then be sure to upgrade to an organic milk source to avoid any added hormones.

The most consumed milk in the world today is goat's milk. Okay, so you may not be ready for goat's milk, but it is a much healthier option than cow's milk. Goat's milk is easier to digest than cow's milk and contains the antifungal compound caprylic acid.

There are also many wonderful, great tasting, plant-based milk options available. I recommend them to everyone. They are easy to digest, more alkalizing for the body, and taste great. My personal favorites are almond, cashew, coconut, oat, and hemp milk. Plant-based milks can also be made easily right in your own kitchen. The best ones to choose are the ones with the fewest ingredients closer to the source.

Juice and Juicing

As our lifestyle continues to speed up, more and more people are juicing as a way to get more fruits and vegetables into their diets.

Drinking juice is an easy way to get a variety of valuable vitamins, minerals, and antioxidants into your diet. Personally, I find it challenging at times to get healthy nutrients in my body and use a juice extractor or go to our local juicer to help fill in the gap. My favorite juice recipe is a combination of beets, celery, carrots, and apples. It tastes great and is extremely alkalizing. I also enjoy the taste of pomegranate and dark cherry juice. I use 1-2 ounces of juice with 1-2 tablespoons of flaxseeds or chai seeds as an afternoon snack.

When drinking juice, I recommend diluting it with water. Use a ratio of 4 cups of water to ½ cup of your favorite juice. There are no substitutions for eating whole fruits and vegetables. However, 100 percent, high-quality juices can be the next best thing and fit nicely into a focused nutrition plan.

Alcohol

We have all heard that one glass of wine is good for you, but are some alcoholic beverages better than others? Nutritionally speaking and calories aside, red wine is your best choice, followed by white wine, spirits, and beer. Red wine is less acidic and has more antioxidants.

Is there a recommended limit on the number of alcoholic beverages to consume each week? Now I am not anyone's alcohol police, but for most people I recommend 4-5 alcoholic beverages or less per week. Too much alcohol can put a great deal of stress on your liver and kidneys, and decrease glomerular filtration rate (GFR), a kidney function measurement. So, feel free to enjoy an alcoholic beverage of choice and drink alcohol in moderation.

Sports Drinks

Sports drinks are being consumed in record numbers, especially among teenagers and young adults. In the gym, at a sporting event, or just hanging out, these drinks have exploded onto the beverage scene. Every major manufacturer now has its own line of sports drinks. Many of these sports drinks are promoted as a healthy alternative, but in many cases, they are loaded with artificial ingredients, colored dyes, processed sugar, or sugar substitutes.

There are alternatives to traditional sports drinks that can provide electrolytes without a bunch of unhealthy ingredients. My personal favorites are organic coconut water or water with lemon and orange slices. I add a splash of apple cider vinegar with a little local honey or maple syrup. It tastes great and keeps me hydrated.

Smoothies

Adding a healthy and delicious smoothie recipe to your nutritional routine can be easy. My favorite smoothie recipe is the Chocolate Chip Mint Smoothie in our *Target to Table* cookbook. It consists of coconut water, organic coconut flakes, hempseeds, Brazil nuts, dates, banana, spinach, mint leaves, and cacao nibs. Just blend for 30-45 seconds for a delicious and nutritious breakfast or midday energy boost.

Water

Water is essential for life and keeping the body healthy. The body depends on water to survive. Every cell, tissue, and organ in the human body needs water in order to work properly. The body is 70-75 percent water. Think about that. The human body is made up for 70-75 percent water. One of the most important things to pay attention to from a nutritional standpoint is water, including water quality and the amount of water to drink.

Drinking enough water throughout my day is my greatest nutritional challenge. I know I need to drink more water, so each day I create a water environment that makes it easy to do. I place a water bottle on my nightstand, in my car, on my desk at work, in the gym, and in my gear when traveling. Wherever I go, I try to make sure I am drinking enough water and staying well hydrated.

Water is the body's cleansing and waste removal fluid. Water carries nutrients and oxygen, cushions joints, and protects organs. Water also aids in digestion, metabolism, and energy.

A common problem for many people is fatigue and lack of energy. Water composes over 90 percent of our blood. As the body becomes dehydrated, blood is the first place the body looks for more water. When the body pulls water from the blood, blood volume decreases, leading to a drop in energy due to a drop in cardiac output. Staying properly hydrated is essential for great energy.

Over 80 percent of emergency room visits can be attributed to unintentional chronic dehydration. Chronic dehydration may be the root cause of many health problems such as asthma, hormonal imbalances, low kidney function, high blood pressure, dizziness, arthritis, osteoporosis, ulcers, digestive problems, gout, kidney stones, constipation, restless leg, muscle cramps, low back pain, memory loss, and obesity to name just a few.

Don't Let Hydration Sneak Up on You

I used to play a lot of golf with my dad. We always had a great time together. He was a ton of fun to be around.

But he was not a healthy guy. Dad was notorious for being chronically dehydrated. It would be late morning or early afternoon, hot and humid outside, and there in the cup holder of his golf cart sat a large cup of coffee. If I asked if he had had any water, his answer was always the same. There is water in my coffee. He knew his answer would make me crazy.

Then I would do the pinch test on the skin of his hand. Squeezing the skin between the index finger and the thumb is a great indicator if someone is properly hydrated or not. Properly hydrated skin should bounce right back.

> *For my dad it would sometimes take 30 seconds or more to come back. Then I would ask if he would drink some water to make his son happy. I would place a large glass of water next to his coffee, and he would drink it. Many people never think about dehydration being a problem, until it is.*

How Much Water Do You Need?

I believe most people, including me, overestimate how much water we consume. Ideally, we should drink half our body weight in ounces of water per day. For a 160-pound person, that amount would be approximately 80 ounces of water per day. The body's need for water may increase due to exercise or living in a warm or dry climate. The goal is to get into a habit of consuming more water.

It is also important to spread water consumption throughout the day. Start each morning by consuming 6-8 ounces of water. Drink again multiple times throughout the day and also in the evening. When using the bathroom in the night, drink some water. Drinking water multiple times per day and night leads to greater absorption of the water we consume.

Upgrade your beverage choices, whether it is milk, coffee, tea, juice, or water. Drink 6 ounces of water every hour.

Track your water consumption over a 2-day period to determine how much water you normally drink per day.

How much water do you drink per day? ______________________

Water Quality

Keeping the body properly hydrated is not just about drinking the right amount of water. It is also important to understand water quality. There are significant differences in the types of water we drink.

Tap Water

Many sources of tap water may contain high levels of chlorine and other toxic ingredients. Chlorinated tap water destroys beneficial bacteria in the body, which can weaken and damage the immune system. High levels of chlorine in the drinking water have also been linked to heart disease and cancer. My first recommendation is to get your tap water checked for high levels of chlorine and other toxic ingredients. If you suspect your tap water to be unhealthy, you may want to look into buying some type of filtration system.

Ionized Water Filtration System

Maintaining a balanced pH is critical for your health. This was discussed in detail back in chapter 8. Finding a good water source is critical in your quest for balancing your pH and overall health. Using an ionized water filtration system can be extremely beneficial in your journey to greater health.

Ionization simply means the gain or loss of electrons. Water that has been ionized becomes either alkaline or acidic, meaning the pH has been adjusted up or down. Back in the early 1950s, two Russian scientists discovered a way to split a stream of water into two parts: one acidic and one alkaline. The process uses a series of magnets to create an electrolysis process. The result is negatively charged "ionized" water that is reconstructed for enhanced absorption and hydration and is high in antioxidants and minerals.

There are three main benefits of consuming ionized water. First, it is a powerful antioxidant. Second, it is extremely alkalizing for the body. Third, it is much more hydrating and detoxifying than normal or conventional water.

If you want a great water source in the convenience of your own home and are tired of buying bottled water and the impact of all those bottles on the environment, I highly recommend buying an ionized water filtration system. I have owned a water ionizer for years. It is well worth the investment. It attaches easily to a water source and is affordable. One more thing—my dog Floyd always chooses ionized water over conventional tap water if he has an option.

Mineral Water

One of the easiest ways to improve health is to drink mineral water on a daily or weekly basis. I personally consume approximately 50 ounces of mineral water per week. Mineral water is highly alkaline and helps maintain essential minerals in the body. Choose only mineral water with natural occurring carbonation. There are also sources of mineral water that do not have the carbonation. Add a slice of lemon, lime, or orange or a shot of juice for a great refreshing taste.

Bottled Water

Today, bottled water is big business with over 80 brands available in the United States alone. Back in the 1970s when bottled water first hit the market, I remember thinking, "Are you kidding me? Do you think people are really going to pay for water that they put in a bottle?" Yet today, bottled water is big business.

The important thing to remember when purchasing bottled water is to choose only natural spring or artesian water. What about purified or reverse osmosis water? Creating healthy water means removing the harmful ingredients while keeping the beneficial minerals. Purified water sounds healthy but is missing some important ingredients, namely minerals. Stripping the water of harmful toxins is good but removing all the minerals from the water is not good. Drinking purified water over time can leach valuable minerals out of the body. Avoid drinking purified or reverse osmosis water for any length of time.

Distilled Water

More and more people are interested in the cleansing benefits of drinking distilled water. Consumption of distilled water in large quantities washes waste products and toxins from the body due to its acidic nature. There are some real benefits of drinking distilled water on an occasional basis for detoxifying benefits. However, drinking distilled water on a regular basis leaches minerals from the body and causes dehydration.

> ***Unable to Pee***
>
> *Many bodybuilders drink distilled water two or three days prior to a contest in attempt to get rid of the excess water and create that ripped look. Many years ago, one of the contestants I was competing against was so dehydrated he needed to wait over six hours to come up with enough urine to be drug tested.*
>
> *I asked him later what he was doing to cause this excessive dehydration. He said he drank two gallons of distilled water two days in a row, and then he did not drink an ounce of water for the next 36 hours. The only water he received was from the food he ingested. This may be an extreme case, but remember, distilled water is not to be ingested on a regular basis.*

Let Water Be Your Drink of Choice!

Start slowly and build the habit of drinking more high-quality water daily. Give your body the water it needs. Use the Beverage/Condiment Target as a tool to guide you on upgrading your beverage choices.

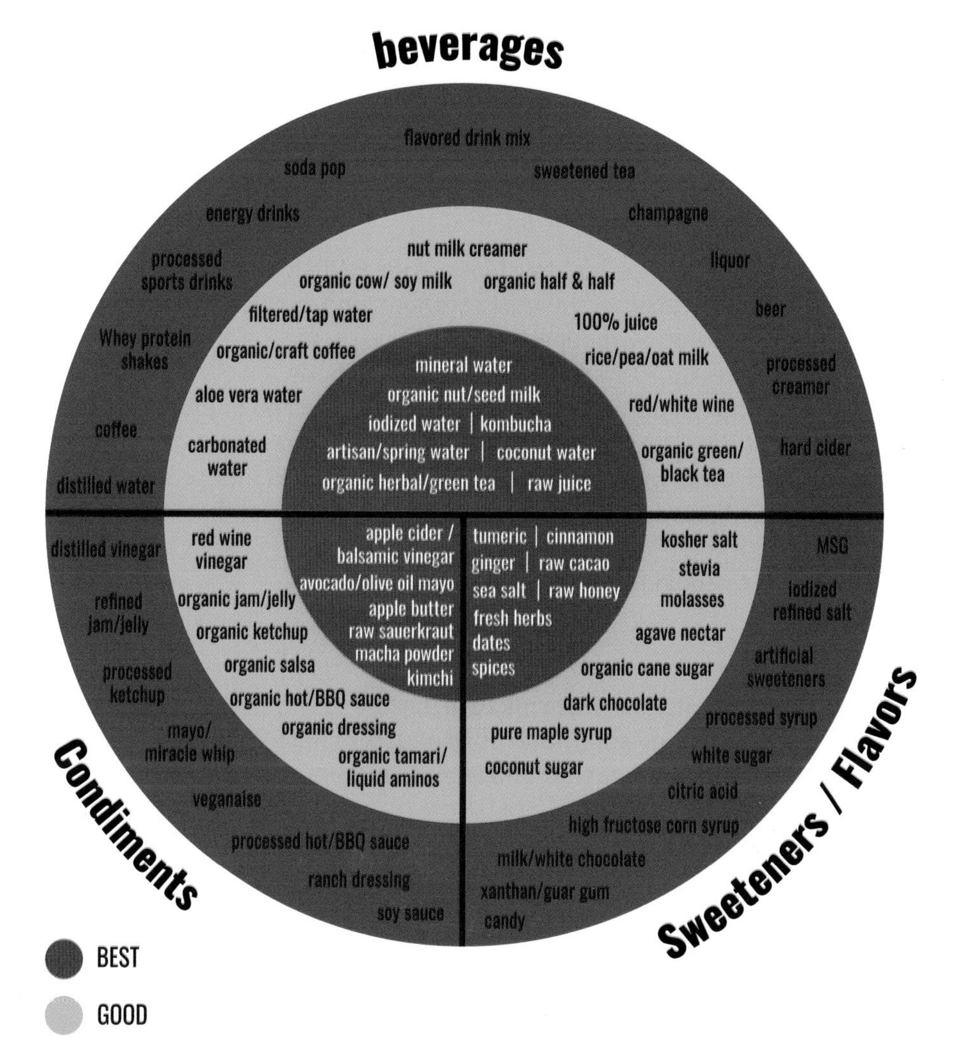

beverage/condiment target

Hydration Essentials

Big Picture

- The EAT Pyramid includes six nutritional building blocks for optimal health.
- Hydration is the first building block of the EAT Pyramid.
- You can survive for several weeks without food, but you will die within a few days without water.
- Water makes up 70-75 percent of the human body.
- Water is energizing and detoxifying for the mind and body.
- Unintentional chronic dehydration may be the root cause of many serious diseases including asthma, endocrine and kidney problems, high blood pressure, heart disease, arthritis, ulcers, low back pain, and obesity.
- Water is essential for life.

Ask Yourself

- How much water do you drink each day?
- Are you drinking a minimum of 50 ounces of water each day?
- How can you upgrade your beverage choices?

Small Steps

- Build your EAT Pyramid slowly.
- Drink 6 ounces of water every hour or half your body weight in ounces of water each day
- Put water in front of you at home, at work, in the car, and at the gym.
- Add lemons, limes, or ginger to your water.
- Let water be your drink of choice.

17 Superfoods

Now that we are well hydrated, we can focus on the second building block in the EAT Pyramid—Superfoods.

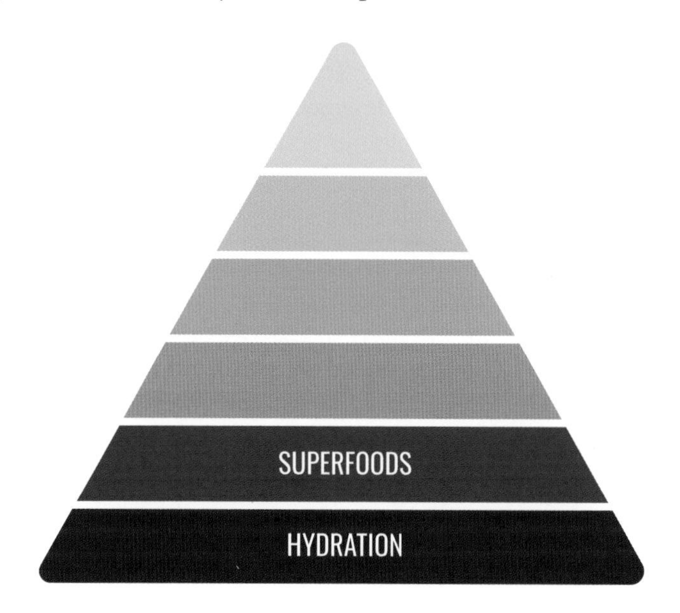

Foods Can Heal the Body

Imagine a food, not a typical food that gives you a few vitamins, minerals, and energy, but a potent superfood. Imagine a food—not a drug—powerful enough to balance your cholesterol, lower your blood pressure, improve your digestion, balance your hormones, improve brain health, decrease inflammation, decrease your risk of heart disease, cancer, and type 2 diabetes, and help you feel and be your best. Where do I sign up?

One frustration I hear on a daily basis is how challenging it can be to know what foods, supplements, or herbs to use in the quest for better health, energy, and vitality. I find many people want to target their specific needs or problems with a specific food, supplement, or herb. They want to decrease the risk for catching a cold, so they take vitamin C. To improve digestion, they take a probiotic. To lower cholesterol, they take niacin or a statin medication. To decrease inflammation, they take an aspirin, ibuprofen, or bromelain. To improve immune function, they take quercetin. For hot flashes, they take evening primrose oil, borage oil, or black currant seed oil. For increased energy, they consume the latest energy drink or more caffeine. If they cannot sleep, they take melatonin. To improve bone health, they take calcium, magnesium, and vitamin D.

First, we have to change our mindset around the healing process. The human body does not heal in isolation. Everything is connected. If we improve our gut health, our sleep improves. As sleep improves, hormones come back into balance. As hormones come back into balance, the body starts to thrive. As we build and improve our health, everything starts getting better.

Second, the human body is not designed to consume nutrients in isolation. Remember it is not what we put into our body, but what our body can break down and absorb.

What is a Superfood?

Superfoods are nutrient-dense whole foods that offer many powerful health benefits. Many people believe they are eating healthy but may be missing important nutrients. Finding the highest quality nutrients can be challenging and confusing. That is the beauty of many superfoods. They can fill large gaps by consuming just a few.

I have found that most people are missing high-quality forms of omega-3 essential fatty acids, high-quality forms of chlorophyll, and many vitamins and minerals. Adding a few superfoods to our nutritional plan is a simple and efficient way to get the basic nutrients our body needs. Once our nutritional pillars are in place, then specific foods, spices, or herbs can be added to target individual needs. A healthy diet incorporating a variety of superfoods can make our cells healthy, balance our pH, control our body weight, rejuvenate our immune system, improve our energy, and help us feel and be our best.

There are so many superfoods to choose from. In fact, just about every brightly colored vegetable or fruit, ancient grain, nut, seed, bean, herb, or spice can be classified as a superfood. I recommend beginning with just one or two superfoods. Build a habit and then add another superfood. Start slowly and experience the amazing benefits superfoods provide. Here are a few of my top superfoods.

Omega-3 Essential Fatty Acids

One of the first superfoods I recommend is omega-3 fats. They are called essential fatty acids because they are essential to our health. Omega-3s are the superstars of healthy fats and make the body strong and healthy. Unfortunately, today over 95 percent of the American population, as well as the rest of the world, are deficient in omega-3 essential fatty acids.

Studies show that omega-3s are linked to immune function, energy, metabolism, decreased inflammation, hormonal balance, brain health, cell health and nerve health. Because omega-3s have been shown to improve chemical messaging and cell structure inside the body, these essential fats help us respond better to immune challenges, enhance recovery after injury or overexertion, and even manage stress. Omega-3 fats are powerful superfoods.

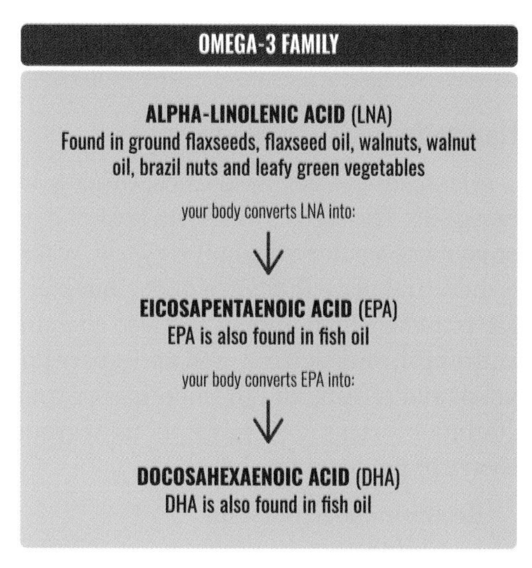

The primary fatty acid in the omega-3 family is alpha-linolenic acid (ALA). ALA can be found in many plant sources such as leafy greens, flaxseeds, chia seeds, walnuts, and pecans. Most nuts and seeds coming from the source have some omega-3s.

Flaxseeds and chia seeds are the richest sources of ALA. There are several levels of omega-3 breakdowns or conversions in the body. ALA converts to one or two other types of fatty acids, depending upon its breakdown pathway. Stay with me just for a minute this will all start to make sense. ALA can be converted to eicosapentaenoic acid (EPA) and then into docosahexaenoic acid (DHA). EPA and DHA are found in wild cold-water fish such as salmon, trout, mackerel, and herring, and in cod liver oil and fish oil.

People often ask whether they need to consume wild cold-water fish, cod liver oil, or fish oil even if they also consume omega-3s such as flax or chia, which are high in ALA. The answer is yes.

The conversion from ALA to EPA and then into DHA is not efficient in many adults and children. The labels on infant formula advertise that they are high in DHA, which is essential for brain development in infants. If DHA is such an important nutrient for brain development and the health of our babies, what about the brain health of our adults?

It can be a challenge to get enough omega-3s in our diet unless we know where to look. We must search for omega-3 fats. Omega-3 fats are extremely unstable and spoil quickly. Most products in the grocery store most likely do not contain omega-3 fats. There are, however, many excellent sources of omega-3 fats.

Good Sources of Omega-3 Fats

Flaxseeds

Flaxseeds are tiny hard seeds, either gold or brown, that are loaded with omega-3s. The seeds themselves are not digestible and must be ground up or you will see them again. Every few weeks I grind up flaxseeds in a coffee grinder and place them in a dark container in the refrigerator. Flaxseeds are extremely high in fiber and also contain lignans, which have antiviral, antifungal, antibacterial, and anticancer properties. Flaxseeds may be used on salads and cereals, and in smoothies or your favorite juice. One of my favorite afternoon snacks is 1-2 tablespoons of ground flaxseeds in 1-2 ounces of dark cherry or pomegranate juice.

Recommended Serving
Children: ½-1 tablespoon, 2-7 times per week
Adults: 1-2 tablespoons, 2-7 times per week

Chia Seeds

Chia seeds, like flaxseeds, are also high in omega-3 fats (ALA). Chia seeds are dark in color, easy to digest, help with food cravings, and decrease inflammation. They are also extremely heart-healthy, high in fiber, and loaded with the relaxation mineral magnesium. Chia seeds do not have to be ground up and can be eaten raw, soaked in juice, added to a salad, used in baking, or in a smoothie. My favorite way to consume chia seeds is to add 1-2 tablespoons to an ounce or two of almond, coconut, or cashew milk, a dash of cinnamon or nutmeg, place in the refrigerator overnight for a pudding like snack. Yum!

Recommended Serving
Children: ½-1 tablespoon, 2-7 times per week
Adults: 1-2 tablespoons, 2-7 times per week

Cod Liver Oil

As a nation, we have a major omega-3 deficiency, especially EPA and DHA. EPA and DHA can be manufactured in small amounts by healthy cells from ALA, however, the conversion from ALA to EPA and then into DHA is small and can be impaired by degenerative conditions such as diabetes. To get enough EPA and DHA directly into your body, take advantage of the wonderful benefits of fish oils.

The richest sources of EPA and DHA are cod liver oil, anchovies, sardines, herring, mackerel, and wild Alaskan salmon. To get the health benefits that fish oil provides, I recommend a daily serving of cod liver oil. Yes, I said cod liver oil! Don't be afraid of the taste. This is not grandmother's cod liver oil. It has a nice lemon flavor, and the health benefits are off the charts.

The reason I recommend cod liver oil over fish or krill oil is that cod liver oil contains a naturally occurring spectrum of omega-3 fatty acids, including bioactive pro-resolving mediators (PRMs). These PRMs play a powerful role in immune system support. Also, cod liver is naturally high is vitamin A and vitamin D3, which are essential for cellular health, improved calcium absorption, immune function, and healthy eyes and skin. Cod liver oil has a smooth texture and tastes like a lemon drop.

Recommended Serving

Children: 1-2 teaspoons per day

Adults: 1-2 tablespoons per day (1,500-3,000 mg of EPA/DHA per day)

Chlorophyll

The second nutrient most people are missing from their diets is chlorophyll. Chlorophyll is the green pigment in plants. The darker the green color, the more chlorophyll the plant contains. Foods high in chlorophyll include leafy greens, parsley, broccoli, kale, spinach, bok choy, collard greens, and mustard greens to name a few. Chlorophyll is extremely detoxifying and energizing. It is loaded with vitamins and minerals, promotes the production of red blood cells, and is fantastic for gut health and immune system support.

Wheatgrass

One of the highest sources of chlorophyll is wheatgrass. Not only is wheatgrass high in chlorophyll but it is also the highest raw source of minerals in the world, with over 90 minerals. Yes, you read this right—90 minerals!

Wheatgrass is a powerful, raw, living food. The grass itself comes from a common wheat plant when it is young, vibrant, and full of rich green chlorophyll. Wheatgrass grown outdoors has many nutritional benefits over wheatgrass grown hydroponically due to natural air, rain, sun, and soil. Wheatgrass is harvested when the grass reaches its nutritional peak, just before the jointing stage, when the plant is between 7-11 inches tall. There is no gluten in wheatgrass.

After wheatgrass is juiced, it is immediately flash frozen to maintain the life force without compromise. Frozen wheatgrass has a high mineral and chlorophyll content and is extremely detoxifying and energizing. It also has an alkalizing effect, supports the immune system, improves gut health, reduces inflammation, and improves mental clarity. Wheatgrass is a powerful superfood that improves overall health.

It tastes like grass, clean and refreshing. Wheatgrass is best taken first thing in the morning on an empty stomach for optimal absorption. Most people prefer to place a few cubes of wheatgrass in a glass of water, let the cubes melt, and then drink it down the hatch.

Recommended Serving

Children:	1-2 cubes
Adults:	3-5 cubes

Spirulina/Chlorella

The second form of chlorophyll is spirulina/chlorella. These two freshwater micro algae are extremely high in chlorophyll, high in antioxidants, and powerful detoxifiers. They improve digestion and help rejuvenate and build the immune system. These amazing superfoods are high in protein, nucleic acid, GLA, folic acid, beta carotene, B vitamins, calcium, magnesium, iron, zinc, and fiber—making spirulina/chlorella one of the most powerful superfoods in the world. Due to their potency, they are known as survival foods. Start slowly and try to spread consumption throughout the day. Spirulina/chlorella tablets are inexpensive and easy to take. No chewing, just swallow the tiny tablets with water.

Recommended Serving

Children:	3-10 tablets per day
Adults:	10-50 tablets per day

More Superfoods

Organic Virgin Coconut Flakes/Coconut Oil

Coconut is a healthy saturated fat high in lauric, capric, and caprylic acids. These acids have antiviral and antifungal properties that contribute to a healthy digestion. Coconut also contains medium-chain fatty acids that can aid in healthy metabolism.

Aim for 1 tablespoon per day. Add to cereal, smoothies, and trail mix. Use in cooking or baking. Use coconut oil as a spread for a healthy, great tasting butter replacement. It can be used to cook eggs, sauté meats and veggies, and make great popcorn.

Cacao

Cacao is the raw unprocessed form of chocolate and is high in magnesium, manganese, zinc, and iron. Cacao has many benefits including brain health, mood enhancement, support of heart health, boost of weight loss, and improved energy. It can also enhance relaxation and promote a better night of sleep. Because it is high in magnesium, it has also been shown to build muscle and aid in muscle recovery.

Take 1 tablespoon of cacao nibs or powder per day. Mix in oatmeal, smoothies, or simply with coconut or almond milk in a blender to make a healthy version of hot chocolate.

Nuts and Seeds

Nuts and seeds are packed with fiber, vitamins, minerals, healthy fats, and protein. Try to get a variety of nuts and seeds into your daily diet, including almonds, walnuts, Brazil nuts, hempseeds, pecans, pistachios, hazelnuts, cashews, and macadamia nuts as well as pumpkin and sunflower seeds.

Add to salads, smoothies, and trail mix, or simply eat as is for a healthy snack.

Super Fruits

Fruits are packed with flavor and are high in vitamins, minerals, fiber, cancer-fighting antioxidants, and are extremely alkalizing. Try to get a variety of super fruits in your daily diet including dark cherries, strawberries, blueberries, raspberries, lemons, limes, apples, and bananas. Dried fruits like figs, dates, goji berries, bananas, and raisins are high in the calming mineral magnesium helping to quiet the mind and relax the body.

Add to salads, smoothies, and cereal/oatmeal, or simply enjoy as nature's candy.

Super Vegetables

Vegetables provide many nutrients including potassium, folate, vitamins A, E, and C, and are extremely alkalizing. Try to get a variety of super vegetables into your daily diet including leafy greens, bok choy, broccoli, asparagus, kelp, sea vegetables, mushrooms, sauerkraut, red cabbage, beets, celery, carrots, peppers, onions, and garlic. Leafy greens, sea vegetables, and broccoli are especially high in the iodine, calcium, and vitamin C needed to keep your immune system healthy and prevent illness. Beets and celery are extremely detoxifying. Garlic is part of the onion family and contributes to a healthy immune system and lower inflammation. Starchy vegetables like red skin, yellow, purple, and sweet potatoes are also a great addition to your diet and provide the brain with healthy levels of serotonin needed to feel happy and satisfied.

Aim for multiple servings of vegetables per day.

Ancient Grains

Ancient grains include oats, teff, amaranth, spelt, quinoa, chia, buckwheat, wheat berries, kamut, freekeh, bulgur, barley, sorghum, millet, wild rice, and farrow. These complex carbohydrates are energizing, alkalizing, and extremely high in protein, vitamins, minerals, and fiber. These grains are also high in energizing B vitamins and are helpful in reducing inflammation.

Add a source of grains to your diet several days a week.

Super Spices and Herbs

Super spices and herbs can decrease inflammation and improve digestion, brain health, and immune function. Try to include a variety of super spices and herbs in your daily diet including turmeric, ginger, cinnamon, mint, and alfalfa. Cinnamon is especially beneficial for balancing blood sugar and keeping energy levels steady. Alfalfa is high in vitamins and minerals and can help treat digestion, kidney issues, joint problems, high cholesterol, and blood pressure. Mint is very energizing and soothing on the stomach.

Adding just a small amount of these super flavors to dishes is a great way to add antioxidant-rich flavor.

Make Superfoods a Habit

I recommend starting out with one or two superfoods, develop the habit, and when ready add another. The first superfood I added to my diet was flaxseeds, and that was more than 35 years ago. I started slowly and over time added a few more superfoods. Today superfoods are big part of my daily nutritional routine.

Superfood Starter Plan

1. Cod Liver Oil: 1-2 tablespoons per day
2. Spirulina/Chlorella: 10-30 tablets per day

Top Superfoods

1. Frozen Wheatgrass Ice Cubes: 3-5 cubes per day
2. Cod Liver Oil: 1-2 tablespoons per day
3. Spirulina/Chlorella: 10-30 tablets per day
4. Flaxseeds, Chia Seeds or Hempseeds: 1-2 tablespoons 3-5 times per week

Superfoods Essentials

Big Picture

- Enjoy the power superfoods can bring to your health.
- A superfood, sometimes called a "functional food," is a nutritionally dense food that can powerfully impact the health of the human body in a very positive way.
- The human body does not heal in isolation.
- Do not take nutrients in isolation.
- We have to break away from the mindset of taking supplements or medications for isolated needs. The human body is designed to eat food.
- The top superfoods are cod liver oil, spirulina/chlorella, wheatgrass, flaxseeds, chia seeds, and hempseeds.

Ask Yourself

- Do you consume an omega-3 fat on a daily basis?
- Do you consume foods high in chlorophyll?
- Do you take supplements that come from the source?
- Can you better meet your nutritional needs through quality food?
- How can you fit a few superfoods into your EAT plan?

Small Steps

- Take one serving of omega-3 fats every day.
- Get in 1-3 servings of chlorophyll each day.
- Start slowly. Add one or two superfoods into your daily nutrition plan to feel like a "Superhero."

18 Food Quality

In chapters 16 and 17, we discussed Hydration and Superfoods as the first two building blocks of our EAT Pyramid. Let's continue to build the EAT Pyramid by discussing the third building block—Quality.

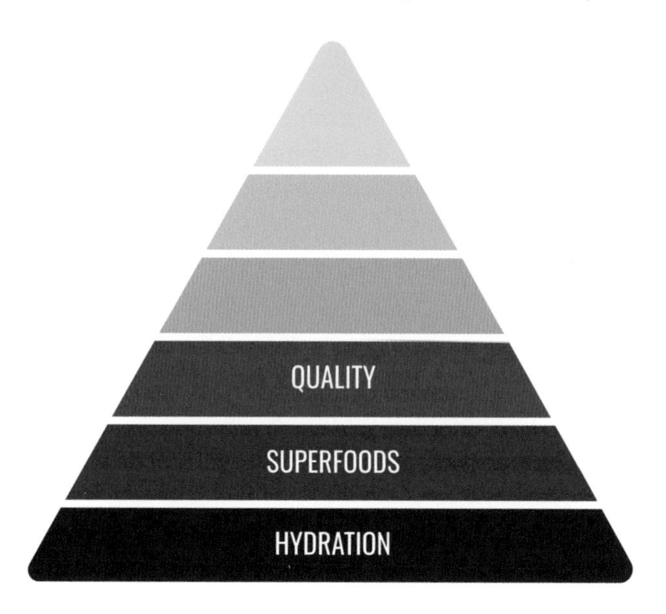

We have all heard the saying, location, location, location when buying real estate. When it comes to food, it is quality, quality, quality.

Many people ask what they should eat to improve their health and energy, to expand their capacity, and to feel and be their best. I tell them to focus on eating high-quality macronutrients:

- **Carbohydrates to fuel the body**
- **Proteins to build the body**
- **Fats to heal the body**

Quality and Balance

Learning to improve the quality of the food and beverages we consume is the essence of the On Target Living lifestyle. To help people learn more about the three macronutrients, eating in greater balance, and improving the food and beverage quality, I developed an easy-to-use guide called the Food Target. The Food Target focuses on a balance of carbohydrates, proteins, and fats, and incorporates an assessment of their nutritional quality. The foods with the lowest nutritional value are on the outside of the Food Target. They contribute the least nutrition to the body and can even be detrimental to your health. The most beneficial and most nutritious foods, those that make the body stronger, are closer to the center.

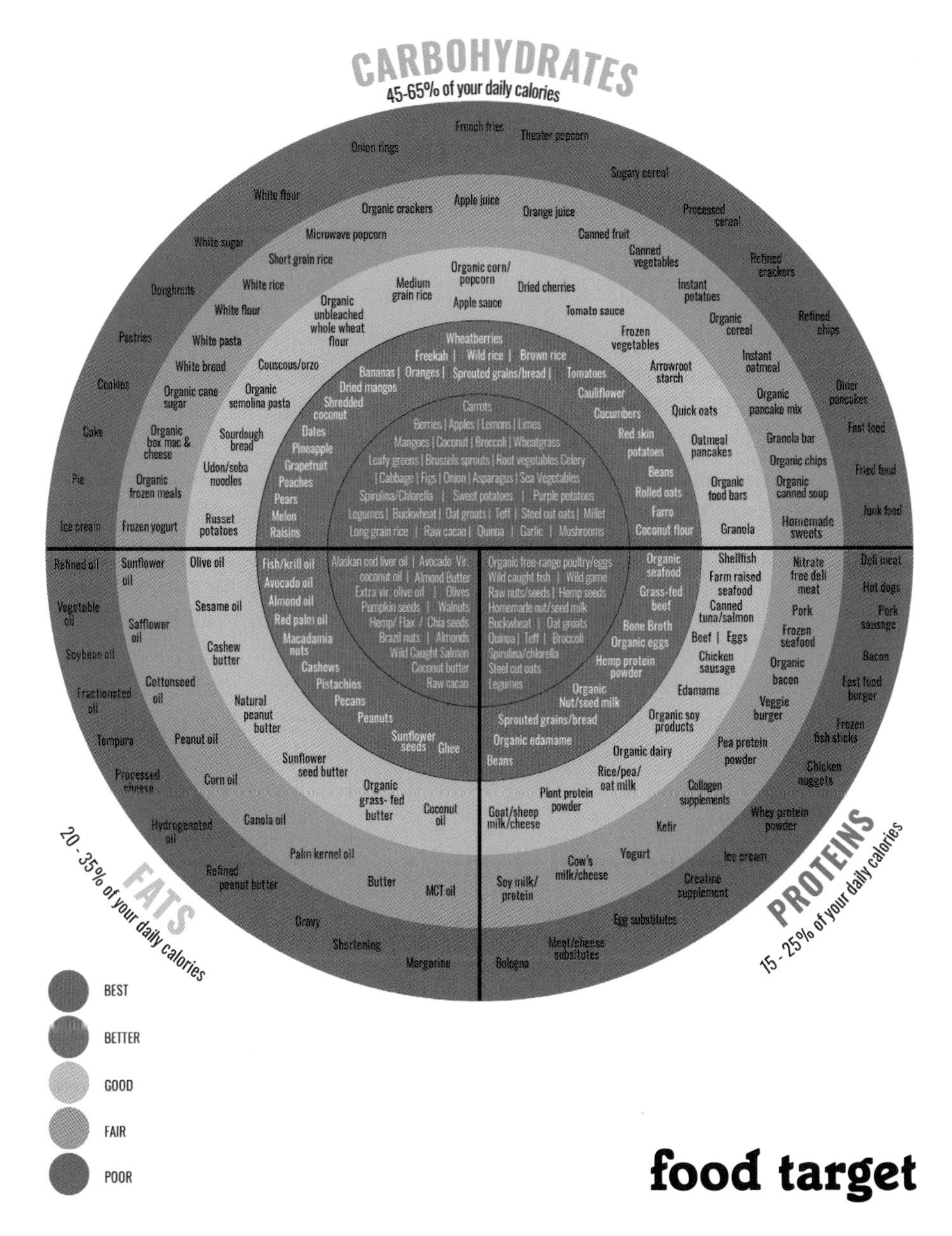

*The Food Target can be downloaded at ***ontargetliving.com***

The idea behind the On Target Living Nutrition Program is to encourage consuming foods and beverages in the green and yellow sections that identify good, better, and best choices closer to the source.

The goal is to slowly move towards the center by upgrading the foods and beverages consumed the most. Like peanut butter? Get a healthier version of peanut butter. Like coffee creamer? Use a better creamer. Upgrade from instant oatmeal to old-fashioned oatmeal that is closer to the source. Our Brand Favorite Shopping List helps make it easy to upgrade. It can be found on our website ***ontargetliving.com***.

Use the Food Target as a learning tool and lifelong guide for eating. Place the Food Target on the refrigerator and refer to it on a daily basis as a guide to upgrading food and beverage choices.

Quality Carbohydrates Fuel the Body

Carbohydrates are simply sugar chains linked together. The shorter the sugar chain, the more processed or refined the carbohydrate. The more refined or processed the carbohydrate, the less fiber, vitamins, minerals, phytochemicals, and antioxidants the carbohydrate contains. The longer the sugar chain, the greater amount of fiber, vitamins, minerals, phytochemicals, and antioxidants. Longer chain carbohydrates create better health and performance.

We often are asked if sugar is bad. Our response is that it depends on the source of the sugar. Is the sugar the processed white version or is it in its most natural state like a piece of fruit or a sweet potato? A doughnut and asparagus are both in the carbohydrate family. That is where their relationship ends. Doughnuts have short sugar chains, are nutrient deficient, lack fiber, and cause a quick spike in blood glucose. Asparagus, on the other hand, has a long sugar chain, is nutrient-dense, high in fiber, and causes little change in blood glucose.

Benefits of Consuming High-Quality Carbohydrates

The health benefits of consuming high-quality carbohydrates, such as fruits, vegetables, ancient grains, starchy carbohydrates, and legumes, include greater gut health, pH balance, greater energy, regular elimination, better sleep, lower blood pressure, decreased inflammation, lower oxidation, heart health, brain health, improved mood, and greater health. High-quality carbohydrates are essential for greater health and performance.

Over the years carbohydrates have been getting a bad rap, with most carbohydrates lumped together in one overarching nutrient category. This is a problem. Lumping all carbohydrates together is like comparing any consumer product. There are higher and lower quality products.

Take for an example two cans of paint. On the outside both cans of paint may look and feel similar except for the price, but let's take a deeper look. The higher quality paint contains 100 percent acrylic resin and a high load of titanium ingredients that create a long lasting, stain resistant, easy to scrub paint that retains its color for years. The lower quality paint contains a vinyl acrylic resin with substitute fillers such as clay to replace titanium. Bottom line, it is an inferior paint that fades, chips, cracks, and shows dirt and stains. The higher quality paint costs more upfront, but the value is clear. This is the same conversation we should have about putting quality foods and beverages into the body.

It is necessary to learn how to distinguish between the quality carbohydrates that come from the source and the processed unhealthy carbohydrates that do not. I want to make it clear that high-quality carbohydrates are essential for greater energy, balancing pH, detoxification, gut health, brain health, better sleep, and immune and nervous system support. Carbohydrates also provide the body with valuable fiber, vitamins, minerals, phytochemicals, and antioxidants. All are important for overall health and feeling your best.

Today many people today believe the best way to lose weight is to cut back on carbohydrate intake without fully understanding the role high-quality carbohydrates play in keeping the body fit, healthy, and happy. With the growing demand for weight loss diets, many carbohydrates have been lumped together as foods to avoid to lose weight.

Bananas—Friend or Foe?

Years ago, a woman approached me in my hometown grocery store and asked if I was that nutrition/fitness guy. I told her that yes, I write books on nutrition, fitness, health, capacity, and speak around the world about the On Target Living lifestyle. Then she asked if I ate bananas. Looking down at the bananas in my grocery cart, I said yes.

She then said, "I am a little surprised that you eat bananas. Don't you know that bananas are high on the glycemic index?" "Yes," I answered, "I know that." The glycemic index rates how fast a food can be broken down in glucose. She then said, "Oh, I didn't think you would eat bananas due to their high glycemic index." She then walked away with a demeaning smirk on her face.

Caught off guard, I felt like I had just been scolded. I decided to walk after her and could not let this go. Now it was my turn. "Excuse me," I said. "Since when does a banana become an unhealthy food choice? Did you know that a banana is one of nature's perfect foods, beautifully packaged, convenient to

> *eat, a natural prebiotic, high in fiber, and full of vitamins and minerals such as magnesium and potassium? Oh, and by the way, they taste great." She was not buying into the benefits of eating a banana. In her mind bananas raise your blood glucose quickly and make you fat. I do not think the high obesity levels in the United States are caused by eating too many bananas!*

Many people think that if you want to lose weight, you cut out carbohydrates. In many of the today's most popular diets, the first thing people are asked to take out of their diet are carbohydrates, especially fruit. Since when does a banana, blueberry, apple, raspberry, or an orange make you fat?

There are many processed carbohydrates that cause poor health and weight gain. Let's start with a better understanding of all carbohydrates.

Here is the bottom line. Do not be afraid of the Big Bad Carbohydrate Wolf. Remember, not all carbohydrates are created equal. Try to focus on eating macronutrients closer to the original source. These are found in the two green circles in the center of the Food Target.

Quality Carbohydrate Sources

Fruits

Most fruits are sweet, naturally detoxifying and alkalizing, high in fiber, and loaded with vitamins, minerals, and antioxidants. They also improve gut health. Examples include berries, apples, kiwis, prunes, figs, mangos, lemons, limes, grapefruit, watermelon, peaches, melon, pears, cherries, bananas, avocados, apricots, goji berries, and plums, to name just a few.

Vegetables

Most vegetables are low in calories, alkalizing, and loaded with fiber, vitamins, minerals, and antioxidants. They too improve gut health. These include broccoli, cauliflower, asparagus, sweet peppers, celery, cucumbers, kale, spinach, sprouts, cabbage, sauerkraut, parsley, leafy greens, Brussels sprouts, onions, garlic, sea vegetables, spirulina/chlorella, and wheatgrass, among many others.

Ancient Grains

Most ancient grains are calming for the mind, serotonin boosting, alkalizing, and high in fiber, B vitamins, and minerals, as well as improve gut health. These include oat groats, steel cut or rolled oats, teff, amaranth, quinoa, millet, wheat, rye, spelt, barley, and rice.

Starches

Starchy carbohydrates are calming for the mind, improve gut health, and are high in fiber, vitamins, minerals, and antioxidants. These include root vegetables, sweet potatoes, purple potatoes, red skin potatoes, white potatoes, carrots, squash, rutabagas, parsnips, and beets.

Legumes

Legumes are high in fiber, low in calories, and high in protein, vitamins, and minerals. These include lentils, red beans, edamame, chickpeas, navy beans, black beans, and yellow or green peas.

Sweeteners

Sugar is a major life force. Sugars in whole foods are balanced with fiber and minerals. Here are a few healthier sweetener options to choose from:

- Fresh or frozen fruit
- Local raw organic honey
- Organic maple syrup
- Organic molasses
- Organic cane sugar
- Organic coconut sugar
- Organic agave nectar
- Organic stevia leaf

Removing Quality Carbohydrates Harms Health

If we take high-quality carbohydrates such as fruits, vegetables, ancient grains, starches, and legumes out of our diet, our body will start talking back to us and not in a good way—with poor gut health, pH imbalance, acid reflux, constipation, problems sleeping, high blood pressure, headaches, increased inflammation, irritability, poor skin, and brittle hair. High-quality carbohydrates are also necessary to help balance neurotransmitters in the brain. Without healthy carbohydrates the brain has a difficult time slowing down. These are just a few of the side effects of taking high-quality carbohydrates out of the diet.

Choose carbohydrates closer to the source. These are found in the green areas of the Food Target. Our goal each day would be to consume approximately 50 percent of our total calories from high-quality unrefined carbohydrates.

And remember, next time someone says they are going on a low-carbohydrate diet, think about what that truly means. Are they cutting out the processed carbohydrates or are they cutting out the high-quality carbohydrates like fruits, vegetables, ancient grains, starches, or legumes?

Removing a macronutrient from the diet will eventually create a macro problem!

Quality Proteins Build the Body

Our second macronutrient is protein. Proteins are the building blocks of life. Proteins play a vital role in every cell in the human body. They create hormones, maintain the immune system, build muscle, transport vitamins, and maintain our blood, skin, and connective tissue.

Proteins are simply amino acids. Our bodies break down protein into smaller nitrogen-containing units called amino acids. The body cannot manufacture essential amino acids, so we must get them through the foods we eat.

Benefits of Protein

In addition to keeping the body strong and healthy, there are many wonderful benefits of eating high-quality proteins, such as cell development, building, and repair. Proteins stabilize blood glucose leading to consistent energy throughout the day. If blood glucose levels are stable, insulin will not be overproduced, leaving us with greater energy. Add a piece of salmon or chicken to a favorite salad or a few nuts to cereal in the morning. Both are excellent ways to stabilize blood glucose levels to help maintain that needed energy required to feel our best.

Proteins also help reduce cravings for refined carbohydrates. By adding protein to your daily diet, cravings for the refined carbohydrates, those in the red area of the Food Target, will slowly go away.

Another benefit of consuming high-quality protein is improved brainpower. Adequate amounts of protein can improve cognitive skills, memory, focus, and alertness.

Is Protein the Golden Child?

The benefits of consuming high-quality proteins are well documented in keeping the human body functioning at its best.

Have we have tipped the scales too far in our demand for more protein? I believe protein has now become the "Golden Child" of the three macronutrients. How often do you hear, "Protein! Protein! Protein! How do I get more protein in my diet?" Many people believe that more protein will lead to a lean, mean, health-conscious machine. We seldom hear people say they want more carbohydrates in their smoothie, more carbohydrates on salad, or a high carbohydrate bar. Powerful marketing is selling the idea that higher protein or higher fat with little or no carbohydrates is the one true way to achieve greater health, lose weight, and increase human performance.

Drinks, energy bars, smoothies, and jerky to name a few are now advertised as high in protein with few or no carbohydrates. What's next? A healthy beer option? Strip away the carbohydrates, add protein, some healthy fats, and fiber, and voilà! Fitness Beer! I bet someone is currently working on this idea. Who would have guessed the energy drink market would become a multi-billion-dollar business. Maybe the next multi-billion-dollar industry is the Fitness Beer industry. I can see it now!

Having enough high-quality proteins in our diet is essential for optimal health and greater performance in all aspects of your life. Just like our discussion about carbohydrates, the real focus should begin with quality proteins, not overloading on them. Just like carbohydrates, not all proteins are created equal.

How Much Protein is Enough?

Protein has tremendous nutritional benefits when balanced correctly in our diet. The goal should be to consume 15 to 25 percent of our daily calories from high-quality protein sources spread evenly throughout the day. The more physically active we are, the higher amount of protein the body may need. Rarely does one need more than 30 percent of their daily calories from high-quality proteins.

What happens if we eat too much protein? Consuming more than 30 percent of our daily calories from protein may cause our body to become too acidic, leading to an increase in inflammation. When proteins are broken down, they must be neutralized by buffering minerals, namely calcium, magnesium, and iodine, to offset the high acid levels in the body. If our protein intake is too high, our buffering minerals may become depleted over time and lead to poor bone health, low thyroid function, and digestion problems. Eating too much protein also places excess stress on the liver and kidneys.

Protein Sources

Most people think of protein sources as meat, eggs, and dairy. These proteins come from animal sources. For years, we focused our attention on animal sources of protein to reach our protein requirements. We need to understand that our daily protein requirements can be met from animal sources, but also from plant-based sources of protein.

Where is the Beef?

During one of my seminars, a member of the audience asked me what I ate for breakfast. I replied that my typical breakfast consisted of organic rolled oats, a few walnuts, almonds, pecans or macadamia nuts, frozen dark cherries or berries, a few raisins, cacao nibs, shredded coconut, and a dash of cinnamon with cashew, coconut, or almond milk. I mix all these ingredients together and let it sit overnight in the refrigerator. This is our Oatmeal on the Run Recipe—no cooking required. I love the taste. It is quick and easy, well balanced, high in quality carbohydrates, proteins, and fats. And it gives me great energy to start my day.

Then a member of the audience asked about the protein in that breakfast. It seemed low in protein. I then explained in greater detail the actual amount of protein in my breakfast: organic rolled oats—8 grams of protein, nuts—5 grams of protein, and plant milk—1 gram of protein for a total of 14 grams of protein. I think many people in the audience were surprised by the amount of protein. This breakfast is just one example of getting high-quality protein from plant-based sources.

Protein Debate

There is a growing debate over the best type of protein for the human body. Is it animal-based or plant-based? From an environmental standpoint, eating plant-based protein is a great deal more efficient and healthier for our environment. It takes over 50 grams of grain to make one gram of protein from beef.

Here is my take on the protein debate. Animal protein is more acidic for the human body than plant-based protein. When you choose to eat animal protein, eat less and make it better quality. Maybe choose to eat animal protein for only one meal each day or designate a meatless day or two each week. I am not a vegan. I enjoy many sources of animal protein, but I believe eating less animal protein is not only good for the human body, but it is also good for our environment.

Animal Proteins

Eggs

When buying eggs, choose only organic, free-range eggs, which come from chickens that are raised in a healthier environment, creating a healthier egg in return. Eggs can fit nicely into a diet. Melt one tablespoon of organic extra virgin coconut oil in a pan. Scramble two or three eggs, including the yolks, with a few vegetables. Add some sliced avocado. In just four or five minutes, it is an easy, great tasting meal.

Fish

Fish is a high protein food that can provide a range of health benefits. White fleshed fish are lower in fat than any other source of animal protein. Fish such as salmon, trout, herring, mackerel, and sardines contain substantial quantities of healthy omega-3 fats. Though generally a good source of protein, not all fish are created equal. The best fish choices are always fish caught in the wild, such as wild Alaskan salmon.

What about farm-raised fish? Farm-raised fish is slowly becoming the future of our fish industry, whether we like it or not. We are starting to see a greater separation in the quality of farm-raised fish practices, similar to the methods being used today in raising organic animals. If you have an opportunity to buy wild Alaskan salmon or rainbow trout caught in the mountain streams of Colorado, thank your lucky stars and enjoy the great taste and wonderful health benefits. If you do not have access to fish grown in the wild, then farm-raised fish may be a good source of protein.

Poultry

As when choosing eggs, the best choices of poultry are organic.

Lean Red Meat

Choose grass-fed beef whenever possible. I am also a big fan of bison. Throw a few bison burgers on a grill along with some grilled vegetables and a few sweet potatoes. Or cook a bison roast in a crock pot with a bunch of root vegetables on a cool autumn day. Yum, yum.

Dairy

Choose 100 percent organic sources of dairy products such as cow's milk, cottage cheese, yogurt, cheese, or butter whenever possible.

Personally, I do not recommend cow's milk to anyone due to the size of the protein molecule and the challenges it may create for the digestive system. Cow's milk can be extremely difficult for the human body to break down and absorb. Cutting back on dairy is one of the first steps in helping improve digestion, skin health, allergies, and asthma. Many people may also be allergic to lactose found in cow's milk and are looking for alternatives.

Another option to traditional cow's milk is goat's milk. Goat's milk is the most widely consumed dairy beverage in the world. Over 65 percent of the world's population consumes goat's milk on a regular basis. Those who have digestive problems may truly benefit from consuming it. Goat's milk is easy to digest and absorb due to the small size of its protein molecule.

Okay, maybe I lost a few of you by recommending goat's milk. There are many plant-based milks that I would highly recommend that are alkalizing, easy to absorb, and taste great. Milk is also made from almonds, cashews, coconut, hemp, and oats to name a few.

Plant Proteins

I think many people are confused over plant-based proteins. I receive numerous questions as to whether a food is a carbohydrate, protein, or fat. I have to explain that most foods have a mixture of the three macronutrients. For example, broccoli, which is a vegetable, is part of the carbohydrate family but also contains protein. In fact, one cup of broccoli contains four grams of protein, which represents over 40 percent of its calories by weight.

Here are a few other examples of plant-based proteins. A half cup of oat groats contains 12 grams of protein. Hempseeds contain 8 grams of protein per tablespoon. Rolled oats contain 6 grams of protein per half cup. One slice of sprouted grain bread contains 6 grams of protein. Almonds contain 6 grams of protein per ounce. A serving of 10 spirulina/chlorella contains 4 grams of protein. So, the next time you are looking for high-quality protein, don't forget your plant-based protein sources.

Protein Supplements

I am asked on a regular basis what protein supplements I recommend. The answer is I do not use or recommend protein supplements. When I want to add protein to a smoothie, I use hempseeds, Brazil nuts, pumpkin seeds, macadamia nuts, and almonds as my protein sources. These nuts and seeds are high in protein, fiber, and healthy omega-6 and monounsaturated fats.

Food Bars, Energy Bars, Protein Bars

Today, there are hundreds of food bars available. I believe the quality of many of these new bars coming into market has greatly improved. Nonetheless, there are still too many that are heavily marketed as healthy but are not. Many manufacturers now use high-quality, whole food, organic ingredients in their bars along with providing great taste. Like smoothies, food bars can be beneficial as a quick and easy nutritional snack when traveling, during a busy schedule, or on the run.

When choosing a food bar, many people make the mistake of first looking at the total number of calories in the bar. Second, they look at the number of protein grams in relationship to the carbohydrate and fat grams. They believe that if the bar is high in protein and low in carbohydrates, it must be a good choice. Remember getting adequate high-quality protein in your diet is important, but high-quality carbohydrates and fats are also important.

When choosing a food bar, be sure to read the label and pay close attention to the number of ingredients, the quality of the ingredients, and the balance. Choose a bar that is balanced with high-quality carbohydrates, proteins, and fats. There are many bars that are healthy and taste good.

Upgrading protein choices can be simple and can make a big difference in overall health and performance. Protein is essential for life!

Quality Fats Heal the Body

Our third macronutrient category is fats. Fats heal the human body. One of the fastest ways to improve our overall health is to blend a variety of healthy fats into our diet.

Despite what we may have heard growing up, healthy fats can actually lower blood pressure, improve our cholesterol profile, balance hormones, decrease inflammation, improve mood, control body weight, improve immune and cognitive function, and reverse and prevent type 2 diabetes. Bottom line: healthy fats heal the body.

Why is eating healthy fats so essential to good health and improved performance? The human body is made up of over 50 trillion cells. Each cell has a specific job to do and is in a constant state of change. On the most basic level, fats help form the membranes that surround each of our cells. The cell membrane, as I talked about in chapter 8, controls nutrients that enter and exit the cell. This is one of the major functions of the body that is threatened by eating unhealthy processed foods and unhealthy fats. Unhealthy fats, such as trans fats and processed omega-6 fats, interfere with normal fat metabolism by crowding or pushing essential fatty acids out from the cell membrane. This makes the cells less fluid and less permeable. Consumed over time, unhealthy fats cause the cell membranes to become stiff and rigid like an M & M candy shell.

When working with a person with type 2 diabetes or anyone who wants to become healthier, one of the first goals is to get their cells healthier. This includes getting the cell membrane soft and permeable. When insulin approaches the cell and tries to open it up to allow nutrients to enter, it has a tougher time doing its job if unhealthy fats and processed foods and beverages have made the outer membrane of the cell rock hard. Over time, the cells become insulin resistant and type 2 diabetes may soon follow. The type 2 diabetes epidemic which has exploded around the world has little to do with genetics and everything to do with how we **REST**, **EAT** and **MOVE**.

Replacing unhealthy fats with healthy fats is the first step to cellular health. Eating healthy fats also satisfies hunger due to the release of two hormones that help control appetite, leptin and cholecystokinin (CCK). Without sufficient healthy fats, we are more likely to overeat. Healthy fats also slow down the digestion of carbohydrates and proteins so there is more sustained release of nutrients into the blood, resulting in stable energy and better health.

If the goal is to lose weight, improve cholesterol profile, lower blood pressure, lower blood glucose, lower inflammation, or just feel great, start by replacing unhealthy fats with healthy fats.

Types of Healthy Fats

Learning to distinguish between a healthy and unhealthy fat is critical for good health and better performance. There are four categories of fats to learn more about: saturated, monounsaturated, omega-3, and omega-6 fats.

Saturated Fats

Can saturated fats be good for us? It depends on the quality of the saturated fat. As consumers, we have been told for years that saturated fats are unhealthy and are responsible for heart disease, cancer, obesity, and a host of other degenerative diseases. Do we need saturated fats in our nutritional program if we want better health and performance? The answer is yes.

Healthy saturated fats give our cells structural integrity. Just as we need a variety of fruits and vegetables to fill many of our nutrient requirements for fiber, vitamins, minerals, and antioxidants, the same is true when consuming healthy fats. Ideally, we want a variety of healthy fats in our eating plan to achieve the nutrient requirements our body needs.

How do we know if a saturated fat is healthy or unhealthy? Look for saturated fats in their most natural state, back to the source. Most nuts and seeds are excellent sources of saturated fat, protein, and fiber. One of the healthiest fats for the body just happens to also be a saturated fat, coconut. For years, we have been told that because coconut is high in saturated fat, we should avoid it at all costs. Is the coconut that I am discussing found in a refined candy bar or is it the coconut that fell from a tree? The fact is coconuts have nourished humans for thousands of years. From skin problems to an upset stomach, coconut was the remedy of choice.

Organic coconut is rich in lauric and caprylic acid, both loaded with antiviral and antifungal properties. Some of the wonderful health benefits of coconut include improving digestive disorders such as acid reflux, gout, and IBS. Coconut also aids in weight loss, improves thyroid function, protects against heart disease, promotes great-looking skin, and is high in antioxidants.

Organic coconut or virgin coconut oil has a wonderful flavor and can be used as a butter replacement. It also is excellent for cooking and baking due to its high heat tolerance. Spread some extra virgin coconut oil on a piece of toast or use it as a cooking oil. Add one tablespoon of shredded organic coconut to a bowl of oatmeal or smoothie recipe. Coconut is one of my go-to healthy fats.

Healthy saturated fats include organic coconut flakes, extra virgin organic coconut oil, and most nuts and seeds.

Monounsaturated Fats

Our second healthy fat category is monounsaturated fats, also known as omega-9 fats. Monounsaturated fats play an important role in a balanced diet and contain a fatty acid known as oleic acid. Oleic acid helps protect arteries, reduces the risk of breast cancer, accentuates the effect of omega-3 fats in the blood, and helps the formation and development of all cell membranes.

One of the main reasons monounsaturated fats are so protective against heart disease is that they help to balance cholesterol, creating a balanced lipid profile along with helping blood vessels relax. No other fat has this effect.

Monounsaturated fats are preferred over polyunsaturated fats for cooking because they have a single double bond between their carbon atoms, making them more stable at high temperatures and not easily oxidized. Anytime a recipe calls for oil, the best choices are monounsaturated fats or extra virgin organic coconut oil.

Healthy monounsaturated fats are found in olives, extra virgin olive oil, avocados, avocado oil, almonds, almond oil, almond butter, peanuts, natural peanut butter, macadamia nuts, macadamia nut oil, pecans, cashews, hazelnuts, and pine nuts.

Polyunsaturated Omega-3s

The first polyunsaturated fat, omega-3 essential fatty acids, is essential for greater health and must be obtained through the foods we eat. In the past, it was believed that any type of polyunsaturated fat was healthy with little distinction between types and processing of polyunsaturated fats. We now understand that polyunsaturated fats fall into two distinct groups. Omega-3 and omega-6 essential fatty acids each address specific functions in the body. The type and processing are important with regard to the quality and benefit of these fats.

With all the processing and refinement taking place in our food industry, approximately 95 percent of United States adults and children are now deficient in these essential fatty acids. In the past our entire food chain—the greens, eggs, meat, nuts, seeds, and fish we ate—all contained these wonderful essential fatty acids. Unfortunately, this is not the case. Today, we have to search for these wonderful fats.

Benefits of Omega-3 Fats

Omega-3 fats are the superstars of healthy fats and make the body strong and healthy. There are many health benefits of consuming these omega-3 fatty acids.

Brain Health. Our brain needs EPA and DHA for brain development and sustainable brain health. Low levels of EPA and DHA have been associated with depression, memory loss, dementia, ADHD, and visual problems. Low levels of DHA have been linked to low serotonin levels. Serotonin is the "feel-good" neurotransmitter that is boosted by consuming omega-3 fats, especially DHA. Low levels of EPA and DHA have also been linked to an epidemic rise in many brain diseases such as Parkinson's, Alzheimer's, and multiple sclerosis. These omega-3 fats are the raw material that feed and nourish the brain for optimal health and performance.

Heart Health. Omega-3 fats aid the cardiovascular system by reducing constriction of blood vessels and decreasing the stickiness of the blood, making it less likely to clot. Omega-3 fats also help balance cholesterol, decrease oxidation, lower inflammation, and improve the sensitivity of the cell membrane. This allows healthy nutrients into the cell and unhealthy waste out of the cell.

Reduced Inflammation. We all know what inflammation is. A bee sting or a sprained ankle causes swelling, hence, inflammation. What about the chronic inflammation that affects millions of people on a daily basis? Ever wondered why some people have more inflammation than others? Want to experience fewer aches and pains? The answer is not another pill, but in consuming omega-3 fats.

One of the worst things to put into the human body on a daily basis is some form of anti-inflammatory medication. Taking medication for a toothache, bee sting, or sprained ankle is not a problem. Taking anti-inflammatory medications day in and day out is a problem. It is a killer to the gut and the overall health of the human body. Most people do not link inflammation to their diets, and most people do not realize that omega-3 fats have a natural anti-inflammatory benefit. To decrease inflammation start taking omega-3 fats.

Hormonal Balance. Omega-3 fats are important for creating hormonal balance in the body. Both omega-3 and omega-6 fats work by forming short-lived, hormone-like substances called prostaglandins. Prostaglandins regulate metabolic processes throughout the entire body at the cellular level. They control cellular communication and are essential in regulating the immune, reproductive, central nervous, and cardiovascular systems. Omega-3 along with omega-6 fats are also the raw materials necessary in building sex hormones such as DHEA, growth hormone, testosterone, and estrogen.

Now you have it. Omega-3 fats are foundational for optimal health and feeling your best. Omega-3 fatty acids can be found in flaxseeds, chia seeds, hempseeds, walnuts, pecans, Brussels sprouts, salmon, trout, mackerel, halibut, oysters, herring, anchovies, sardines, and cod liver oil.

Flaxseeds are high in fiber and contain anti-cancer lignans. Buy a cheap coffee grinder and grind enough flaxseeds for a couple of weeks. You can put your flaxseeds in a few ounces of dark cherry or pomegranate juice, in your favorite smoothie, or on your oatmeal. Chia seeds are the sister of flaxseeds, and also high in fiber and the mineral magnesium. Chia seeds do not need to be ground to be consumed.

Cod liver oil is a better choice than fish oil or krill oil because it is naturally high in essential omega-3 fats (EPA and DHA) and is the also one of the highest sources of vitamin D3 of any food in the world. Taking 1-2 tablespoons of cod liver first thing in the morning is an easy habit to develop. It has a smooth creamy texture and tastes like a lemon drop.

Flaxseeds, chia seeds, and cod liver oil along with many other forms of omega-3 fats are magical in the health benefits they bring to the body. These wonderful omega-3 fats can truly improve high cholesterol or triglycerides, hormonal balance, diabetes, inflammation, ADHD, depression, poor energy, and weight loss.

Polyunsaturated Omega-6 Fats

The second type of polyunsaturated fat is comprised of omega-6 essential fatty acids. The primary fatty acid in the omega-6 family is linoleic acid (LA). Vegetable oils such as corn, soybean, cottonseed, safflower, sunflower, pumpkin seed, and sesame seed oil all contain linoleic acid. It is also found in many nuts, seeds, and leafy greens. Animal sources of omega-6 include lean meats, organ meats, and mother's breast milk.

Like the omega-3 family, which converts ALA to EPA and DHA, the primary omega-6 fatty acid LA converts into two fatty acids, gamma-linolenic acid (GLA) and arachidonic acid (AA).

Unlike omega-3 fats, which are universally healthy fats, there are great differences in the quality and health benefits of omega-6 fats. Arachidonic acid (AA) is the end product of omega-6 fat conversion (LA-GLA-AA). The body needs some AA to function optimally, but too much can promote poor health. Refined oils, such as corn oil and soybean oil, along with too much animal protein can lead to AA overload. To correct this, try to consume only unrefined oils and consume less animal protein. Also, the consumption of omega-3 fats helps by blocking the conversion to AA, keeping essential fats in balance.

Benefits of Omega-6 Fats

There are many benefits of consuming high-quality omega-6 fats. Two benefits are prostaglandin health and maintaining brown fat.

Prostaglandin Health. Omega-6 fats are necessary for production of many hormones including prostaglandins, the short lived, hormone-like substances that regulate many of the body's life-sustaining systems. The body produces prostaglandins from essential fatty acids we consume from food each day.

The Metabolic Power of Brown Fat. Our bodies have two types of fat cells: white fat and brown fat. White fat is the fat under our skin (subcutaneous fat) that insulates the body and is used for energy. This is the fat most of us are trying to lose. Brown fat (visceral fat) is the fat surrounding our organs and differs from white fat in many ways. Brown fat acts as a thermostat and helps the body acclimate to hot and cold temperatures. It aids in weight loss by helping the body convert calories into heat via thermogenesis. Brown fat helps burn 25 percent of all fat calories. In this regard, brown fat is an important element in metabolism.

As we age, brown fat begins to decline. Think about the difference between seniors, who are often sensitive to cold and gain body fat (white fat) later in their years, and youngsters, who can tolerate cold temperatures easily. Most young children have metabolically active brown fat. I remember going to see my grandparents as a kid. The heat in their house was always cranked way up. I never understood why they were always cold, even when the heat was on high.

So how can we increase brown fat? Gamma-linolenic acid (GLA), like its cousins from the omega-3 family (EPA and DHA), helps fight heart disease, cancer, diabetes, inflammation, arthritis, and also promotes weight loss. GLA in our daily diet provides the raw material needed by prostaglandins to stimulate brown fat. Dietary deficiencies and disease may block or slow the conversion of linolenic acid (LA) into GLA.

Just as we must search for omega-3 fats, we must also search for high-quality omega-6 fats. The best sources of omega-6 fats are hempseeds, pumpkin seeds, Brazil nuts, sunflower seeds, sesame seeds, evening primrose oil, borage oil, black current seed oil, and leafy greens. Most raw nuts also contain omega-6 fats. Do not cook or heat omega-3 or omega-6 fats. Heat destroys the benefits of these healthy fats.

There is no other nutrient available that can heal the body and keep it healthy from infancy to old age like HEALTHY FATS!

Food Quality Essentials

Big Picture

- Use the Food Target as your nutritional guide.
- Job one when it comes to nutrition is to focus on improving the quality of what you eat and drink. Get closer to the source.
- There are 3 macronutrients: carbohydrates, proteins, and fats.
- If you take a macronutrient out of the diet you will develop a macro problem.
- Carbohydrates fuel the body.
- Proteins build the body.
- Fats heal the body.

Ask Yourself

- How many fruits and vegetables do you eat per day?
- Do you eat any type of ancient grains on a regular basis?
- What types of plant-based proteins do you eat?
- If you eat animal protein, how can you make it better?
- Do you consume omega-3 or omega-6 fats on a daily basis?
- What upgrades can you make with your carbohydrates, proteins, or fats?

Small Steps

- Focus on food quality and a balance of the three macronutrients: carbohydrates, proteins, and fats.
- Over the next 30 days begin to upgrade the foods you currently eat the most.

19 Meal Patterning

We continue to build the EAT Pyramid with building block number four—Meal Patterning.

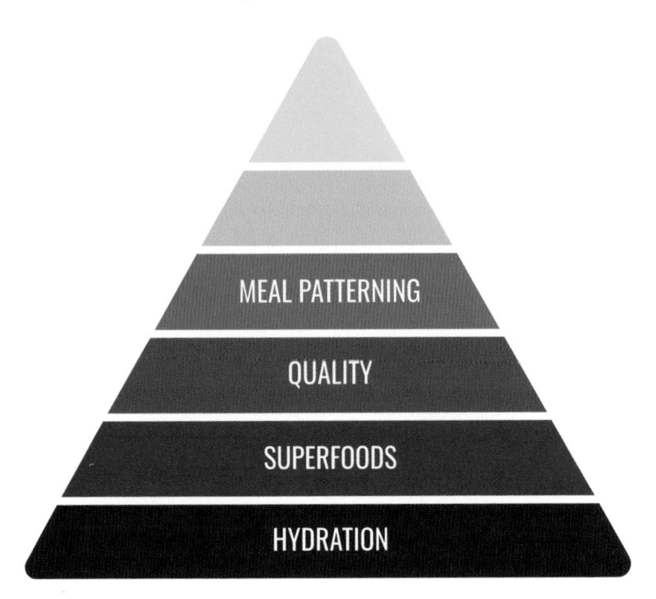

What is Meal Patterning?

Does it truly matter how often and when we eat? Should we eat three meals each day and have a snack between meals? Is eating breakfast the right thing to do? Is fasting healthy for the mind and body?

My first book was titled *Meal Patterning.* For many years I had watched and listened to how people eat—their patterns of eating. While working at the Michigan Athletic Club, one of the largest health clubs in the world, I become fascinated by how many people were in constant pursuit of losing weight. I heard all the typical conversations around weight loss: high carb/low fat, high protein/low carb, high fat/no carb diets, cut calories, and exercise more.

In 1992 I read an article on sumo wrestlers, the largest human beings on the planet. It focused on something that is seldom discussed, patterns of eating. A sumo wrestler's success depends on his weight. The bigger the wrestler, the better chance he has in competition. The article went deep into the science of how they gain their weight, A sumo wrestler's diet is aimed entirely on the ability to gain weight as quickly and efficiently as possible.

Sumo wrestlers have learned that it is not just what they eat that makes them gain weight, but also how and when they eat, as well as what they do after eating. To gain weight, they become gorgers. Most eat one or two large meals each day consisting of 3,500 to 6,000+ calories per meal. They also eat a high nutrient packed stew called "Chankonabe." Immediately after eating, they take a 2-4-hour nap.

One budding sumo wrestler initially weighed in at 350 pounds and ate 6,000 calories a day spread over three meals: 2,000 calories for breakfast, 2,500 calories for lunch, and 1,500 calories for dinner. To gain more weight, he decided to change his approach to eating or patterns of his meals. At the end of 18 months, he gained 150 pounds while cutting his calorie intake by 1,000 calories a day. How did he do it? He simply adopted the life of established sumo wrestlers. He decreased the frequency of eating and changed from eating three daily meals to one. He increased the quantity by eating 5,000 calories at his single meal, and he went to sleep immediately after eating.

5,000 calories x 1 meal/day + nap = 150 pounds of weight gain in 18 months!

By the way, many sumo wrestlers develop type 2 diabetes by their mid-thirties, and many die by the age of 50.

What can we all learn from the sumo meal patterns? Obviously, the sumo wrestlers eat an extremely high number of calories. This is a big part of their weight gain strategy. Too much food at one meal floods the body with the fat storing and hunger hormone insulin. To further enhance their weight gain, sumo wrestlers focus on skipping meals to increase the sensitivity of lipoprotein lipase. Then they take a nap after they eat to slow down their metabolism even more.

Reducing Calories and Frequency May Lead to Weight Gain

How is it possible to reduce the total calories consumed and the frequency of meals and still gain weight? It is possible because of two processes the body uses to protect itself from starvation—lipoprotein lipase and insulin.

Lipoprotein Lipase

First, the human body protects itself from skipped meals by increasing lipoprotein lipase. Lipoprotein lipase is the key enzyme that stores fat to protect the body from starvation. When we decrease the frequency of meals or snacks, our lipoprotein lipase enzymes become more sensitive to storing calories. As the frequency of meals decrease, the lipoprotein lipase enzymes begin to work overtime in an effort to store extra calories in the form of fat throughout the body.

Insulin

Second, after we eat, blood glucose levels rise initiating a release of the hormone insulin. Insulin's job is to open the cells to receive and use nutrients. Once the needs of the cells are met, the rest of the nutrients may then be stored as glycogen (stored carbohydrates) and body fat. The increase in insulin levels leads to an increase in body fat stores as well as greater insulin resistance.

Better Meal Patterning

Now let's reverse engineer this strategy of gaining weight to become leaner. We begin by eating high-quality foods spread throughout the day by eating three to four smaller meals. We also move a little bit after each meal. This is the opposite approach to the sumo eating patterns.

Frequency of Eating

When and how often we eat is a critical component in keeping our body healthy, strong, and feeling our best. One of the first things many people do when they want to lose weight is cut calories. They believe that the easiest way to do this is to skip meals. Unfortunately, this is just the opposite of what we need to do.

Skipping meals slows down our metabolism. This is just one reason why eating breakfast is so critical to our success. It is important to break the overnight fast and fuel the body properly. Skipping meals also alerts the body to release more of the fat-storing enzyme, lipoprotein lipase. Remember, skipping meals is a strategy the sumo wrestlers use to gain weight. When people begin to skip meals, it can become more difficult to get the necessary nutrients to keep the body strong and healthy. By skipping breakfast, we lose out on valuable vitamins, minerals, and fiber that can be found in an ancient grain like oatmeal, or in fruit and nuts.

Eating smaller meals more frequently throughout the day allows the body to properly break down and absorb their nutrients. This trains the body to be a fat burning machine. Also, eating more frequently throughout the day decreases the chances of overeating. If you are not hungry within 3-4 hours after eating, you most likely ate too much at your last meal.

The 3-4 Hour Rule

When I trained for my first body building contest, I consumed smaller meals more frequently. Spreading calories throughout the day can rev up metabolism. The rule I followed was to eat every 3-4 hours. Eating smaller meals more often helps to:

- Increase our metabolic rate, allowing the body to burn more calories
- Improve energy by maintaining a steadier blood glucose level
- Make better food choices because we are not as hungry
- Control portion sizes

CHRIS'S SAMPLE DAY

6:30am	**Wake up**: Drink 6-8 ounces of water and take my dog Floyd for a walk
7:00am	**Morning Routine**: Water with lemon and orange slices (10 oz), frozen wheatgrass ice cubes (5 cubes), cod liver oil (2 tbsp)
9:00am	**Breakfast:** Oatmeal on the Run (2/3 cup rolled oats, ½ cup of almond or cashew milk, 1 tsp each cinnamon, cacao nibs, and shredded coconut, 1 tbsp raisins or frozen fruit (make and refrigerate the night before)
12:30pm	**Lunch**: Leftovers or a large salad with veggies, hempseeds, and homemade vinaigrette or a smoothie with frozen berries, coconut water, hempseeds, ginger, beet, flaxseeds, banana, spinach, and a few dates, and 15 spirulina/chlorella tablets with water
3:30pm	**Snack**: 15 spirulina/chlorella tablets with water, smoothie or an apple with Brazil nuts
6:15pm	**Water:** 1 glass of mineral water with lemon/orange slices while preparing dinner
6:30pm	**Dinner**: Organic chicken, wild salmon, or bison burgers with sweet potatoes with coconut oil and baked broccoli with extra virgin olive oil
8:00pm	**Evening Chill Time:** Herbal tea with a slice of ginger, popcorn with coconut oil, or 3 cubes of frozen wheatgrass

Do you eat breakfast? Yes or No

How many meals do you eat per day? ____________________

How much time elapses between meals? ____________________

Miracle of Fasting

There is nothing better to keep the human body healthy and performing at its best than fasting. Fasting involves a controlled voluntary abstinence from caloric intake to achieve a physical, mental, or spiritual outcome. Although fasting may appear to be the latest buzz in the health and fitness arena, fasting has been a practice throughout human evolution. Ancient hunter-gathers did not have the luxury of supermarkets, refrigerators, or food available year-round. Sometimes they could not find anything to eat. As a result, we all carry that feast-or-famine genetic code, even though most cultures of today now eat more consistently with two to four regular meals each day, plus snacks and desserts. As a result, our digestive tracts stay full most of the time, unable to allow our bodies to experience the beneficial effects of temporary emptiness and the natural cleansing process fasting creates.

We now know one of the simplest, yet most effective strategies for improving our overall health is fasting. Fasting has been shown to improve:

- Gut Health
- Immune System
- Energy
- Brain Health
- Heart Health
- Longevity and Aging
- Improved Awareness and Relationship to Food
- Body Weight
- Overall Health

With so many incredible benefits of fasting it is no wonder the popularity of fasting has exploded.

Why Fast?

I think most people want to begin a fast with one thing in mind—to lose weight. This may be a great goal and can be effective, but I believe the greatest benefit of fasting is that it allows the body enough time to clean, build, and repair itself.

One way the body detoxifies, builds, and repairs is the process of autophagy. Autophagy is the body's way of cleaning out damaged cells in order to regenerate newer healthier cells. "Auto" means self and "phagy" means to eat. So, the literal meaning of autophagy is "self-eating." Essentially, this is the body's mechanism of getting rid of all the broken down, old cell machinery when there is no longer enough energy to sustain it. It is a regulated, orderly process of cleaning, building, and repairing the body.

Nutrient deprivation is the key activator of autophagy. As mentioned earlier, when we eat, insulin goes up. When insulin goes up, glucagon goes down. When we do not eat (fast), insulin goes down, and glucagon goes up. It is this increase of glucagon that stimulates the process of autophagy. In fact, fasting provides the greatest boost to autophagy. Not only does fasting stimulate autophagy, fasting also stimulates growth hormone, one of the key hormones that tells the body to start rebuilding and repairing. The human body is amazing in its ability to heal and self-correct if given the right tools.

How to Fast

There is no one right way to fast. It all comes down to our own personal goals. If you have a medical condition, you should consult a health professional before trying any form of intermittent fasting. Here are few simple ways to begin the fasting process.

Overnight Circadian Rhythm Fast (12-14 hours)

One of the easiest and most effective ways to keep our mind and body functioning at its best is a daily overnight circadian rhythm fast. Fasting 12-14 hours overnight on a daily basis is a fantastic way to keep the body clean and feeling its best. If our last meal or snack ended at 8:00 p.m., then we do not eat again until 8:00, 9:00, or 10:00 a.m. Go 12-14 hours without eating. It is simple and effective and does not feel like a diet. This is my recommended fasting plan for almost everyone including myself.

Intermittent Fasting. One of the hottest crazes today is intermittent fasting. It is an eating pattern that cycles between periods of fasting and eating. During the fasting periods, very little or nothing at all is eaten. There are several different ways of intermittent fasting. All involve splitting the day or week into eating and fasting periods.

16/8 Method. This method involves restricting the daily eating period to 8 hours and fasting the other 16 hours. Most people who follow this method skip breakfast, start eating around noon, and end their eating at 8 p.m. This is the most popular type of intermittent fasting. It is simple and easy to sustain.

24-Hour Fast. This fasting method involves not eating for an entire 24 hours. This may be practiced once per week, once per month, or once every other month. It is a more advanced type of fast and is not recommended as a starting point.

Thoughts on Fasting

There are hundreds of methods of fasting. Fasting on a regular basis can have tremendous benefits. Here are a few thoughts to keep in mind when fasting.

- Start slowly. Begin a fasting plan with a 12-14 hour overnight fast. It is safe, easy, and effective, and will not feel like a diet. It is easy to develop a habit of going 12-14 hours without eating. Most of this fast occurs overnight when sleeping. The best part is that this type of fasting can be followed for life.
- Be careful to not cut out food groups and nutrients by skipping meals.
- When skipping meals, many valuable nutrients will be missed. Make sure to drink enough water to help in the detoxification process.
- Break the fast with nutritious, easy to digest foods close to the source. Wheatgrass juice, cod liver oil, ancient grains such as oatmeal, and fruit are generally the first foods that go into my body after my 12-14 hour overnight fast.
- Experiment with the different approaches of fasting and find something that you enjoy and fits your goals.
- If you have a medical condition, consult with a health professional prior to fasting.

Fasting can be an extremely powerful method to keep us feeling and being our best!

Focused Eating

Any diet is primarily a focused eating program. Where we go wrong is when the program cannot be sustained over time, or when we do not enjoy the process. When we put our energy and focus into enjoying the process, it provides us with a roadmap for success. Noom, Weight Watchers, Keto, and Paleo are all exercises in focused eating. The same can be said for focused relaxation and focused movement. We need to be aware of what we are consuming so that mindless eating does not derail us.

At On Target Living, we offer a 21-day EAT Challenge that anyone can join at any time. The program provides a focused eating plan that centers on the middle two circles of the Food Target. It is just one tool to stretch your focused eating muscles and gain control over your daily eating plan and to help you reach your goals.

21-Day On Target Living EAT Challenge

Dive in with our 21-Day EAT Challenge. It is extremely simple to follow, but it is not easy. This is why it is called the EAT Challenge.

- Eat strictly within the two inner circles of the Food Target for 21 days.
- This plan creates a routine of eating healthy for life.
- During the 21 days new habits and routines are built and old habits get broken.
- Use the Food Target and the challenge-friendly Eat Guide below.

Challenge yourself and the returns will be amazing.

EAT GUIDE

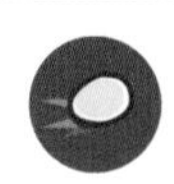

FRIENDLY FATS

Avocado
Chia Seeds
Cod liver Oil
Extra Virgin Olive Oil
Flaxseeds
Hempseeds
Nut Butters
Organic Virgin Coconut Oil
Pumpkin Seeds

BEVERAGES

Almond Milk
Alkaline Water
Coconut Milk
Coconut Water
Herbal Teas
Mineral Water
Nut Milk Creamer
Organic Coffee/Tea

SATISFYING STARCHES

Purple, Blue & Red Skin Potatoes
Root Vegetables (Beets, Turnips, Parsnips, Carrots, Onions)
Sweet Potatoes

VEGGIE VITALITY

Asparagus
Bok Choy
Broccoli
Brussel Sprouts
Cabbage
Cauliflower
Celery
Collard Greens
Cucumber
Kale
Peppers
Spinach

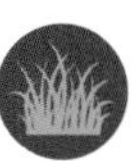

SUPERFOODS

Cod Liver Oil
Flaxseeds
Hempseeds
Spirulina Chlorella
Wheatgrass

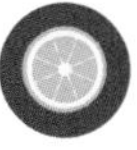

FRUIT FRENZY

Apples
Banana
Berries
Citrus Fruits
Cherries
Grapefruit
Grapes
Kiwi
Melon
Peaches
Pineapple
Pomegranate
Raisins
Tomatoes

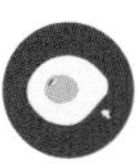

POWERFUL PROTEINS

Beans
Bison/Buffalo
Chia Seeds
Flaxseeds
Hempseeds
Lentils
Organic Free-Range Eggs
Organic Grass-Fed Beef
Organic Poultry
Venison
Wild Caught Fish

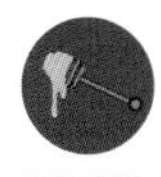

NATURAL SWEETS

Agave Nectar
Cacao Nibs
Dates/Figs
Pure Maple Syrup
Raw Local Honey

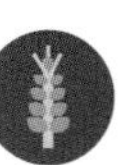

BRAIN GRAINS

Coconut Flour
Farro
Millet
Oat Groats
Organic Polenta
Quinoa
Rolled Oats
Sprouted Grains (bread, wraps)
Steel Cut Oats
Teff
Wheatberries
Whole Grain Rice

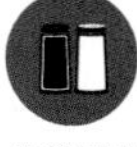

CONDIMENTS

Sea Salt
Black Pepper
Herbs & Spices
Apple Cider Vinegar
Balsamic Vinegar
Red Wine Vinegar
Liquid Aminos
Chicken/Veg. Broth

Find more information about the 21-Day On Target Living EAT Challenge on our **app at **ontargetliving.com.***

Cleansing

In addition to fasting there are many powerful ways to clean and detoxify the body on a regular basis. As discussed in chapter 15, it is important to keep the 5 Superhighways of Elimination (BULLS) functioning well. Diaphragmatic breathing, good sleep, daily movement, and hydration are all essential to keep the body clean and healthy.

Cleansing Foods and Beverages

Here are some of the top foods, beverages, and herbs that keep the body clean and functioning at its best.

- **Chlorophyll and Cruciferous Vegetables:** Wheatgrass, spirulina/chlorella, spinach, kale, broccoli, cabbage, leafy greens, basil, and cilantro
- **Fruits:** Lemons, apples, bananas, blueberries, avocado, pomegranate, kiwi, berries, and cacao
- **Vegetables/Starches:** Beets, ginger, sweet potatoes, parsnips, tomatoes, carrots, and onions
- **High Fiber Foods**: Flaxseeds, chia seeds, beans, legumes, and ancient grains
- **Beverages:** Green tea, ginger tea, herbal teas, wheatgrass juice, celery juice, and apple cider vinegar
- **Herbs:** Turmeric, cayenne pepper, cilantro, sage, dandelion, nettles, red clover, milk thistle, slippery elm, comfrey, burdock root, cardamom, alfalfa, and lemon peel

3-Day Smoothie Cleanse

An easy way to jumpstart and reset the body is with a 3-day smoothie cleanse. Smoothies are heartier than a juice cleanse and are easy to prepare and taste great. For three consecutive days, consume a smoothie for breakfast, lunch, and dinner.

Here is a guide to build a perfect smoothie. Simply start with a liquid, toss in fruit, throw in greens, build in protein, and add healthy fats. Bump up the nutrition even more by adding superpower superfoods.

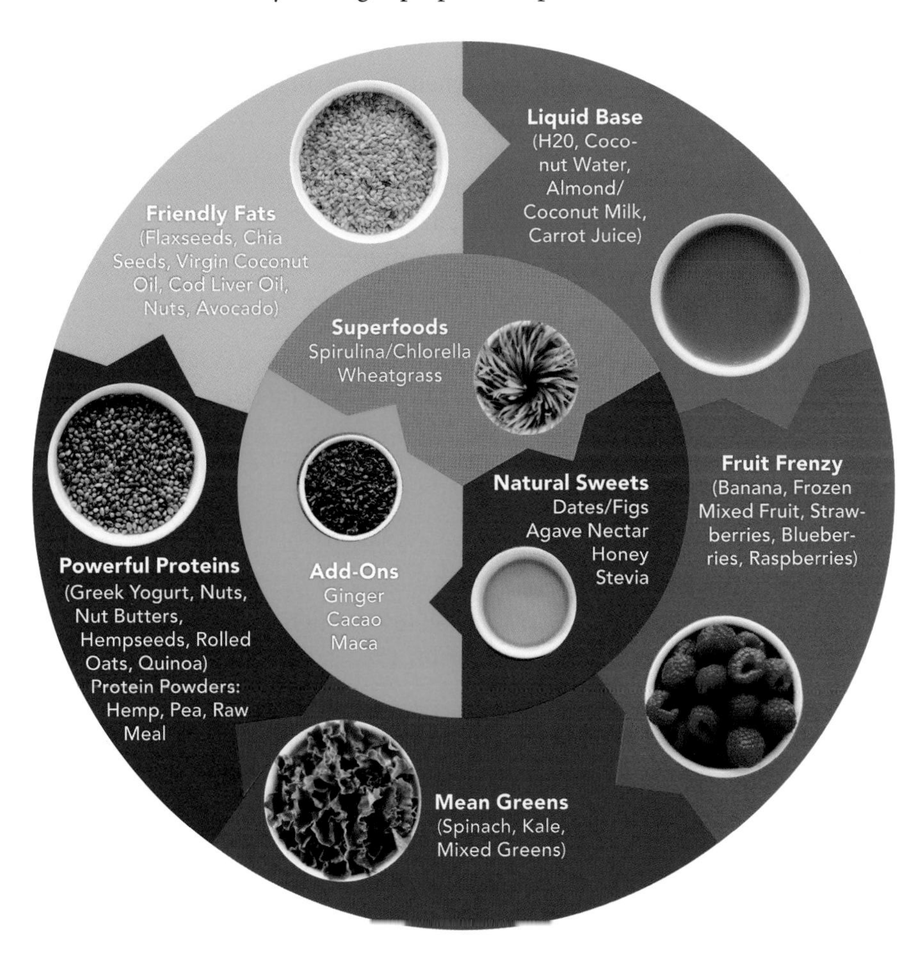

Find Your Rhythm

What we eat, when we eat, how often we eat, and what we do after we eat—**Your Meal Patterns**—all play a large role in our overall health and feeling our best.

Meal Patterning Essentials

Big Picture

- What you eat, how you eat, and when you eat all play a critical role in your overall health and feeling your best.
- Sumo wrestlers gain their weight by skipping meals and eating one large meal followed by taking a long nap.
- Lipoprotein lipase is a fat storing enzyme.
- Insulin is a hunger and fat storing hormone.
- Overeating or eating the wrong types of foods can overstimulate insulin.
- The miracle of fasting (autophagy) allows the body enough time to clean out the trash and repair the body. While you sleep is part of a 12-14 overnight fast.

Ask Yourself

- How long do you fast most nights?
- Do you currently eat breakfast?
- What time do you normally break your overnight fast?
- How many meals do you consume on a typical day?

Small Steps

- Fast for 12-14 hours most nights.
- Eat breakfast.
- Eat smaller meals more frequently—every 3-4 hours.
- Find your rhythm of eating.

20 Quantity

We continue building the EAT Pyramid with building block number five—Quantity.

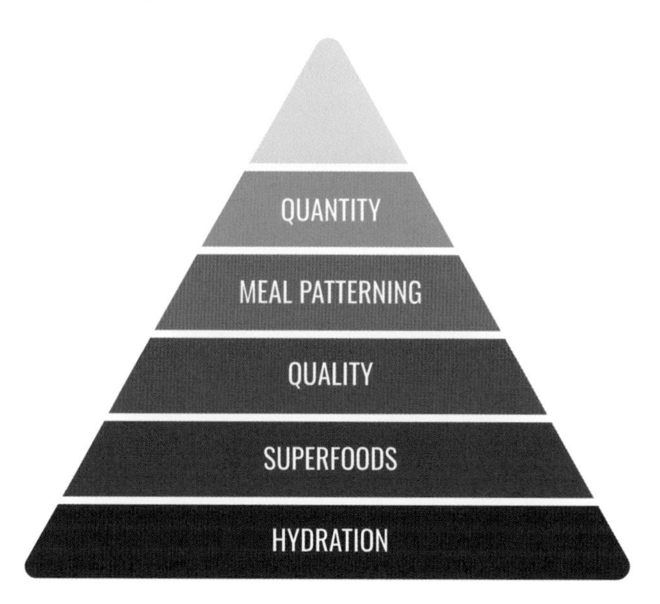

All Calories are Not Equal

Now that we have a better understanding of food and beverage quality, meal patterns, and fasting, it is time to turn our attention to quantity and calories, because calories do count.

Ask most people how to lose weight and they often say to eat less and move more. One belief I find hard for many people to change is their belief that a calorie equals a calorie.

Do you believe 100 calories of a processed bag of chips or cookies equals 100 calories of broccoli or an apple? Yes or No

Do you think your cells would be affected by these foods in the same manner? Yes or No

Do you believe the impact on your pH would be the same? Yes or No

Does the amount of sleep and stress make a difference in how many calories you consume each day? Yes or No

Let's begin this discussion on the calorie. A calorie is a unit or measurement of energy. All foods and beverages contain calories, and calories give us energy. If we consume too many calories at any one time (gorging) over the course of the day, week, month, or year, regardless of high food and beverage quality, one or more of these problems may arise:

- Overproduction of insulin
- Drop in energy
- Hormonal imbalance
- Poor digestion
- Increased body fat
- Poor health

It is easy to understand why many people believe that by limiting calorie intake and moving the body more, losing weight will just happen. In fact, many people believe it does not really matter what we eat as long as we do not eat too many calories. This type of thinking is not going to get us very far. The results will be short term at best. Calories are important, but the quality of foods and beverages is key.

How Many Calories to Consume Each Day

The number of calories a person needs each day depends on many factors including activity level, lean muscle mass, stress, frequency of meals, and food and beverage quality.

Activity Level

Factors, such the amount of daily exercise or movement we get each day, how sedentary our lifestyle is, and whether we have a physical job, will help determine how many calories we need in a day. If we routinely walk, jog, bike, climb stairs, strength train, dance, practice yoga, or play, we may need more calories to sustain energy.

Lean Muscle Mass

Having more lean muscle mass burns more calories at rest and throughout the day. There are over ten times more mitochondria in a muscle cell than a fat cell. The mitochondria act as the car engine of the cell. To keep the body burning calories, we must keep the mitochondria healthy and active. This is just one reason why strength training is so important in maintaining a healthy metabolism.

Stress

Do not underestimate the role of stress and its effect on how the body burns calories. Remember the stress response is physical. The human body is designed to handle acute response with fight-or-flight. We are not designed to handle chronic stress and the overproduction of the stress hormone cortisol. If cortisol levels go up, the hormones that make us healthy and lean, growth hormone and testosterone, go down. Chronic overproduction of cortisol can break down the body and increase body fat.

Frequency of Meals

When we eat more frequent small meals, our body does not overproduce insulin, making it easy for the body to break down and absorb nutrients more efficiently. It also makes it difficult to overeat.

Food and Beverage Quality

High-quality carbohydrates, proteins, and fats along with proper hydration keep the body running at its best.

Our daily calorie needs may vary depending on how the day unfolds. We need to listen to the body to predict its nutritional needs. If you are truly hungry, eat, but challenge yourself first. Are you truly hungry? When was the last time you ate? Could you just be bored or stressed and looking for some relief? It takes time to develop meal patterns.

Too Much of a Good Thing

Years ago, when I began training with Michael, he asked me about eating nuts. I explained the many benefits that nuts provide and gave him a few options including a few of my favorites, such as almonds, macadamia nuts, Brazil nuts, pecans, pistachios, and walnuts.

A month later Michael told me that he had been gaining weight. I asked what he might be doing differently. He reported eating macadamia nuts as an evening snack and loving the taste of them. You probably know where this conversation is going. When I asked how many nuts, his answer was approximately a half cup. Every night? He said yes. I had to inform him that he was consuming over 500 calories each night just before bed.

Michael had no clue that there were so many calories in these healthy nuts. The choice of macadamia nuts was a good one, but only a few at a time. We had a good laugh together and now he is aware that nuts are extremely healthy but are also nutrient and calorie dense.

Below is a range of calories to work with. Remember, this is just a range. While the goal is not to count calories, it is important to be aware of the quantity of food and beverages we consume. Because there are so many variables when it comes to how many calories we need per day, these ranges are just guidelines. Listen to your body and its nutritional needs.

Calorie Ranges for Adults

Adult Female:	**1,200-2,500 calories per day**
Adult Male:	**1,500-3,000 calories per day**

Our body needs quality food and water in adequate amounts in order to stay healthy and feel our best. We may exceed the high-end calorie range based on our activity level, lean muscle, stress level, and frequency and quality of meals. Lumberjacks have been known to consume over 11,000 calories per day in an attempt to maintain their body weight.

How Many Calories Should We Consume at Each Meal?

This may vary depending on the time of day, the last time we ate, or when our next meal comes. Eating more than 600-1,000 calories per meal, depending on nutritional needs, may be too many calories. This is one of my greatest challenges when it comes to food. Many times, I eat too much at one meal.

Think of the stomach as a washing machine. My daughter Kristen loves to pack the washing machine so full that the clothes can barely move. Her clothes get wet, but do her clothes get clean? We must be kind to our stomach. Do not stuff it full. Leave room in the stomach for it to digest and process food properly.

It is not necessary to count calories. In fact, I do not recommend counting calories for anyone. I do recommend having an awareness of how many calories foods and beverages contain. Having this awareness is essential for optimal health and feeling our best. Remember, all calories are not created equal, but calories do count!

Food Quantity Essentials

Big Picture

- Make your calories count!
- Calories are important, but the quality of foods and beverages comes first.
- The number of calories you eat per day depends on many variables: activity level, lean muscle mass, stress, sleep, frequency of eating, and food quality.
- Counting calories is not important, but calories do count.
- Caloric Range for Women: 1,200-2,500 calories
- Caloric Range for Men: 1,500-3,000 calories
- Just as you avoid overloading the washing machine to allow space for the clothes to get clean, take the same approach to eating. Eat to 70 percent full to allow optimal breakdown and absorption of food.

Ask Yourself

- Does a calorie = a calorie?
- How much physical activity do you get on a daily basis?
- Do you do any form of strength training each week?
- How many meals do you eat each day?
- How many hours of sleep do you get each night?
- How many calories do you eat on a typical day?

Small Steps

- Focus on food quality first.
- If you are hungry, eat, but ask yourself first if you are truly hungry.
- Be aware of how much you are eating.
- Don't fill the washing machine to capacity.
- Be aware of the caloric content of what you like to eat.

21 80/20 Rule

The last building block in the EAT Pyramid is the 80/20 Rule.

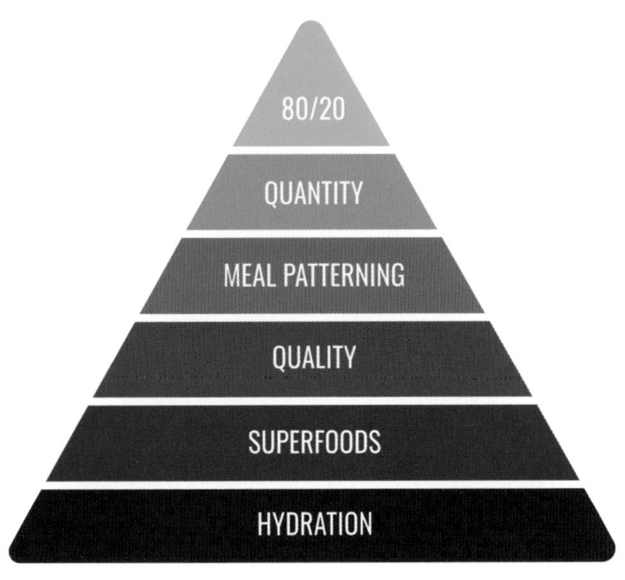

80/20 Rule

We have previously covered hydration, superfoods, quality, meal patterning, and quantity. All are essential in developing a successful eating plan. As we wrap up this section, Let Food Be Your Medicine, we need to include the best kept secret for living healthy without making sacrifices. It is the 80/20 Rule.

The 80/20 Rule is a sustainable lifestyle plan that can be maintained and enjoyed forever. The 80/20 Rule allows us to make room for the things we love without giving up our health and still see the results we are looking for.

Here is how it works. For **80 percent of the time,** focus on eating the highest quality foods found within the two center circles of the Food Target. The other **20 percent of the time** allows room for some of the things we love like birthday cake, dinner and wine out with friends, and mom's home cooking. After all, a healthy lifestyle is about balance with a mix of eating for purpose and eating for pleasure.

Following the 80/20 Rule we become more mindful of the eating experience which allows us to pivot when needed. This is the biggest reason why diets do not work. The reason birthday cake is so special is because we only have it on special occasions.

The next time you are thinking about going on a diet ask yourself:

- **Does this program make sense?**
- **Can I really live on 1,200 calories per day?**
- **No fruit? No potatoes? No oatmeal?**
- **Eating only apples for the day? Only raw foods?**
- **No liberties?**

Most of us at one time or another have tried some type of diet, only to abandon ship after a specified period of time or specific result. Then we immediately go back to our old ways or patterns of eating. A better option is to follow the 80/20 Rule. For 80 percent of the time, focus on eating healthy. For 20 percent of the time, we can "splurge" a bit. The plan allows 4 meals per week or 6 days per month to splurge a bit.

80/20 SAMPLE WEEK

MONDAY	TUESDAY	WEDNESDAY	THURSDAY	FRIDAY	SATURDAY	SUNDAY
BREAKFAST	BREAKFAST	BREAKFAST	BREAKFAST	BREAKFAST	BREAKFAST	BREAKFAST
LUNCH	LUNCH	LUNCH	LUNCH	LUNCH	LUNCH	LUNCH
DINNER	DINNER	DINNER	DINNER	DINNER	DINNER	DINNER

Mindful Eating Rules to Live By

Mindful eating is about paying attention to eating with purpose. It is a nonjudgmental practice of eating in a way that makes us feel healthy and happy and uses our intuition or common sense to make choices. We should not have to rely on science, diets, trends, programs, books, or technology to tell whether a food is truly healthy. We already know. So, let's start with the number one rule to mindful eating.

Rule 1: Use common sense.

There is so much information out there that sometimes we can lose our common sense when it comes to eating. Do we really believe that adding butter to our coffee will boost metabolism? Is it smart and sustainable to completely give up carbohydrates? Where will we get our energy? How long will this no-carbohydrate diet really last? Does energy really come in a can? Remember that we do not eat nutrients, we eat food. Food is the most powerful medicine on earth.

The behavior we choose should be sustainable for life. We should not give up carbohydrates during the week only to binge out on the weekend. We need to build a lifestyle that sticks. A key factor to a long-term healthy and sustainable lifestyle is recognizing that it must be done with pleasure.

Rule 2: Extremes and food restrictions do not work.

Yes, being too healthy is absolutely a thing. When we live "too healthy" we take the fun out of eating, and when we live too unhealthy we take the fun out of life. The more we restrict, the more we want. Life is about freedom, especially when it comes to our eating choices. Find balance. It is more fun. Do not give anything up. Just make everything better.

Rule 3: Be aware of how much and how often you indulge.

We do not get pleasure when we overdo things. Perhaps that piece of chocolate cake will bring instant gratification, but it will not bring long-term health and happiness. Think about it. That ice cream we love so much will be much more rewarding if we do not eat it every day. Do not overdo anything. Add variety to life and practice moderation. Everything can fit into a healthy lifestyle.

Rule 4: Pause before giving in to cravings.

Most cravings only last 10 minutes. To distract from the craving, we can go for a walk, take a stretch or breathing break, or drink some water. Revisit the craving after 10 minutes. If it is still there, think about how that particular food will make you feel after you eat it. Does it energize you or make you lethargic? Does it contribute to your long-term goal? Is it really worth it? How could you make it better?

We need to become aware of our food choices and the reason behind them. Is boredom or stress creating the craving. It is okay to give into those cravings from time to time, but not all the time. Start to build that muscle to say no or not now. It does not mean we can never have it. It is that just now may not be the right time.

Rule 5: Allow for special occasions.

Look at the relationship and bigger picture. One meal of splurging will not ruin your long-term health goals. My wife comes from a large Lebanese family where food is definitely the center of every occasion. We get pleasure by feeding people because food is love. It connects us and is meant to be shared. Food is social, and our social interactions also contribute to long-term health and happiness.

We do not remember the things we buy, but we do remember the meals we eat and with whom we share them.

Rule 6: Find things that make you live more mindfully.

These things can include traveling, wine, dinner, home-cooked meals, Sunday brunch, coffee dates, adventures, and yoga. Traveling allows us to be present and soak in new experiences. It is a state of complete engagement. Be strategic about meals when traveling. We do not travel all the way to France to eat a packaged croissant on the airplane. Save this experience for that little café where a freshly baked croissant and a cappuccino can be enjoyed while people watching. Plan ahead and take some time to scope out the best food spots. Be present and take in the full experience.

Rule 7: Stop worrying about being perfect.

There is so much more to food than eating to lose weight or be healthy. It is an experience that is meant to be enjoyed in every way. It is not about being perfect. It is about being better. A key factor to long-term sustainable weight loss is recognizing that it must be done through pleasure.

Rule 8: Do not take short cuts.

Short cuts do not work, and they will never work. When we build a lifestyle over time, it will become effortless. I promise. Will power and motivation will run out. It is our lifestyle and our daily habits and rituals that will always pick us back up again.

Remember to be intentional about choices and mindful about how much and how often to indulge. Food is an experience, and it is meant to be enjoyed in every way.

80/20 Rule Essentials

Big Picture

- 80/20 Rule: For 80 percent of the time, focus on high-quality foods and beverages. For 20 percent of the time, make room for things you love like birthday cake or mom's home cooking.
- Mindful eating is paying attention to eating with purpose.
- Use common sense to make healthier choices.
- Understand that extremes and food restrictions do not work.
- Food is an experience to be enjoyed.

Ask Yourself

- Is food on your mind 24/7?
- During a typical week how often do you indulge?
- Are there certain trigger foods that get you going? Like the slogan for Lay's potato chips claims, "You can't eat just one!"?
- What are some of your trigger thoughts?
- How can you become more mindful with your eating experience?

Small Steps

- Develop consistent eating patterns.
- Plan your meals.
- Think ahead and ask yourself if that piece of cake is really worth it.
- Your goal is to make small changes and slowly develop an eating plan that you enjoy and can sustain.

22 Dieting and Weight Loss

Before we wrap up our final chapter on eating, I want to devote some conversation to dieting and weight loss. With the obesity epidemic in full swing around the globe, more and more people are looking for ways to lose weight.

Why Diets Do Not Work

Today, approximately 100 million people in the United States are currently on some type of diet to lose weight and spend upwards of $60-70 billion a year on weight loss-related products and services. Here is the craziest statistic of all. The weight loss industry has a failure rate of over 95 percent. People may lose weight, but most have not learned how to develop a lifestyle that they can sustain and enjoy.

After spending more than 35 years in the health and fitness industry, I have watched numerous nutritional strategies come and go. What can we learn from the past? We know diets do not work, which is why there is always some new diet on the market and another one on the way. Let's take a quick journey back in time. Some of these strategies are scary, and some may even look a little familiar.

1820s: Lord Byron popularized the Vinegar and Water Diet, which entailed drinking water mixed with apple cider vinegar. Lord Byron would be happy to see apple cider vinegar making a powerful comeback.

1920s: The Lucky Strike cigarette brand launched the "Reach for a Lucky instead of a Sweet" campaign which tried to capitalize on nicotine's appetite-suppressing superpower. Did people really believe that smoking would be the answer to losing weight? I believe many did.

1950s: The Cabbage Soup Diet promised people could lose 10-15 pounds in a week by eating a limited diet including cabbage soup every day. People must have been in the bathroom a lot.

1960s: Weight Watchers made its debut with the Point System. It is a great way to keep people aware of the quantity of food they consume. Weight Watchers has been upgraded over the years, and today is a pretty solid program that provides a focused eating plan.

1970s: New diets included the Scarsdale Medical Diet, Slim Fast, and one of my favorites, the Cookie Diet. The cookies were made with a blend of amino acids (high protein) designed to curb the appetite. Hollywood ate it up.

1980s: The High-Carbohydrate/Low-Fat movement began. If a food was fat-free or low-fat, it was a go. McDonald's introduced the McLean Deluxe low-fat burger. Other products included Snackwell Cookies, Less Bread, Entenmanns low-fat coffee cake, muffins, bagels, and no-fat frozen yogurt. There even was a Seinfeld episode on the no-fat yogurt craze where Jerry's pants were getting tight. Obesity and type 2 diabetes began to explode. What were they thinking?

1990s: The High-Protein/Anti-Carbohydrate movement hit the United States. The Atkins and South Beach era took hold. High protein became the answer, and carbohydrates became the villain. Eat all the protein possible—eggs, dairy, bacon, hot dogs, beef, chicken, jerky, meat, meat, and more meat. Just stay away from the bun. If the food or beverage was high in protein and low in carbohydrates, it got a green light. On this diet, hair became thin and brittle. Skin felt like sandpaper, and breath smelled like nail polish. People experienced low mood, trouble sleeping, constipation, and acid reflux. But hey, look at me, I lost weight and look great!

2000s: The FDA banned diet drugs and supplements containing ephedra after it was linked to heart attacks. A nonprescription drug "Alli" hit the market. By sprinkling this powder on food, the body would not absorb much of the food, resulting in weight loss. Seriously gang, this was not that long ago.

2010s: The HCG Diet combined a fertility drug with a strict 500-800 calorie a day regimen and no exercise to lose one pound a day for 30-days. Imagine what truly goes on inside the body following this plan.

Ketogenic Diet

There are many diet trends currently on the market today. One in particular that I think needs better understanding is the Ketogenic Diet (Keto). Keto has been around for decades as a very specific treatment plan for epilepsy. Over the last few years, this diet has been gaining in popularity for its claims for quick weight loss, gains in energy and mental clarity, and decreased food cravings. The Ketogenic Diet severely reduces carbohydrate intake while increasing fat intake.

Let's dive into this a little deeper. Our body uses energy to simply stay alive. This is called our basal metabolic rate (BMR). As we move throughout our day or add exercise to the mix, the need for more energy increases. Most of our energy usually comes from the food we eat.

The bulk of our energy comes from the three macronutrients: carbohydrates, proteins, and fats. This is where the chemistry lesson begins, and we see how amazing the human body is designed. When we eat carbohydrates, they are broken down into glucose and used for immediate energy. If our energy needs are already fulfilled, carbohydrates may then be stored as glycogen in our muscles and liver. If our energy demands are met and glycogen reserves are already at capacity, carbohydrates may then be stored as fat. Glycogen capacity hovers at approximately 2,000 calories. This is a reserve that can be used immediately as the energy demand rises. This process is call glycolysis (a breakdown of glycogen into glucose).

The goal of the Ketogenic Diet is to severely restrict carbohydrate intake, deplete the body's glycogen stores, and force the body to draw on its own fat reserves for its primary fuel source. If there is not enough glucose available to meet energy demands, the body will adopt an alternative strategy in order to meet those demands. This process is called gluconeogenesis (a generation of glucose from non-carbohydrate food sources).

As the body begins to breakdown fat stores to provide glucose, ketone levels in the blood begin to rise. Ketones are a potentially toxic by-product of partially burned fatty acids that the body has used as an alternative fuel source when carbohydrates are not available. These acids slowly build up in the blood and are eliminated in the urine and through the breath. In small amounts, they serve to indicate the body is breaking down fat. However, high levels of ketones can poison the body, leading to a process called ketoacidosis. As the body begins to breakdown fat stores to provide glucose, ketone levels in the blood begin to rise. This is known as ketosis.

Health and Performance

Take a macronutrient (carbohydrates, proteins, or fats) out of the diet and macro problems will develop. The human body needs a balance of all of three of these macronutrients for optimal health and performance.

Ideally, the human brain needs approximately 100 grams (400 calories) of carbohydrates per day for fuel. When any of the three macronutrients becomes compromised, the brain neurotransmitters that regulate mood, serotonin, dopamine, GABA, and adrenaline, may get out of balance. Serotonin and GABA cool or relax the central nervous system. Dopamine and adrenaline on the other hand stimulate or rev up the central nervous system.

One of the Ketogenic Diet claims is that a diet high in fat and low in carbohydrates clears up brain fog and helps concentration. This may be true if people have been consuming a lot of processed, unhealthy sources of carbohydrates that cause lethargy and lack of focus. What is not being discussed is the quality and quantity of the carbohydrates currently being consumed before cutting them out.

Imagine what is taking place inside the brain when a person eats a diet deficient in high-quality carbohydrates. Serotonin and GABA become compromised leading to problems quieting the brain. The mind begins to race. Staying asleep becomes a major problem, and anxiety starts to climb. On the other side of the ledger, a diet primarily consisting of processed carbohydrates, with little protein or fat, causes dopamine and adrenaline to become compromised, leading to a lethargic mind and body.

Removing carbohydrates from our nutritional plan may cause other imbalances to occur. A diet low in carbohydrates like fruits, vegetables, ancient grains, and starchy carbohydrates will cause the body to be deficient in valuable vitamins and minerals. It is a shift in pH balancing, moving to the acid side of the pH scale. This leads to a depletion of precious buffering minerals such as calcium, magnesium, and potassium, as they try to bring pH back into balance. This high acid level also begins to wreak havoc on gut health, digestion, blood work, and the immune system, leading to allergies, asthma, acid reflux, gout, and high blood pressure. High acid levels may also elevate homocysteine and highly sensitive C-reactive protein, two blood tests that measure oxidation and inflammation, key risk factors for heart disease and cancer.

Expanding Human Capacity

Taking carbohydrates out of the diet not only compromises our health but limits our "capacity." My son Matt and I co-wrote the book *Capacity* a few years ago. Its underlying theme is that human capacity can be expanded by building greater health. As health improves so does capacity, providing more fuel in the tank when it is needed.

The human body at its greatest demand will move to the most efficient fuel source, and that, my friends, is carbohydrates. Fat is a great fuel source for walking in the woods or working at a computer. For greater performance and expanded capacity, carbohydrates are the high-octane fuel needed.

Getting Leaner

In today's world of nutrition, the word "carbohydrate" has become demonized. The word on the street is that if we want to get leaner, have greater mental clarity, and perform at our best, we need to cut the carbohydrates.

As was mentioned earlier in this section many people have been led to believe that when we cut out carbohydrates, we will lose weight. This may be true in the short term, but it is not sustainable. Many people believe that when we increase fat or protein intake and decrease carbohydrate intake, we teach the body to burn fat as the major fuel source. Many believe that consuming carbohydrates and the ability to burn fat do not go together.

The truth is we can burn fat while also consuming carbohydrates. My exercise physiology professor Dr. Kwok Ho told his students over and over that "fat burns in a carbohydrate flame." Not only do carbohydrates provide energy for working muscles, but they also assist in enabling fat metabolism.

Fat Burns in a Carbohydrate Flame

I have personally competed in many Natural Bodybuilding contests starting back in 1985. My most recent contest was in 2013 at the age of 56. For my first contest, I followed the traditional bodybuilding diet of bulking up and then cutting down. My eating plan consisted of a diet high in protein and moderate in fat. During the last six weeks leading up to the contest, I began to carb-deplete. I took out oatmeal, fruit, and starchy carbohydrates. I began to eat only vegetables, salads, healthy fats, meat, and fish. Three days prior to the contest I began to carb-load, adding carbohydrates back into my diet to fill the muscles with glycogen and water.

I may have looked good up on stage, but I was miserable. I was dehydrated, my skin was dry, sleep had become a problem, I developed acid reflux, and I was grouchy and tired most of the time. I never wanted to experience this misery again. I understood this type of eating was not healthy. There had to be a healthier way to get in great shape.

Remembering the words of Dr. Ho, I made it my goal for my next contest to get in great shape and also have vibrant health. So, I changed my approach. I ate in the center of the Food Target for three months leading up to the contest with a balance of high-quality carbohydrates, proteins, and fats. I brought oatmeal back for breakfast with fruit. Apples, bananas, raisins, and potatoes were all back as part of my plan. I fasted overnight for 12-14 hours and ate every 3-4 hours. The results were fantastic. I got in great shape with the vibrant health I was looking for.

Get to Your Goal

To achieve greater energy, a lean attractive body, and, most importantly, vibrant health, follow these simple principles.

- **Water:** Drink ½ your body weight in ounces of water each day.
- **Superfoods:** Add a few superfoods to your current nutritional plan. These include omega-3 fats, frozen wheatgrass, spirulina/chlorella, greens, cacao, coconut, colorful fruits and vegetables, sweet potatoes, ancient grains, nuts, and seeds.
- **Quality:** Slowly upgrade the quality of your food choices by using the Food Target as your guide.
- **Balance:** Eat a balance of high-quality carbohydrates, proteins, and fats.
- **Meal Patterning:** Pattern your meals by experimenting with fasting and frequency.
- **Fasting:** Fast for 12-14 hours each day (7 p.m. to 8 a.m.) to allow the body to clean itself.
- **Frequency:** Slowly increase the frequency of your meals. Try to eat 3-4 small meals every 3-4 hours.
- **Quantity:** Be aware of the quantity of the food you consume.
- **80/20 Rule:** Develop a plan that you can enjoy and live with.

Move Daily

One of the keys for sustainable weight loss is daily movement or exercise. It is not the calories burned during a workout, but the engine being built. Approximately 75-80 percent of our daily calories burned comes from our basal metabolic rate (BMR). BMR is the engine. The bigger the engine, the more calories the body burns to keep it running. This is why exercise, especially strength training, is so beneficial in building a higher metabolic engine. Strength training can also stimulate youthful, lean hormones. More will be said on this topic in Section 5: Movement: The Fountain of Youth.

Learn how to pivot and enjoy the journey. This is your plan. Make mistakes and try new foods. Most importantly, enjoy the process.

As my daughter Kristen likes to say, "Use common sense when it comes to new diets and food trends. If you would not consider feeding a food to five-year old child, it is probably not a healthy option for yourself. If you can eat as much bacon as you want but cannot eat a bowl of oatmeal or a piece of fruit, it is probably not a good thing either. Trust your gut. It is always right."

Make the Decision

When consulting with a man many months ago, I asked him what made him motivated to get healthier and in better shape now. He said, "I stepped on the scale and looked down and the scale read 250 pounds! I was totally shocked. I had no idea that I had slowly gained over 50 pounds. I said to myself enough is enough and made the decision at the moment that I was going to take control of my weight and my health!"

When discussing weight loss with almost anyone, it always comes back to one key point. When did you decide? Once people make the decision, no more second guessing, no more starting next week. Now is the time, and this is what I am going to do!

Are you READY?

Are you ABLE?

Are you WILLING?

Dieting and Weight Loss Essentials

Big Picture

- Obesity levels around the world continue to rise.
- 100 million people in the United States are currently on some type of diet.
- The weight loss industry is a $60-70 billion a year business with a 95 percent failure rate.
- The human body needs a balance of healthy carbohydrates, proteins, and fats for optimal health and performance in all aspects of life.
- If you would not consider feeding a food to five-year old child, it is probably not a healthy option for yourself.

Ask Yourself

- How much do you currently weigh?
- How much would you like to weigh?
- When was the last time you were on a diet? What worked? What did not? What new habit did you develop? What did you learn?
- Before adopting a diet, determine if it is in line with the three principles: Cellular Health, pH Balance and Close to the Source.
- Does your current nutritional plan include a balance of carbohydrates, proteins, and fats?
- How much water do you drink each day?
- Do you fast 12-14 hours overnight?
- How often do you move your body?
- How can you enjoy the process of eating better?

Small Steps

- Choose two or three steps to take to get closer to your desired bodyweight.
- Do a one-day food log to create awareness of what you are eating.
- Have the courage to monitor your bodyweight with a scale, a pair of pants, a belt, or the mirror.
- Build one habit at a time.
- Learn how to pivot and enjoy the journey.

23 Putting Your EAT Plan in Place

Make Mistakes

Making mistakes is critical to success in any endeavor. If oatmeal or a smoothie for breakfast is not exactly hitting the mark on taste, experiment and try new concoctions until it does. Make mistakes by continually upgrading and adapting. This is what makes your EAT plan fun and repeatable. The plan is not a prescription, it is customizable. Own it. It is YOUR plan!

That Smoothie Tastes Like Mud

Years ago, I was training the CEO of a large company. He was concerned about his lack of energy especially later in the day. He said he usually ate breakfast around 9 a.m. and then went the entire day without eating. On most days. His last meal hovered around 8 p.m. I explained that he needed to eat more frequently for greater energy. He felt he had little time to add in meals due to his tight meeting schedule.

I suggested he make a smoothie each morning to take to work. This would allow him to get some healthy nutrients in his body and greatly improve his energy to sustain him through his hectic schedule. He loved this idea.

Here is what I asked him to put in his smoothie: 2 cups of water, 2 tablespoons hempseeds, 2 tablespoons flaxseeds, 1 tablespoon almond butter, 1 banana, and 2 cups of frozen berries. He was pumped to start his new plan.

The following week at our next training session I asked how the smoothie plan was going. He said his smoothie was the nastiest tasting thing he had ever had. It was so thick he could hardly drink it. I asked him to tell me exactly how he made the smoothie. He reported that he did exactly what he was told to do. To 2 cups of water, he added 2 cups of hempseeds. . . Stop right there! Two cups of hempseeds? No wonder it tasted like mud. I said it was mud. We had a big laugh.

He then played around with the recipe, liked the new taste, and loved his improved energy throughout his day.

Create a Healthy Food Environment

Family Dynamics

Taking this journey with a significant other or family members can be a challenge. Getting everyone's buy-in is not always easy. I caution people not to go home and overwhelm the family. It is always best to go slow and let them watch and learn. Additionally, feeding kids or grandkids can be very challenging. Here are a few tips.

Start with being the role model. I remember when my daughter Kristen was growing up, she told all her friends and family members that her dad was a freak. Today, Kristen is our registered dietician as well as an author and speaker for On Target Living. Lead by example and show guidance. Slowly over time let them make those decisions by themselves. You can help and guide them, but you must lead by example. They are watching you.

Get your kids involved. My wife Paula did a terrific job getting our kids involved in meal planning and cooking at a very young age. Today our daughter Kristen and son Matt are both terrific cooks.

Make meals healthier for the family. Start with what the kids eat most often. If they like macaroni and cheese, pop tarts, or pizza, make better mac and cheese, healthier pop tarts, and better pizza with better ingredients. Then build the foundation of superfoods. One very easy superfood to start with is some type of omega-3 fat, such as cod liver oil, flaxseeds, or chia seeds. Omega 3-fats are the foundation of a healthy diet. Have the entire family get on board and start building some of these superfoods into their diets.

Last but not least, don't be the food police. Work with them and guide them. Experiment with new foods and recipes. Remember, I was the guy who grew up on all the garbage and survived to tell about it. Be patient and let your family slowly build their own nutritional habits.

Food Shopping

Creating a healthier food environment begins in the grocery store. Creating a healthy environment at home, at work, or wherever life takes us is critical for supporting a healthy lifestyle. Whether I am on the road, in the office, or at home, I always try to have healthy food and beverage options available to support my goal of feeling my best and being my best.

Learning how to maneuver in the grocery store, health food store, or farmers market is a learned skill that will help in the quest for being our best. I spent over eight years working for Butternut Bread and Frito-Lay. I have watched people in the grocery stores look at labels trying to figure out the healthiest foods available and how to put a healthy meal together on a budget.

Knowing how to maneuver in the grocery store is not easy. A few times each year, we hold shopping trips at our local health food store, **Foods for Living**. It is a beautiful store, pleasing to the senses. It offers a variety of fresh produce, meats, bulk items, supplements, and non-perishables. They also have a terrific staff who are extremely passionate and knowledgeable about healthy eating. At the beginning of each trip, we ask if there are any first-time shoppers. Many are completely overwhelmed. When we tell the group that nobody will have to eat alfalfa or sea vegetables, everyone laughs. They begin to relax and the learning begins.

We conduct the tour by breaking down the store aisle by aisle to show what to look for, how to read labels, how to make easy upgrades, and then determine if some of these foods or beverages can fit into their lifestyles. We explain how they can improve their ketchup, salad dressings, soup, peanut butter, crackers, mineral water, nuts, seeds, produce, meats, milk, frozen food, shampoo, deodorant, lotions, toothpaste, laundry soap, and even food and treats for their pets. We also want them to know why they are making these upgrades.

It is one of my favorite events, and many people look forward to it.

The Taste Factor

It is important to take small steps when developing a nutritional plan. Over time, these small steps become a permanent routine. People may not like the initial switch from a processed, highly sweetened peanut butter to a natural or organic peanut butter or almond butter, but within a week or so, they get used to it. Then they wonder how they ever ate anything else.

People at our events often worry about how things will taste. Whenever I talk about cod liver oil and its wonderful health benefits, many people get a disgusted look on their face. For years we have been trying to get some of our family members to start taking cod liver oil. At a Christmas gathering many years ago, I poured everyone a shot of cod liver oil. Don't you wish you could spend Christmas at our house? Most thought it tasted okay and not as bad as they anticipated. Many decided this was something they could do.

Do you choose foods that taste good or foods that are good for you? Can foods that are good for us taste good too? Absolutely! We must be open and willing to try new tastes and be patient.

Many people have a difficult time understanding how wheatgrass or the lemon cod liver oil can be part of their daily routine. They wonder if my taste buds were out to lunch the first time I tried them. My intention was not that these products were going to taste good. My intention was to achieve the wonderful health benefits they bring. Improving the quality of the foods and beverages we consume makes a tremendous difference in how we look and feel. It will improve overall health and performance in all aspects of life. When you fill your shopping cart wisely, you are well on your way to a healthier you.

Start by ridding the pantry and refrigerator of unhealthy food and beverages. Start fresh. Go shopping with a plan and ask questions. Making upgrades can be easy. Start slowly and experiment with foods and beverages.

Eating on the Run

How can we eat healthy when on the run? In our fast-paced lives, it can be difficult to eat healthy, especially when we get busy or while traveling. It is easy to get out of our normal routines, and this is when many people get in trouble.

I am on a plane many weeks each year. I truly love what I do, but flying can beat me up coping with busy airports, delays, over-booked flights, cramped seating, recycled air, processed nuts, crackers, chips, cookies, soda pop, juice, alcohol, and water. It is like going into the jungle. I must plan ahead and be prepared so that I can feel my best when I arrive at my final destination.

Here is a sample of my travel items, whether by plane or by car. I begin by packing water for my car trip or purchasing water immediately at the airport. I prepare enough individual bags of my personal trail mix consisting of rolled oats, raisins, dried white figs, macadamia nuts, pecans, organic shredded coconut, and cacao nibs to last for the duration of my trip. I love the taste of this trail mix. It travels well, and it is very satisfying to me. Sometimes it is the only meal I have time for during a day of travel. I also like to travel with an apple, banana or orange, a few carrots, and celery. Carrots and celery are great foods for edema when sitting too long. I also travel with spirulina/chlorella. It keeps my gut healthy, helps my immune system to stay strong, helps me to feel my best, and it is easy to travel with.

Plan ahead, come prepared, and maybe you can share a healthy snack with a new friend.

Dining Out

Dining out is one of the most popular leisure activities around the world.

Almost everything we do is centered around food: football tailgating, soccer matches, graduations, weddings, retirements, holidays, entertainment, business meetings, and getting together with family and friends. You name it; we do it with food.

From a health standpoint, eating out can be a bit more challenging than eating at home. Is it possible to eat out and maintain healthy habits? Most restaurants have healthy choices. The choices we make can have a major impact on the waistline, our health, and feeling our best. Here are a few tips for dining out.

Have a plan. Just like grocery shopping, dining out begins with a plan. What do you want to eat? What type of restaurant? What are your options at this restaurant? How much time do you have? Go with a plan.

When I am dining out with people for the first time, they often want to know what I plan to order, then often order the same thing. Granted, I do not get many invitations to dinner, and I try not to be the food or exercise police, but I guess this comes with the territory.

Many times, after we have ordered, I ask the group if they would like to learn more about the menu and how to make healthy choices. We go over the menu and discuss options and how to make upgrades. It generally turns into a fun exchange. Most restaurants allow for substitutions. For example, many times I order a plain baked or sweet potato with extra virgin olive oil on the side, a clear soup versus a thick cream soup, a healthier salad dressing option, or just oil and vinegar, or a fresh bowl of berries for dessert instead of the hot fudge sundae with a cookie. It is the little stuff that makes a big difference over time.

Making better choices when dining out gets down to one thing—focus. You may want to debate me on this statement, but the next time you eat out, take a second and think about what you are focused on. I believe that what we focus on is what we get. Are you focused merely on taste or are there other factors that you want along with that taste? Don't get me wrong, taste is important. I want my food to taste good too. Are you also focusing on other factors that influence your decision-making process, such as your health, your energy, your waistline, and your performance? Every time you eat out, you will be faced with these decisions. Focus on what you want. If you know what you want, your decisions will be much easier.

Choices! Diet soda or a glass of mineral water with a slice of lemon? The bread before lunch or dinner? The salad with bacon, croutons and ranch dressing or a salad with nuts, added vegetables, extra virgin olive oil and balsamic vinegar for the dressing? The pasta with Alfredo sauce or the Alaskan salmon with asparagus? The chocolate cake or a cup of raspberries for dessert?

The instant gratification from food and beverages is extremely powerful and making healthier choices can be challenging at times. As I have said throughout this entire book, change can be difficult, but we can all change. Moving our attention away from just taste to other areas such as health, energy, and controlling body weight takes a little practice.

Food is meant to be enjoyed and shared. Eating out can be healthy and pleasurable experience all rolled into one.

Cooking at Home

When I was a kid, Friday night meant hamburgers on the grill, and Sunday meant pot roast. All real food. Our mom used to make an amazing pot roast with carrots, potatoes, and gravy. It was home cooking. When we cook at home, not only can we control our health, but we also control our family's health. The benefits of cooking and eating at home are very powerful, not just for the health of the human body, but the health of our spirit. Cooking and eating at home have so many incredible benefits: time with family, face time, and creating traditions.

I think we all agree we need to start having more home-cooked meals. My daughter Kristen says it best. "If more people cooked at home, they would be healthier and, in most cases, happier." Let's start to teach cooking in a fun, easy, and healthy way.

Sample Plan

Here is a sample plan to help guide you. I have slowly evolved over the years from my Captain Crunch cereal for breakfast, bologna sandwiches on white bread with Beefaroni for lunch, and Jon's Country Burger, Demarco's Pizza or Kewpee for dinner.

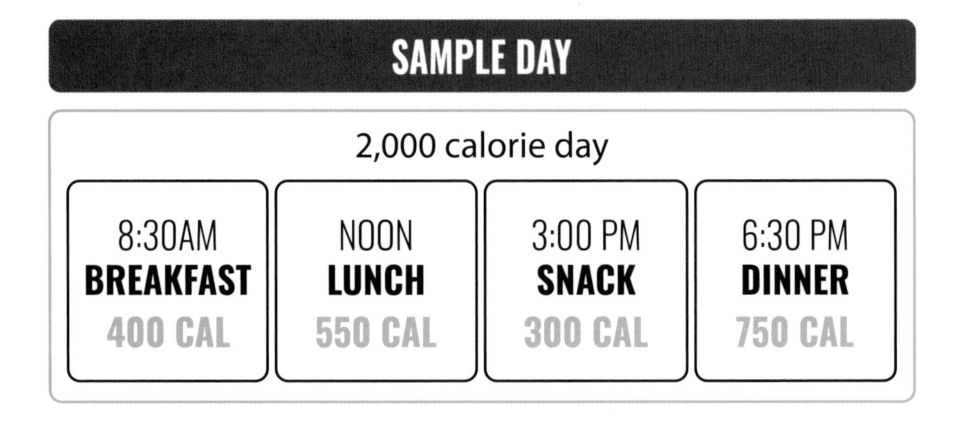

Start experimenting and make mistakes in the kitchen. Getting healthier truly starts with cooking more meals at home!

Putting Your EAT Plan in Place Essentials

Big Picture

- What you eat and drink can change your life.
- Food is medicine, and food is information. Food is love, and food is taste. Food is energy, and food is health. So much of life is centered around food.
- You must make mistakes. Learning how to pivot is essential for success.
- Don't be the food police. Lead by example.
- Create a healthy food environment at home, at work, or traveling.
- If you have to eat on the go, plan ahead and bring water and simple healthy snacks. Use a soft cooler for travel.
- When dining out, go with a plan.
- Eat at home. Getting healthier begins in the kitchen.

Ask Yourself

- When was the last time you tried a new food or new recipe?
- How many of your groceries come from the source?
- Do you know how to read a food label? Products with fewer ingredients are best.
- When traveling, do you pack food, snacks, or beverages?
- Do you have a soft cooler for the car or for work to carry your food and beverages?
- How many meals each week do you eat at home? Eat out?
- Do you have a healthy environment to support your nutritional plan at home, at work, or when traveling?

Small Steps

- Start slowly and build YOUR plan.
- Hydration: Drink one half of your body weight in ounces per day.
- Superfoods: Consume 1-2 superfoods each day.
- Quality: Upgrade the quality of your carbohydrates, proteins, and fats.
- Meal Patterning: Fast 12-14 hours overnight and eat every 3-4 hours.
- Quantity: Calories do count, so be aware of overeating.
- 80/20 Rule: Develop a plan that you can sustain and enjoy.

SECTION

5

MOVEMENT—THE FOUNTAIN OF YOUTH

24 Movement Mindset

In Section 4, we discussed the second pillar of health, **EAT**, and the power of food. Our third foundational pillar is **MOVE**. For centuries, people have been searching for the Fountain of Youth, and the answer has always been right in front of us. The answer is MOVE! When given restorative rest, quality nutrition, and daily movement or exercise, the human body has an amazing ability to heal and self-correct. If we could put movement in a bottle, it would be the most prescribed medication in the world. It can be said that movement is the Fountain of Youth.

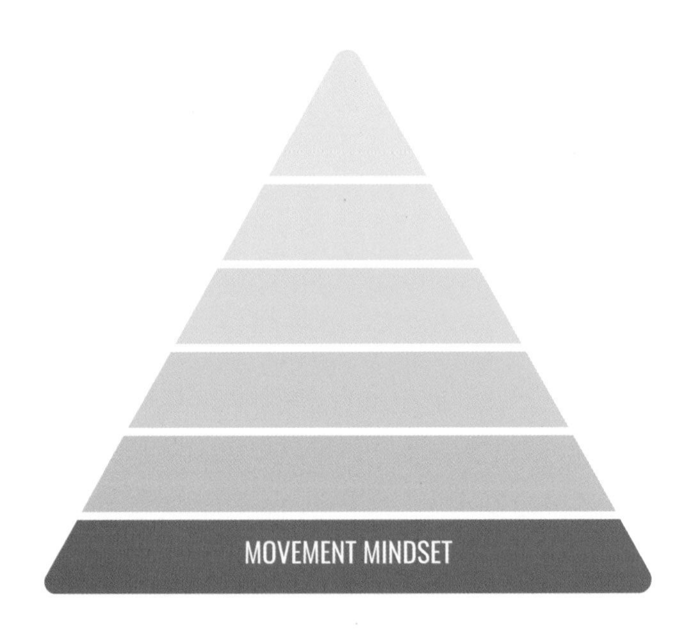

Now it is time to talk about moving our body. As a child I always loved moving my body - running, jumping, climbing trees, working out, and playing sports. As my Grandma Johnson used to say, "If there is a ball involved, that boy is interested in playing." As long as I can remember, I was interested in moving my body. Exercising was fun to me, and I pursued that passion with a graduate degree in exercise physiology from Michigan State University. I have spent much of my life helping people learn how to exercise and move.

I have worked with many clients with varying levels of health and fitness over the past 30-plus years, ranging from professional athletes to people who have had severe health problems. I have worked with people with chronic lung and heart problems, type 2 diabetes, severe obesity, dementia, and cancer, along with physical injuries to the neck, shoulders, hips, knees, and ankles. I truly enjoy watching people grow and get better. Movement and exercise are a big part of what we do at On Target Living. It is also a passion and love of mine.

Developing a **movement mindset** is a critical first step for creating a lifetime of movement. In the following chapters I will provide what I believe are some of the best ways to move the body and get the results we desire.

Before we jump into the basics of movement or exercise, we have to get the mind in a place for optimal success. To successfully adopt a movement mindset, we need to plan it into our life. Daily movement creates compound interest for the mind and body. Moving our body every day provides benefits in reserve. Just a little bit of movement everyday can change our life in so many positive ways.

The human body is designed to move or exercise on a daily basis. I will use exercise and movement in the same context throughout the rest of this book. When I speak of exercise, many people immediately come up with excuses. They do not have enough time to exercise, do not enjoy exercising, do not like to sweat, or find it painful. Basically, the dog ate their homework! There are many reasons why people do not invest in moving their body.

Let's begin with a conversation about the cost of moving or not moving the body. The costs may include time, effort, energy, discomfort, and even money. Now imagine the costs of not moving the body: stress, poor health, and a decrease in mobility, flexibility, and strength. There are many costs associated with not moving our body.

Daily movement plays an important role in maintaining a healthy body weight, but it is the combination of lifestyle factors that contributes to a healthy weight and better health. Having the right information is necessary for success in all areas of life. This is one reason that my recommendation to many people is to hire a health and fitness coach to guide and educate them, and to develop a movement plan that works for them.

What Holds People Back?

Here is a crazy statistic. Eighty-two percent of the American population does not move or exercise on a regular basis. Why are we not moving more if it is so good for us?

With more than 30 years of health and fitness coaching, speaking all over the world, and talking with thousands of people at our events as well as with friends, family, clients, physicians, and colleagues, I believe there are five factors that can influence people to move their body more.

Values and Beliefs

We all have different values and beliefs in all aspects of our lives. I am not here to make judgments about your values and beliefs. My goal is to get you to think about them. Values are different from beliefs. We may value success but believe that to be successful we have to make over a million dollars a year. We may value our health but believe that we must eat perfectly and spend hours in the gym to become healthy.

For many people, movement is low on the priority list and may not even be on the radar screen. I believe most people recognize that movement or exercise is a good thing, but that is where it ends. Many feel that movement is not for them. They may feel intimidated, feel uncomfortable with their body, or fear they may fail.

If we asked our friends and family members if their health was of great importance to them, I am sure they would say yes, that they value their health. Most of us know that when we do not have our health, we do not have much. How valuable is your health to you? If you believe your health is important, what are you willing to do to maintain or improve it? Moving from doing NOTHING to doing SOMETHING is the key. We all have to put some effort into maintaining our health. Make movement a priority. Value your health, and believe you are worth the investment..

Focus on the Now

We have become a world that wants everything now. When I consult with people about movement, it is clear they want to look lean, fit, and healthy. But movement is so much more than just looking great. The real magic occurs when the mind and body connect.

Moving our body on a daily basis is an investment in our future. Simultaneously, it is also an investment in the now. So many amazing benefits from movement can be gained, and the biggest one is in the mind. The benefit of positive emotions that come with movement is priceless. Every time I do not feel like moving my body, I remind myself that in just a few short minutes I will have more energy, greater focus, and in most cases a positive change in mood.

Too many people focus on moving their body as a way to lose weight, improve their blood pressure, or increase their bone density. These are all great goals. However, focusing only on the future is not going to get it done for most people. Finding objective measurements around movement can be extremely powerful. We must pay attention to how our mind and body feel during the movement or activity. We must enjoy the process. This mindset is critical for long-term success.

How do you feel when you move throughout your day?

____

____

What is your energy like after moving your body?

____

____

Do you have fewer aches and pains after moving your body? Yes or No

Do you sleep better after moving your body? Yes or No

Does your mood improve after moving your body? Yes or No

Knowledge

Just as on the nutritional side of the health equation, most people lack the knowledge about what exercises to do, how to start, how much exercise is enough, and how to keep their exercise or movement plans going. There is an unending supply of podcasts, blogs, articles, books, magazines, videos, infomercials, and apps dedicated to movement. As with nutrition, there is so much information that people can be overwhelmed.

Many people may be confused about whether to do high- or low-intensity cardiovascular exercise to lose weight or which strength training exercises to shape or sculpt a certain body part. Should they do yoga, Pilates, CrossFit, swim, or strength train? Should they invest in a Peloton bike or the Mirror?

In addition to these concerns, many people have specific questions about movements that relate to their personal needs, such as bad knees, hips, shoulders, or back pain. Others have health issues such as type 2 diabetes, high blood pressure, neck pain, obesity, or migraine headaches. They do not know which exercises to avoid, and which would be beneficial.

Time

During a recent television interview with a health and fitness expert on the subject of weight loss, the question came up about exercise and how much exercise or movement is necessary to lose weight. The expert recommended 60-75 minutes of steady state cardiovascular exercise per day to lose weight.

I almost fell over in disbelief. I thought to myself, is this person out of their mind? Most people do not move their bodies on a daily basis and now some expert is telling millions of viewers to exercise 60-75 minutes a day. I think many viewers were saying to themselves that they might as well sit back on the couch and eat some chips or cookies. There is no way they were going to do cardiovascular exercise for 60-75 minutes a day. Pass the remote.

Time is a big issue for almost everyone and I want to make this point extremely clear. We can never out-exercise a poor diet. Most people do not need to spend large amounts of time to get in better shape and stay healthy. When training for a triathlon or the Olympics, then yes, we need to invest large amounts of time to reach our goals.

Here is the big mindset shift when it comes to movement or exercise. We need to move our body every single day for at least 5-10 minutes. If you are currently working out 3-4 times a week for 45-60 minutes, great, keep it up. But be sure to move on the other days. We all know the hardest part of exercise is just getting started—the first 2-3 minutes.

At the beginning of each new year, many people desperately try to get in better shape. This is going to be the year! One of the biggest mistakes people make is believing that more time spent exercising will produce greater results. Spending more time on a treadmill or in the gym does not necessarily add up to greater results. What race are we trying to run? Is it the 100-meter sprint or the marathon? What kind of pace can we sustain for a lifetime? This is a big reason why most people slowly abandon their movement plan. It may be too difficult to sustain over time.

It is important to get into the mindset of moving the body every single day. By moving our body every day, the benefits continue to pile up. Just a little bit of movement everyday can change life in so many positive ways.

One last point about time. If there is very little space in our life, chances are we will not have the time to move or exercise. Movement or exercise requires SPACE in our day. No Space = No Exercise!

Do you have space in your life to move your body daily Yes or No

Less Can Be More

Years ago, I was discussing this concept with a new coaching client. He was frustrated with his weight, his health, and his current exercise program of 75-90 minutes, 2-3 times per week. His program included 30 minutes of cardio, 40 minutes of strength training, and some light stretching. By the time he arrived at the gym, exercised, showered, and left, he was spending over two hours on his exercise commitment.

I thought his exercise frequency might be the problem. So, I asked a better question. How often did he exercise? His answer was 2-3 times per week. Then I asked him how many times he exercised in the last year. Was it 100, 150, 200 times? When he had to analyze the frequency of his exercise, he realized he had actually exercised less than 30 times last year. His life was so busy with his job, his family, and other commitments that he felt like he just did not have the time to devote to his movement routine.

I asked him what kind of results he would expect if he moved his body over 300+ times a year. Remember, he had been exercising less than once per week. Now I was asking him to move his body on a daily basis. I told him the two major changes he needed to make were to decrease time and increase frequency. His new program consisted of a 5-minute morning warm up and stretch routine before he showered. He also committed to walking 10 minutes every day, along with doing six strength training exercises twice a week. The frequency of moving his body increased, but the total time now invested was 2-3 hours per week.

Similar to eating more frequent small meals, he was moving more frequently in smaller pieces of time. An additional bonus was he could do most of his movements at home saving even more time. Six months later, he had lost 25 pounds and said he had never felt better. His new movement program created tons of momentum. He became more in tune with his breathing, his sleep, his eating, and his mood. He said he never would have believed a little bit of daily movement would really make this much difference in his life. He now believes.

Enjoyment

In addition to a daily movement mindset, find movement activities that are enjoyable. Consider activities like dancing, swimming, yoga, walking in the woods, strength training in the gym or at home, snow or water skiing, tennis or pickleball. One of the keys for sustainable movement is finding activities we enjoy. Imagine the possibilities when exercise or movement is viewed a little differently. Like the slogan, "Just Do it," view movement as something to do on a daily basis.

Moving could be as simple as a few stretch breaks during the day, yard work, going for a walk over lunch, playing outside with the kids or grandkids, working out at a fitness club, or maybe using a personal coach. The key for a lifetime of mind and body health is a lifetime of daily movement.

Daily movement can be fun and enjoyable, and there are endless ways to move the human body. Here are a few to choose from.

- Baseball or Softball
- Basketball
- Biking
- Dancing
- Football
- Golf
- Gymnastics
- Hiking or Climbing
- Ice Skating
- Jump Rope
- Lacrosse
- Mini Trampoline
- Paddle or Racquet sports
- Roller Blading or Roller Skating
- Skateboarding
- Snow, Cross Country, or Water Skiing
- Soccer
- Strength Training
- Surfing
- Swimming
- Volleyball
- Walking, Jogging, or Running
- Yoga, Pilates, or Tai Chi

What new activity or activities would you like to try?

___

___

FUN—The Great Motivator!

Years ago, I began training Joan and Robert. They had been married for over 40 years and were so cute together. Joan loved coming to the club. She enjoyed lifting weights, Pilates, swimming, and took a few stretch classes. As for Robert, he was not a physical guy, and did not enjoy working out. Slowly this became a rub between the two of them. One day I asked to meet with Robert privately. I began our conversation asking Robert about his thoughts and feelings about working out at the club. Robert said he did not enjoy coming to the club to exercise. I told Robert not everyone enjoys lifting weights, swimming, or many other forms of exercise. The key was finding movements and activities he enjoyed. Now was the time to find something for HIM.

I asked Robert if there was any activity or sport that he would like to try. Out of the blue he said basketball. He would like to learn how to play basketball. Robert was almost 73 years old and said that he never learned how to play basketball, but it looked fun.

The next day we were in the gym learning how to dribble, pass, and do lay-ups, free throws, and even a few 3-pointers. Robert was smiling from ear to ear and was hooked. We even put together a few specific exercises and drills to help him with his new love for basketball. Joan wondered what I had done with her husband. Now all he wanted to do was come to the club to play basketball!

Motion Creates Positive Emotion

As most people are aware, movement has many wonderful benefits including improved bone health, mobility, flexibility, balance, strength, heart health, blood pressure, brain function, digestion and elimination, hormonal balance, increased energy, and better sleep as well as decreased risks of cancer and type 2 diabetes.

But the greatest benefit of moving the body is what it can do for the mind. Daily movement **washes the mind!** How many times have you moved your body and suddenly felt a sense of rejuvenation? Your mind becomes clearer, and your body feels loose and relaxed. You feel energized and alive. Have you ever had a challenging day with too many things on your mind? Then you move your body and the stress that you may have been dealing with magically disappears. No longer do some of the little things bother you as much. Your energy is up, and you feel great. Do not get me wrong. I like the look of a fit trim physique, but it is the experience and feeling I get when moving that keeps me coming back. I cannot say this enough. To improve mental health, begin with moving the body.

You Cannot Out-Exercise a Poor Diet

Before I jump into the specific exercise or movement portion in upcoming chapters, I must discuss weight loss and the mindset associated with successful weight loss. Many people have a specific goal of losing weight and believe that they will lose weight if they exercise more. The truth is, it is just not that simple. We will burn more calories and maybe lose a few pounds by exercising more, but many people who exercise regularly are still overweight due to their poor nutritional patterns. Many folks also believe that long-duration, low-intensity, steady state cardiovascular exercise is the best method to lose weight.

Cardiovascular exercise is an important component of a balanced exercise plan, but long-duration, low-intensity cardio is not the most efficient method for losing weight. A more successful approach to exercise takes into account the hormonal effects that occur with daily movement.

Exercise Paired with Nutrition Gets the Job Done

I have competed in Natural Physique Competitions for many years. My daily movement routine does not change a great deal prior to the contest. It just becomes more focused. Nutritionally, however, everything tightens up. I eat more frequently, have smaller portion sizes, fast every night for 12-14 hours, take no liberties, and eat foods only in the green center of the Food Target for 12-14 weeks.

I move from the 80/20 rule to the 99/1 rule. This 99/1 eating regimen is very strict and difficult to sustain long term, but I can do it for 12-14 weeks. I enjoy the challenge and am extremely focused.

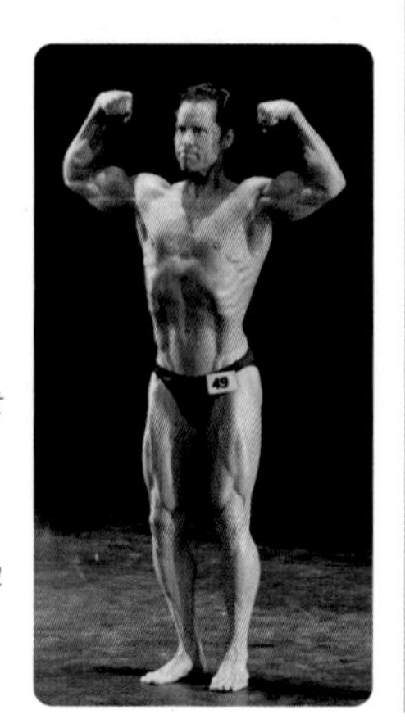

Proper nutrition accounts for 80-85 percent of successful weight loss. To get to our desired weight, we must begin with nutritional changes. Interestingly, while 80-85 percent of initial weight loss begins with nutrition, research shows that maintaining weight loss has to do with a combination of lifestyle factors, namely the big three - restful sleep, proper nutrition, and most importantly daily movement—**REST**, **EAT**, and **MOVE**.

Posture—Posture—Posture

When I was young, my grandmother always told me to stand up straight and tall. She was so right to stress the benefits of good posture. As we age, we are in constant battle with gravity which is trying to pull us out of our ideal posture alignment. Daily stresses of life, sitting, texting, standing, bending, walking, playing, and exercising challenge our posture and body alignment. We all make some type of compromise when it comes to our posture. The challenge is to be aware of the times our posture becomes compromised so that we can make adjustments to reinforce good posture over time.

What is ideal posture alignment and why is it so important? Ideal posture alignment happens when the body is perfectly aligned or in neutral position, starting with the feet and ankles, moving up through the knees, hips, pelvis, arms, shoulders, neck, and head. The five key checkpoints for posture alignment are the ear, shoulder, hip, knee, and ankle.

POSTURE

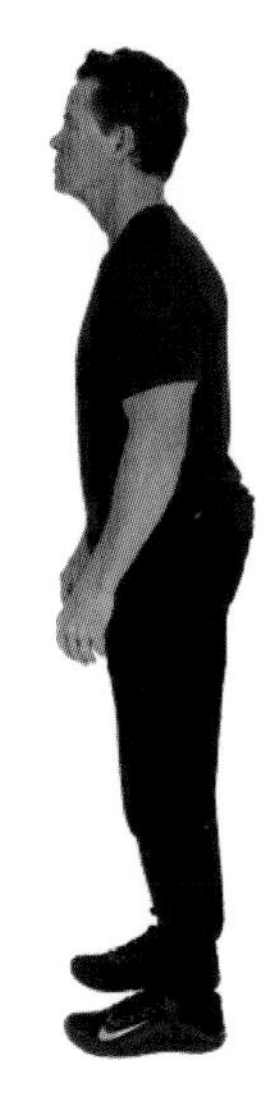

Poor Posture

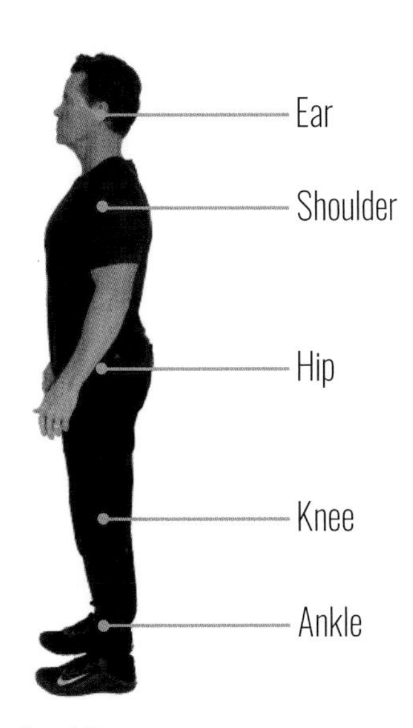

Good Posture

We all get into repetitive movement patterns, which, over time, result in certain muscles becoming shorter and stronger while opposing muscles become longer and weaker. This creates muscle imbalances that can lead to poor posture, injuries, pain, and decreased mobility. Proper movements can improve muscle imbalances and lead to better posture and body alignment.

Having good posture is key to feeling and being our best. Posture and body alignment is the foundation to any exercise plan. I will stress this more in the next few chapters. We must pay attention to our form and technique before trying to make a movement more difficult. Starting with the foundation of posture and body alignment will prevent bad habits that will be harder to fix later. Don't worry. Poor posture can be improved with some simple posture exercises.

Here are some simple posture assessment exercises to help you recognize how your posture stacks up. Practicing these simple exercises will create greater awareness and improve your posture.

Your movement plan begins with good posture.

POSTURE ASSESSMENTS

Standing Posture against the Wall

- Stand against a wall facing away from the wall.
- Put your heels and feet together touching your heels to the wall.
- Touch your rear end and shoulders to the wall.
- Try to touch the back of your head against the wall without tilting you head back.
- Raise your straight arms overhead without bending the elbows and keeping your head against the wall.

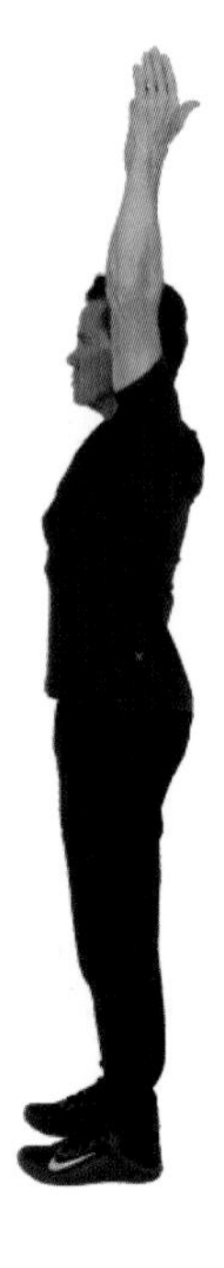

Standing Posture against a Wall

POSTURE ASSESSMENTS

Overhead Squat

- Hold a bar or broomstick over your head with straight arms.
- Face the wall, standing 2-5 inches away.
- Stand with your feet shoulder width apart, toes slightly turned out.
- Keep your body weight in the center of your feet.
- Squat as low as you can while maintaining straight arms overhead.

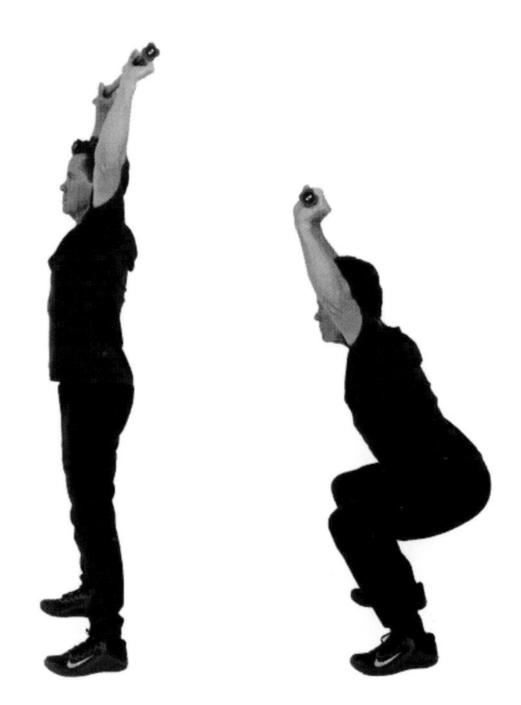

Overhead Squat

POSTURE ASSESSMENTS

Prone Posture

- Lay face down on the floor extending your arms and legs.
- Clasp hands together and reach out as far as you can.

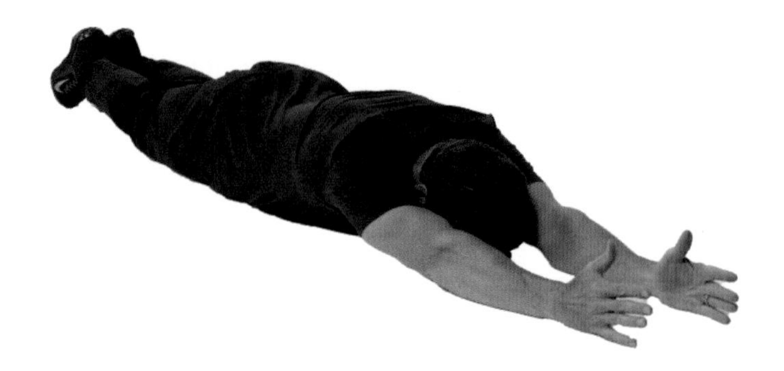

Supine Posture

- Lay flat on your back with hands and feet together.
- Stretch out as far as you can.

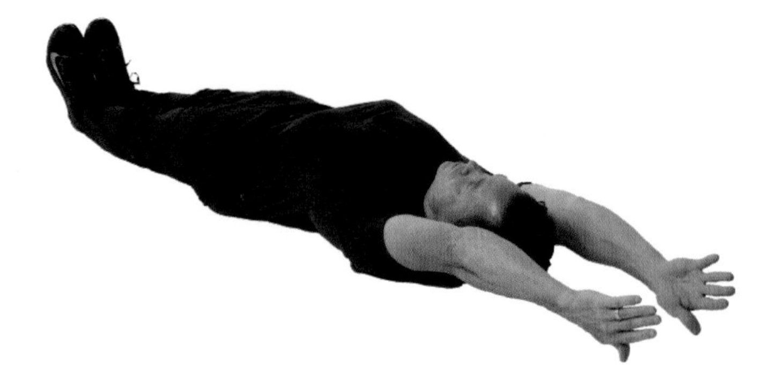

Mr. Posture

Many years ago, a client walked into my office complaining of back and neck pain. For years, he had been working in a hunched-over position. Over time gravity had taken its toll. As part of my evaluation process, I had him stand against the wall with his heels, glutes, and shoulders touching the wall. When asked to put his head against the wall, we were both surprised when he couldn't get it closer than 12 inches away from the wall. No wonder he was having major shoulder and back discomfort. His posture alignment needed help, so we began working on it, starting on his back laying down, and progressing to sitting, and standing posture exercises. We also worked on his nutrition plan and incorporated the use of a foam roller daily and getting massages 2-3 times per month. Over the course of four months, his posture drastically improved, he lost 25 pounds, and he started playing tennis again for the first time in 20 years.

How Much Movement Is Enough?

How much movement is necessary to "move the needle" for any given person at any given point in time? It is a lot less than most people think. When people find their "sweet spot" between what is too easy and what is too hard, movement becomes enjoyable.

On a 1-10 scale (10 being the highest) how important is exercise or movement in your life? __________

Are you currently moving your body on a daily basis? Yes or No

If you are not moving your body on a daily basis, what may be holding you back? ____

Is there enough space in your life to move your body on a daily basis? Yes or No

What do you want to accomplish? ______________________________

What are your goals?

____

____

How would you rate your current fitness level on a 1 to 10 scale? ______

What would you like your current fitness level to be? ______________

What type of investment is it going to take to achieve your health and fitness goals?

____

How can you incorporate more movement in your life?

____

____

I do not want to suggest that there is only one specific way to move the body or that the movements I will explain here are the only means of achieving results. My recommendations are meant to be a starting point for someone new to exercise or movement, or a way to get back to some of the basics for the lapsed or experienced exerciser. With increased knowledge comes a better ability to change or adapt a movement routine. The goal is to find movement activities that are enjoyable. As previously mentioned, this is critical for success both emotionally and physically. Develop a routine and daily movement rituals. Then over time experiment with new forms of movement.

My daily rituals include a series of dynamic warm-up and foundational movements every day. They help improve my strength, balance, mobility, and posture, and they take only 5-8 minutes to complete. I also try to walk daily. On top of these rituals, I like to do 15-20 minutes of cardio exercise and a split strength training routine that takes around 30-40 minutes, followed by 3-10 minutes of stretching. I also like to play ping pong, paddleball, pickleball, tennis, and golf, and to swim, hike, bike, and snow ski. Some days I need to get away from my daily routine and just play. Mixing it up keeps my daily habits fresh.

Start slowly. Choose ways to move your body daily in ways that are smart, fun and enjoyable.

MOVE Target

Use our MOVE Target as a fun guide to help you slowly upgrade and build movement habits into your life!

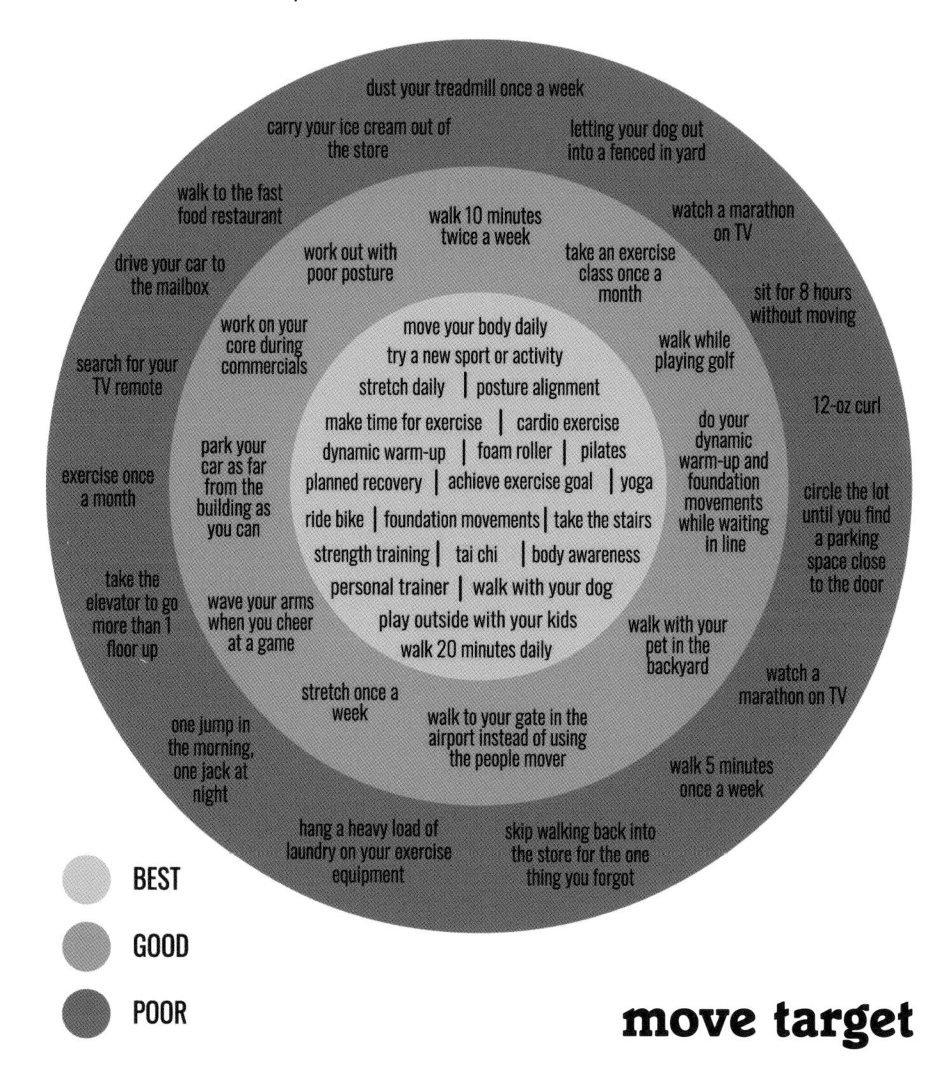

Movement Mindset Essentials

Big Picture

- Movement is the Fountain of Youth!
- If movement came in pill, it would be the most prescribed medication in the world.
- Developing a Movement Mindset is critical to achieving daily movement.
- In the United States, 82 percent of the population does not move their bodies on a daily basis.
- Motion creates positive emotion.
- You cannot out-exercise a poor diet.

Ask Yourself

- How important is your health to you?
- Are you satisfied with your current fitness level?
- How much time do you spend moving your body each week?
- Do you enjoy exercising? If not, what can you do to improve the exercise experience?
- How much exercise or movement is enough?

Small Steps

- Move your body daily.
- Make a list of activities you enjoy and make them part of your daily movement.
- Improve your posture.
- Move more.
- Play more.

25 Dynamic Warm-Up, Foundation and Restorative Movements

Now is the time to get MOVING! The second building block in our MOVE Pyramid includes Dynamic Warm-Up, Foundation, and Restorative Movements.

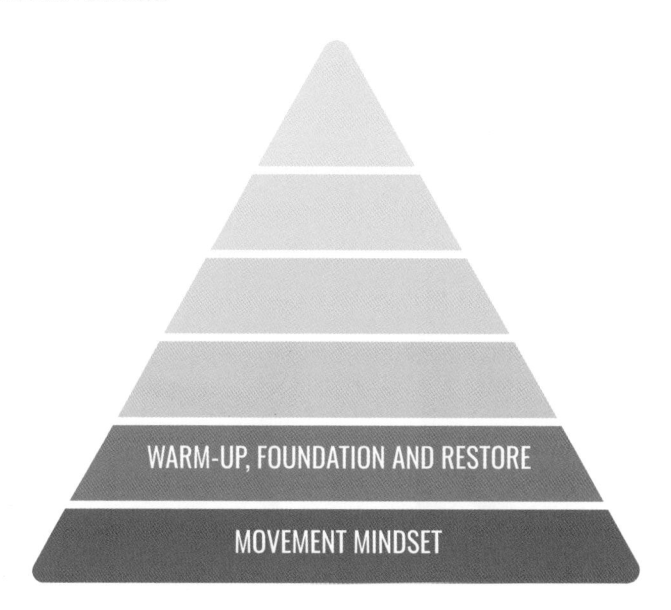

Dynamic Warm-Up: 2-3 Minutes Daily

With every form of exercise or movement, our body needs time to transition from a static or sedentary state into a dynamic or active state. This allows the body enough time to activate the nervous, cardiovascular, and muscular systems. These dynamic warm-up movements engage the entire body, increase synovial fluid to help lubricate the joints, improve balance and flexibility, and are quick, taking less than 2-3 minutes to perform.

Use slow and controlled movements and gradually increase the range of motion as the body warms up. If some of the movements are difficult, modify as needed. Take 2-3 minutes to properly warm up the body before taking a fitness class, strength training, or playing a favorite sport. You will feel better and perform better.

DYNAMIC WARM-UP

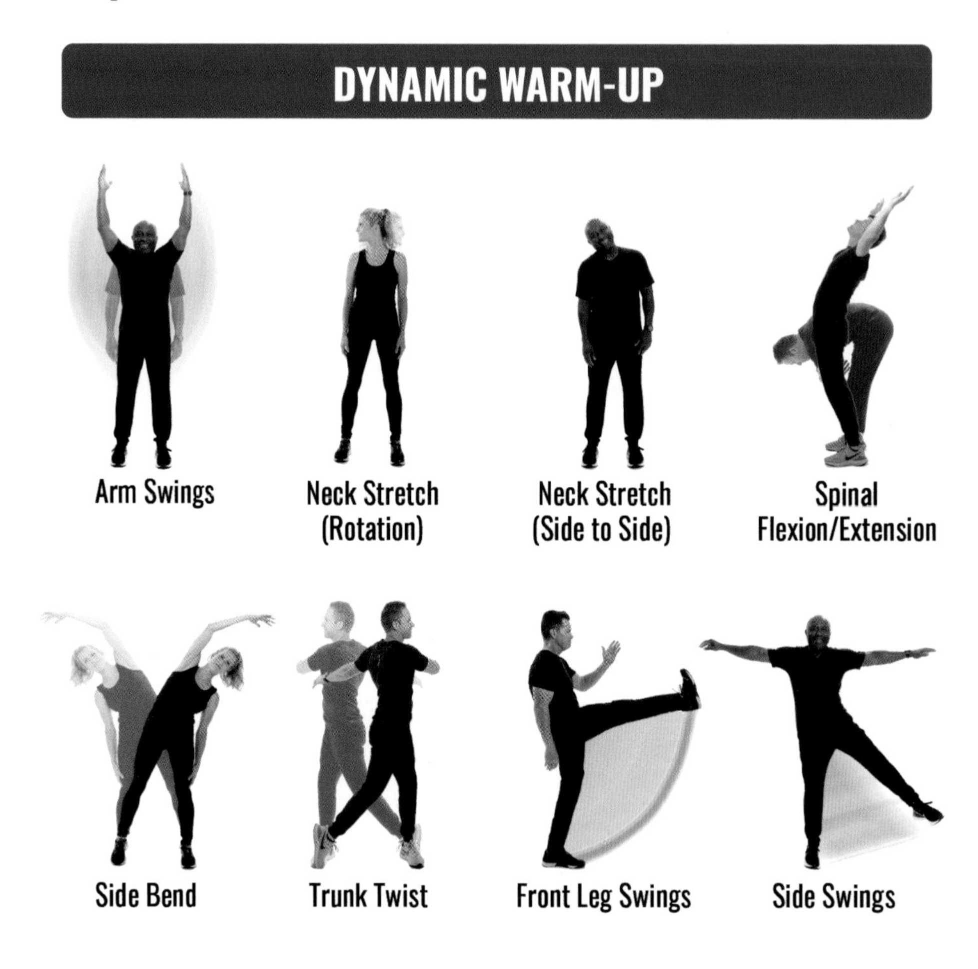

*Find movement videos on our ***app*** at ***ontargetliving.com***

Foundation Movements: 5-8 Minutes Daily

After completing the Dynamic Warm-Up routine, it is time move into Foundation Movements. Foundation movements are exceptionally beneficial to improve posture, balance, mobility, flexibility, strength, and fitness. They take 5-8 minutes to complete. The beauty of these foundational movements is that they take little time, can be done almost anywhere, and require no equipment. Most of all, they work. Individual movements can be added or deleted to fit specific needs. I recommend doing them every day. Hold each movement for 5-15 seconds and focus on perfect form.

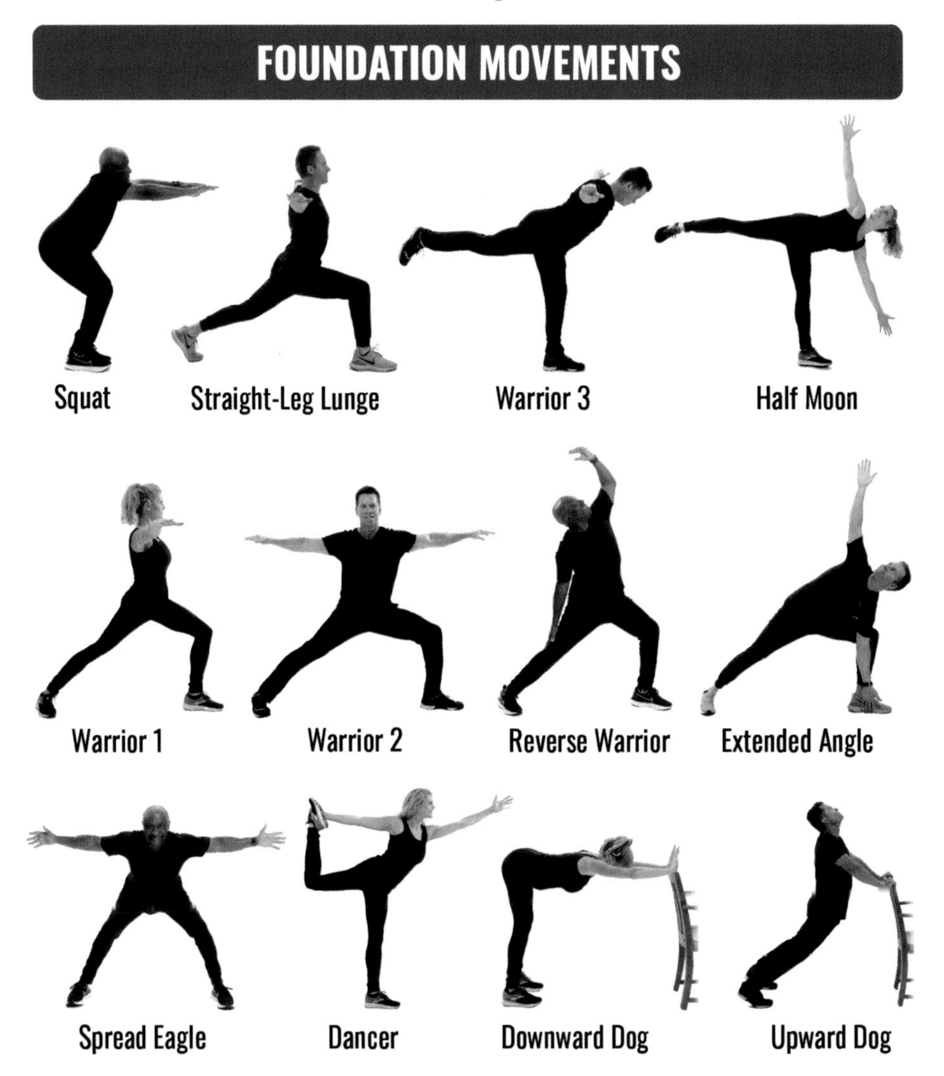

Restorative Movements

Restorative Movements are specific exercises to help maintain or improve our ability to move. On top of restoring our ability to move, we sometimes need specific movements to help us recover from pain or injuries. Restorative movements are specific movements that can also help relax the body and quiet the mind. These movements can be practiced on a daily basis and can also be targeted to specific areas of the body depending on individual needs. Try to move or hold each of these restorative movements for 15-90 seconds while breathing into each movement. Here are a few of my favorite restorative movements.

RESTORATIVE MOVEMENTS—STANDING

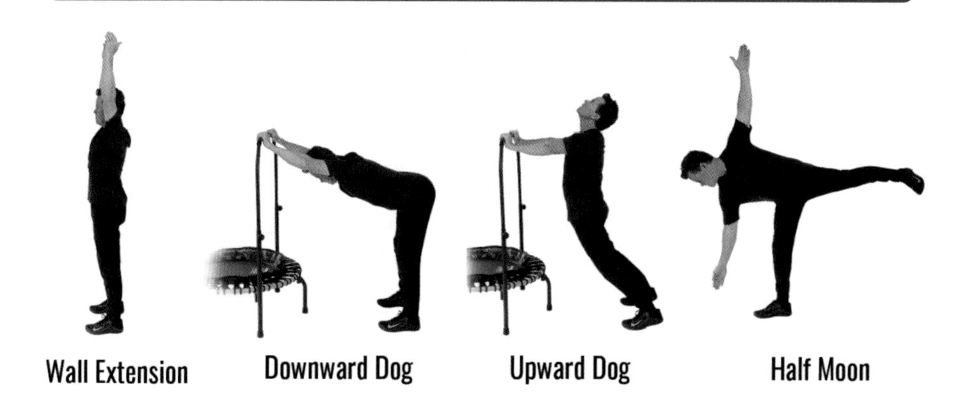

*Find movement videos on our ***app*** at ***ontargetliving.com***

RESTORATIVE MOVEMENTS—FLOOR

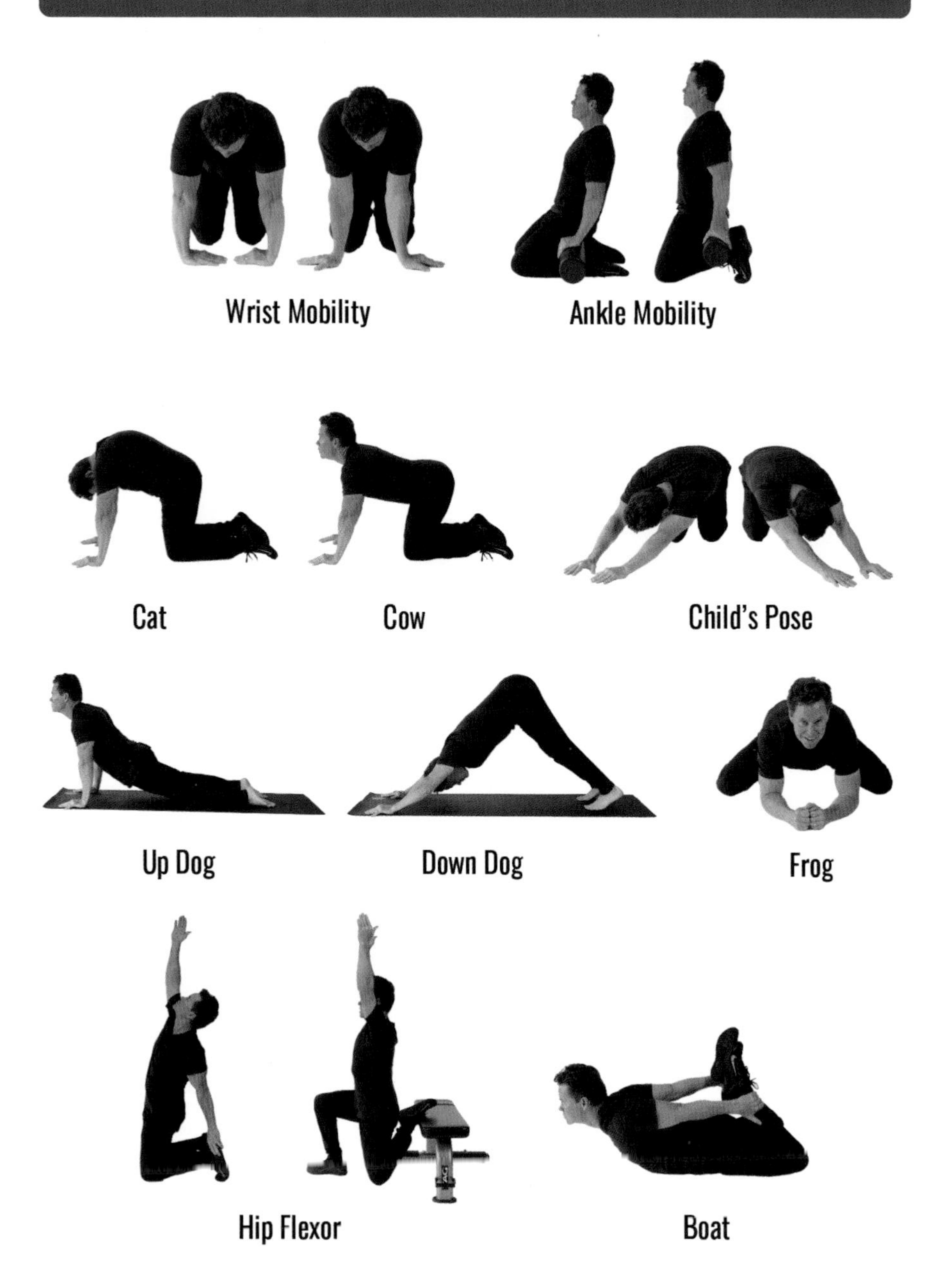

RESTORATIVE MOVEMENTS—FLOOR

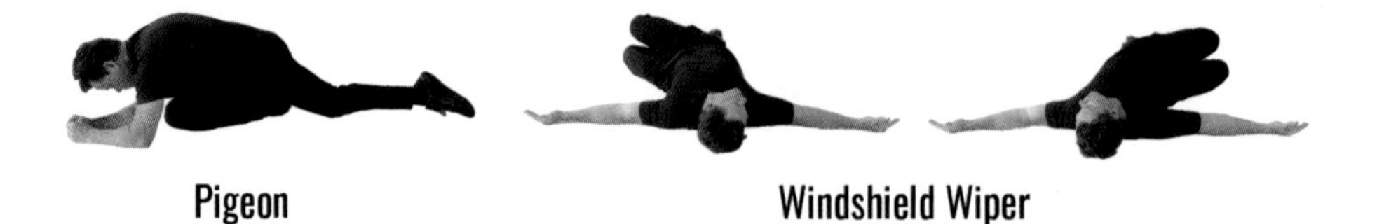

Pigeon

Windshield Wiper

Psoas

Hamstrings

Hip and Back

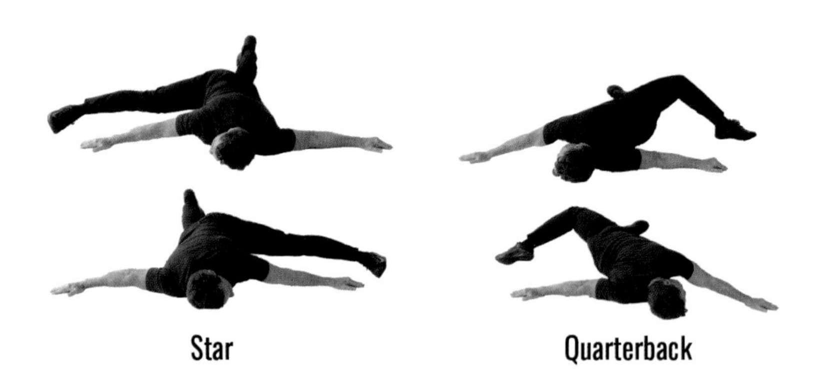

Star

Quarterback

*Find movement videos on our ***app*** at ***ontargetliving.com***

RESTORATIVE MOVEMENTS—FOAM ROLLER

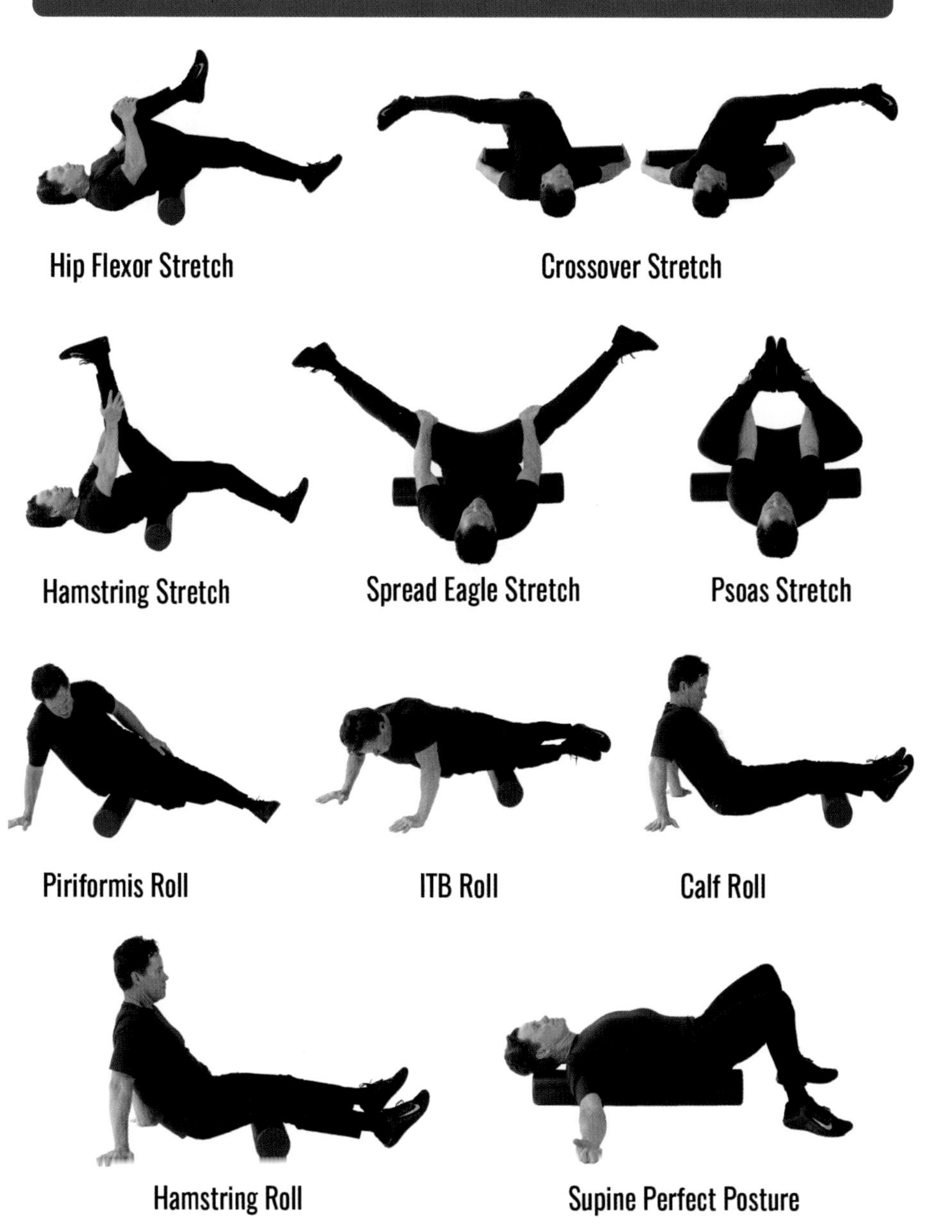

Hip Flexor Stretch

Crossover Stretch

Hamstring Stretch

Spread Eagle Stretch

Psoas Stretch

Piriformis Roll

ITB Roll

Calf Roll

Hamstring Roll

Supine Perfect Posture

RESTORATIVE MOVEMENTS—WALL

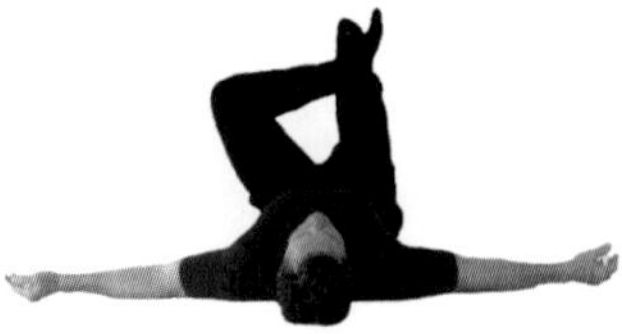

Hip Opener

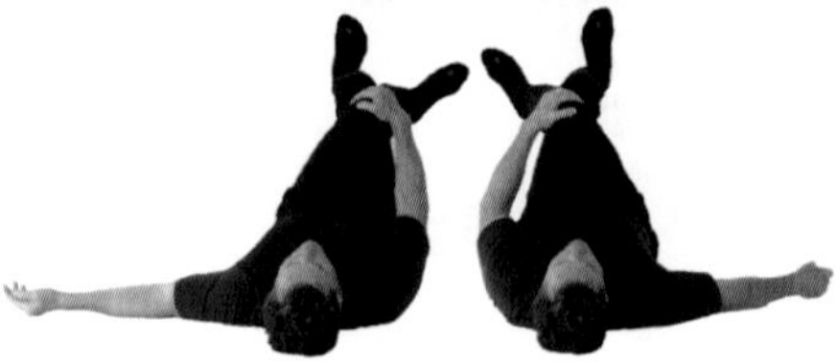

Piriformis

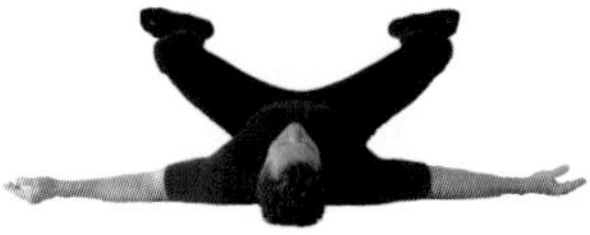

Plie

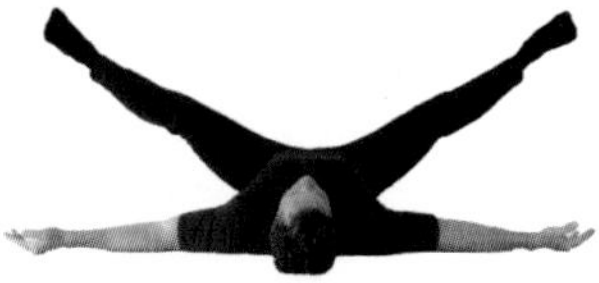

Spread Eagle

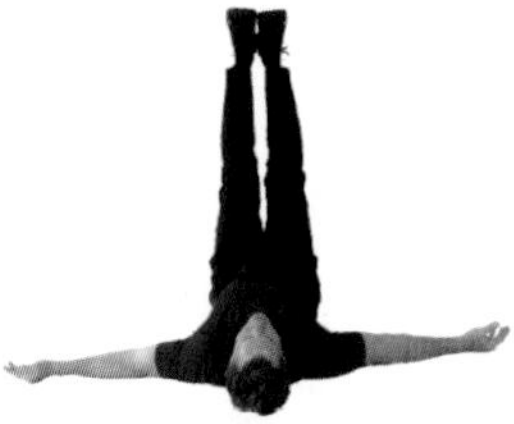

Waterfall

*Find movement videos on our ***app*** at ***ontargetliving.com***

Dynamic Warm-Up, Foundation and Restorative Movement Essentials

Big Picture

- **Dynamic Warm-Up:** Doing 2-3 minutes of movement helps transition the body from a static or sedentary state into a dynamic or active state.
- **Foundation Movements:** Structured movements to improve posture, balance, mobility, flexibility, strength, and fitness can all be rolled into a short 5–8-minute daily routine.
- **Restorative Movements:** These specific exercises are designed to help restore the body and mind, and improve your ability to move.

Ask Yourself

- Do you take time to warm up before you exercise or move?
- Do you spend time working on your posture and body alignment during the day or during your exercise sessions?
- Do you suffer from any nagging injuries? If so, what exercises are you doing to help restore your body?
- How are you going to include warm-up and restorative movements into your daily routine?

Small Steps

- Take 2-3 minutes every day to incorporate Dynamic Warm-Up into your movement plan.
- Spend 5-8 minutes each day to work on your posture, body alignment, balance, flexibility, mobility, and strength with Foundation Movements.
- Pick a few Restorative Movements to practice.
- Taking the time to properly warm up, align, and restore the body are gifts that your mind and body will love.

26 Cardio

The third building block of the MOVE Pyramid is Cardiovascular Exercise.

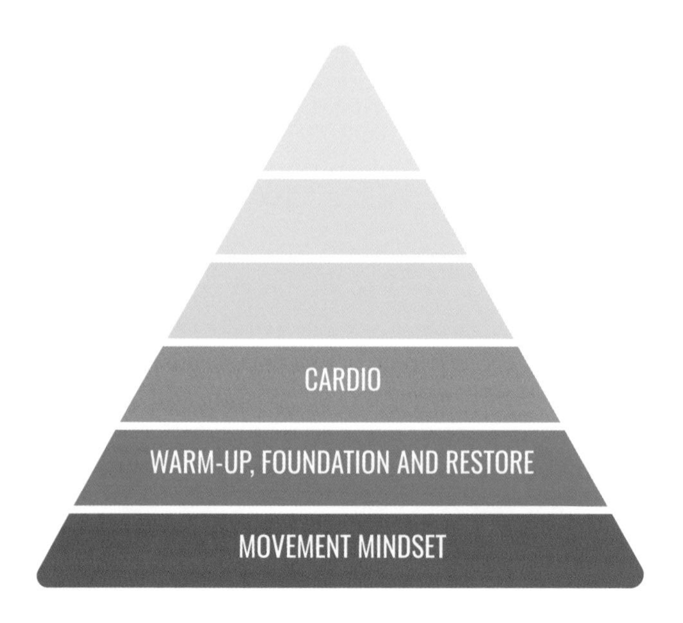

What is Cardio?

Cardiovascular exercise or "cardio" refers to any movement that is rhythmic in nature placing increased demands on the heart, lungs, blood vessels, muscles, and organs. Cardio includes activities like walking, jogging, running, biking, hiking, swimming, cross country skiing, calisthenics, and more. During cardio, breathing becomes more rapid, and heart rate and blood pressure rise. Blood vessels dilate ands muscles contract. Our organs send messages throughout our entire system that the body is speeding up.

Benefits of Cardio

The many wonderful benefits of cardio include stress management, mood elevation, mental clarity, pH balance, and improved cellular sensitivity, blood pressure, glucose levels, lipid profile, detoxification, brain health, and weight control. Cardio also increases strength and efficiency of the heart, lungs, and blood vessels.

How much time do you currently spend doing cardio each week?

____

If you do not do any type of cardio, what may be holding you back?

____

____

What is your favorite type of cardio?

____

Is there a new type of cardio you would like to try?

____

The Science of Cardio

Cardio results in a number of important physiological changes.

Cardiac Output

One of the first changes in the body with regular cardio movement is cardiac output. Cardiac output is the heart's ability to pump blood throughout the entire body. Higher output expands cardiovascular capacity.

Cardiac Output = Heart Rate x Stroke Volume

One of the first and best signs of getting in better cardiovascular shape is a low resting heart rate. As fitness levels improve, resting heart rate begins to slow down. This is due to increased cardiovascular system efficiency, specifically an increase in stroke volume. Stroke volume is the strength of the contraction of the heart. With a higher fitness level, each beat of the heart can push out more blood. One of the greatest indicators of overall health and fitness level is a low resting heart rate.

Low Fitness Level:	Resting Heart Rate **above 72** beats per minute
Moderate Fitness Level:	Resting Heart Rate of **60-72** beats per minute
High Fitness Level:	Resting Heart Rate **under 55** beats per minute

Heart Rate Range

Another great indicator of fitness capacity is heart rate range. Heart rate range is the range between resting heart rate (RHR) and maximal heart rate (MHR). Here are three examples of heart rate range. As fitness levels improve, heart rate range expands.

Low Fitness Level:	75 (RHR) - 115 (MHR) = 40 Heart Rate Range
Moderate Fitness Level:	65 (RHR) - 145 (MHR) = 80 Heart Rate Range
High Fitness Level:	50 (RHR) - 175 (MHR) = 125 Heart Rate Range

Aerobic vs Anaerobic

Cardio can be either aerobic or anaerobic or somewhere in between depending on the intensity level of the movements.

In **Aerobic** cardio, demand **meets** the supply of oxygen.
In **Anaerobic** cardio, demand **exceeds** the supply of oxygen.

It is important to understand the difference between aerobic and anaerobic exercise and how the duration and intensity of an exercise program can impact the heart, lungs, hormones, and, most importantly, increase results.

As aerobic fitness level improves, the goal should not be to continue to increase the amount of time dedicated to cardio, but rather to slowly increase the intensity of the movements or exercise. I believe many people look at cardio as a way to burn calories and lose weight, assuming more is better. This is not necessarily true. If the goal is to lose weight, it is far more effective and more efficient to limit the time spent on cardio to 25 minutes or less and slowly raise the intensity of the movements.

This may challenge some of your current beliefs. I am not asking you to do more. I am asking you to do less and make the movements more focused and intense. A higher intensity can challenge the nervous system, growth hormone, testosterone, estrogen, and muscles, as well as impact the body in many ways including weight loss.

Heart Rate Variability (HRV)

One of the latest measures of stress reduction, heart health, performance enhancement, and overall well-being is Heart Rate Variability (HRV). Many wearables, such as Oura, Whoop, and many others, now have the capability to track HRV.

HRV is a measure of the subtle beat-to-beat changes in the pattern of heart rhythm. HRV is not as common as pulse, blood pressure, or body temperature as a health screening tool. It is, however, becoming widely recognized as a powerful indicator to uncover future health problems. Learning how to control HRV is one of the great practices to reduce stress, lower blood pressure, and improve the quality of our health, our hearts, and our lives.

Heart rate variability is literally the variance in time between heart beats. If a heart beats at 60 beats per minute, it is not actually beating once every second. Within that minute there may be 0.9 seconds between two beats and 1.15 seconds between two others. A normal HRV for most adults can range anywhere from below 20 to over 200 milliseconds. A normal HRV measurement can be established over a few weeks by using a wearable device.

HRV is linked to the autonomic nervous system (ANS) and the balance between the sympathetic (fight-or-flight) and parasympathetic (rest and digest) branches. This was discussed earlier in Section 3. By balancing these two branches, the ANS helps us respond to daily stressors, balance hormones and, regulate heart rate, breathing, and digestion. HRV is one of the most effective methods of monitoring the balance within the ANS.

Low HRV

When we feel stressed, anxious, frustrated, or threatened in any way, the sympathetic nervous system goes into quick action. Heart rate and blood pressure rise, and pupils dilate. Muscles contract and digestion shuts down. It is our sympathetic nervous system (fight-or-flight response) that tells the heart to speed up, limiting space for variability and leading to Low HRV. Think of low HRV as a piece of music where the notes get jammed together, creating little space between the notes. The music would not sound the same. In low HRV, there is little space between the beats of the heart, and in most cases can be a great indicator that the body is out of balance. Low HRV over time may be linked to heart disease, cancer, type 2 diabetes, high blood pressure, sleep apnea, and a variety of other health problems in the future.

High HRV

On the other end of the spectrum is High HRV. This is when there is adequate space between the beats of the heart. Generally speaking, high HRV is associated with the parasympathetic nervous system (rest and digest), leading to more peacefulness, relaxation, and a higher cardiovascular fitness level. There are many health benefits for the heart, mind, and body with a high HRV. Imagine heart rhythms as the waves of a sea. On a beautiful calm day, the waves are long, flowing, smooth, consistent, repetitive, and peaceful looking. But during a storm the waves become large, stressed, spiked, irregular and erratic. They are anything but peaceful looking—the ocean is upset. That is the difference between high HRV and low HRV.

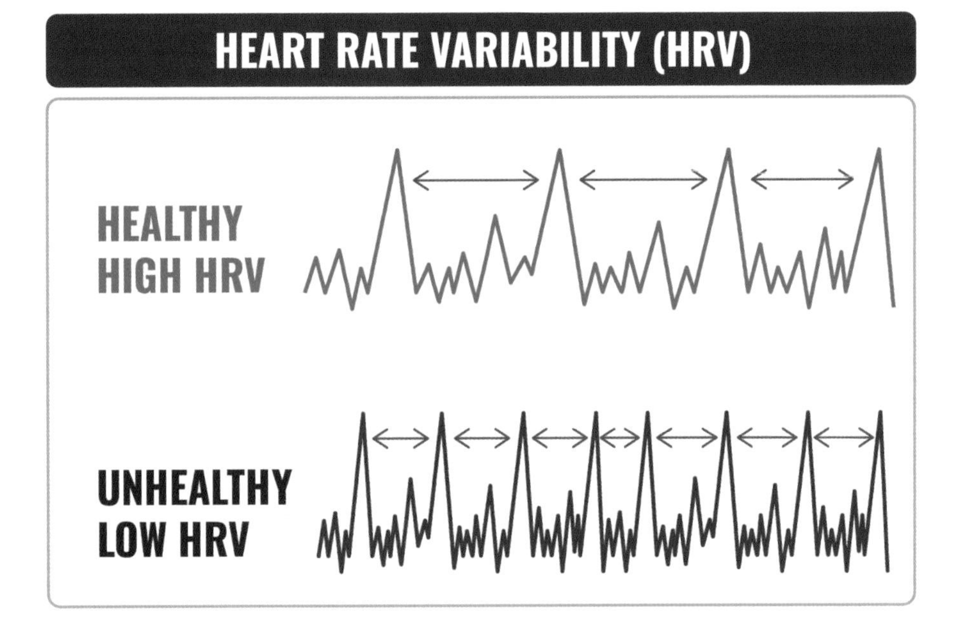

Measurements for high and low HRV are unique for each person. High and low HRV is a highly sensitive measurement that responds uniquely for each person. The key, like most metrics, is to develop baselines that allow HRV to be monitored on a regular basis.

We have the ability to go from a low HRV to a high HRV by improving how we **REST**, **EAT**, and **MOVE**. Improving some simple lifestyle habits can directly influence our HRV: how we breathe, how we sleep, making enough space for recovery, balancing pH, hydrating, consuming healthy foods, and moving our body on a daily basis.

Oxygen Uptake (VO2 max)

Because muscles use oxygen to function, measuring how much oxygen the body uses in a given time provides a way to measure how efficiently the body is working.

Remember the scene in Rocky IV when Ivan Drago, the Russian Boxing Champion and fitness specimen, was sprinting full speed up a severely inclined treadmill, breathing into a mask, wires attached everywhere, and lights flashing on the computer? What were the Russian team of doctors and coaches testing? They were testing Ivan Drago's heart rate, blood pressure, blood gases, and lactate levels. Most importantly they were testing Drago's VO2 max. The Russians were using state of the art science to measure his fitness level instead of Rocky's "old school" method of running up a hill in thigh deep snow with a huge log on his back.

Maximal oxygen uptake, or VO2 max, is widely considered the gold standard as a measure of aerobic fitness. The "V" represents the volume of gas (oxygen, O2) taken up by the body over time. The "Max" represents the maximum amount of work that can be done during high intensity exercise. It is commonly used to test aerobic endurance or cardiovascular fitness in athletes before and at the end of a training cycle.

Maximal Oxygen Uptake Levels

Level of Aerobic Fitness	VO2 max (ml/kg/min)
High	49.0-56.0
Good	39.0-48.9
Average	25.0-38.9
Low	14.0-24.9
Poor	3.5-13.9

Although VO2 max is a great marker of cardiovascular fitness, it has some downfalls. The only accurate way to measure of VO2 max requires expensive clinical equipment, which is why VO2 max is usually a fitness marker reserved for elite and professional athletes. I think Rocky's method of running up a hill in three feet of snow with a huge log on his back is just as effective.

Crushing that VO2 Max Test

When I was in graduate school all of the exercise physiology students in our class had an opportunity to do a VO2 max test. It is a brutal test, and nobody enjoyed taking their turn. Looking back, I remember my lifelong friend and classmate Dan Bender taking his turn on the treadmill. Dan and I have known each other for over 50 years. We played "Pop Warner" football together, worked out together, and happened to enroll in graduate school at the same time. Dan was a beast. He looked like a body builder but was also a runner and a very fit guy.

Many of our classmates did not fully understand the fitness crossover from strength training to cardiovascular fitness. In fact, many teased Dan and me, saying they could not wait to see us take our turns on the treadmill. They had no idea the type of training Dan and I did and believed that strength training had little value when it came to cardiovascular fitness.

I still remember to this day the look on their faces watching Dan crush his VO2 max test. Quads pumping, sweat flying, and treadmill whining, Dan was a sight to see. Ivan Drago had nothing on Dan. Our professor, Dr. William Heusner later reported that Dan had one of highest VO2 max levels that he had ever tested!

The "Training" Effect

Take a moment to consider what happens inside the body when we walk, run, swim, ride a bike, stretch, or do a few sets of push-ups or squats. What goes on inside the mind and body when we play a game of tennis? How is it that the body gets better at specific, targeted movements?

Exercise physiology is the study of the body's response to physical activities as well as how the body adapts to these physical activities over time. When we begin to move our body, acute responses take place. Heart rate and blood pressure increase, blood vessels dilate, digestion shuts down, and an array of other physiological changes quickly take place throughout the entire body. Over time the body moves into chronic adaptations to these specific movements creating specific changes in the muscular, cardiovascular, and neurohormonal systems.

What we do (modality), how hard we do it (intensity), and how long we do it (duration) all are big players in what is called the "Training Effect." When training for a 5K, our workouts are going to be specific to running. If our goal is to swim 100 meters, we need to spend a good deal of our training time in the pool. Both of these activities tax the cardiovascular system differently. Both are goal specific, and the training effect is specific to the activity. This is why a person who is in great cardiovascular shape from running can get gassed from doing a few laps in the pool. Running may create a solid cardiovascular baseline, but swimming is a completely different beast, with a different training effect.

For many years when doing one-on-one training, I asked my clients how they rated their cardiovascular fitness level on a 1-10 scale (10 being the highest). Many rated their cardio fitness at a 7 or higher. Many reported logging steps, minutes, or miles each week by walking, jogging, hiking, biking, or swimming. To get a better indication of their cardiovascular capacity, I asked them to climb up and down one flight of stairs three straight times, rest for 15 seconds, and then repeat this exercise two more times. This entire stair climbing exercise took less than five minutes for most to complete. I think most were shocked that such a simple exercise made them so out of breath.

This stair climbing exercise helped my clients understand training specificity and the differences between aerobic and anaerobic training. Their current exercises might be great for maintaining overall fitness. If their goal was to improve their cardiovascular capacity, then they needed to add in some anaerobic work. My advice was to devote some of their precious workout time to occasional bursts of higher intensity movements. If they enjoyed walking, then change it up. Walk for 30 seconds and then jog or run for 30 seconds. If they enjoyed biking, sprint on the bike for 30 seconds, slow down and recover for 30-60 seconds. Then repeat 3-10 times. If they enjoyed swimming instead of just logging laps in the pool, increase the intensity now and then by swimming faster for two laps, rest for 30 seconds, and repeat. This type of interval training would raise their anaerobic threshold, improve their cardiovascular capacity, and provide their workouts with more intention and purpose.

It may sound simple to lose weight using cardio by increasing the intensity and going like mad, but there are a few other things that must be understood about high-intensity cardio.

Redlining

Performing high-intensity cardio day in and day out is tough and may become extremely challenging to the mind and body. It may turn many people off exercise altogether.

When an exercise or movement routine is teetering on the edge of too much, I call this "Redlining." It may lead to stress and a drop in performance. Participating in cardio that is really hard every now and then is great, but when the intensity is turned up too much, it can crush the mind and body. No longer do we reap the wonderful benefits of cardio. Our cardio routine may have crossed the line. How can we tell if we are redlining? Sleep may become broken. Energy drops and resting heart rate goes up. Digestion may come to a halt or quickly speed up. We may become more irritable or be in a foul mood. The feeling of being burned out both mentally and physically may start to creep in.

Leading up to a few of my bodybuilding competitions early in my career, I knew I was redlining when I began to witness changes in my sleep, energy, resting heart rate, and most importantly when my passion and juice for going to the gym started to disappear. I knew I was overtraining and needed to back it down and bring in some needed rest.

Battle of the Titans

Years ago, several of our health club members put together a two-day contest titled, "Battle of the Titans." It was a contest similar to a decathlon, except there were 13 events spread over just two days. The events were selected by a committee and included events of skill, strength, power, stamina, and most importantly, grit. We were all members of the Michigan Athletic Club, and most were also friends. The group ranged from the typical weekend warrior to former college and professional athletes. This was a tough crowd in many ways. As I learned during the competition, it was a great group of guys.

Looking back, I believe there were three events that stuck out in everyone's mind and pushed us all into redlining.

Squat: *We loaded up a bar with our body weight and tried to squat as many reps as we could within a 2-minute time limit. Just watching our fellow competitors go through this gauntlet of pain was extremely stressful. Not only were we completely gassed during and after the event, but we could barely walk for days later.*

Plate Push: *I think this was the hardest 90 seconds of my life! We took a 45-pound plate, placed it on a towel, placed our hands on the plate, and pushed the plate around a large gym as fast and far as we could in 90 seconds. This event was based on anerobic power. Pushing as hard as possible and in a bent-over position made breathing extremely difficult. I remember members lining up around the gym to watch. The excitement was electric. But when it was their turn, no contestant was smiling.*

StepMill: *We got on a revolving stair machine and climbed as many flights of stairs as possible in 10 minutes. If our hands grabbed the railings, we were deducted an entire flight of stairs. Competitors tried to pace themselves, but in most cases, they started too quickly, crossed into anaerobic pain, and* *then quickly started falling apart. Again, this was a tough event to watch especially if you were up next.*

To this day, I think many of our redlining events left a mark. It was an exciting time. We developed great relationships and friendships, and along the way, we learned a great deal about ourselves!

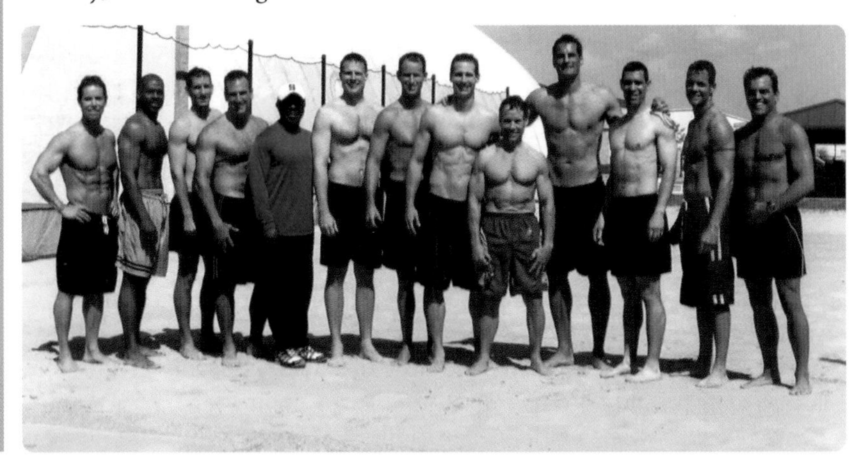

Create a Cardio Plan that Works for You

Creating an effective and efficient cardio plan includes several components: modality, frequency, duration, and intensity. Here are the specifics to consider for each of those components.

Modality

When adopting a cardio plan, it is critical to start with cardio activities that are enjoyable. Whether it is walking, jogging, running, biking, swimming, mini trampoline, calisthenics, or a group fitness class, we must keep searching until we find cardio movements we enjoy. I do not particularly like to swim in the wintertime, but I love to swim in the summer. My favorite cardio activities include the mini trampoline, calisthenics, walking/jogging/running with my dog Floyd in the woods, and the occasional use a variety of cardio machines. I also like to play to improve my cardio. I enjoy paddleball, pickleball, ping pong, snowshoeing, snow skiing, hiking, and biking. Try new activities and keep searching for cardio movements you enjoy.

Sample Cardio Modalities

- Biking
- Calisthenics
- Cross Country Skiing
- Jumping Rope
- Mini Trampoline
- Playing
- Swimming
- Walking/Jogging/Running

Frequency

People often wonder how often they should do cardio. We should develop a cardio plan that fits our time and our schedule. I try to do cardio almost every day. Some days are more intense than others. Consistency is very important. It is the consistency that adds up over time and helps create a habit. Just a few minutes on the mini trampoline or going for a 10-minute walk have benefits. Remember, the benefit of moving the body is not just for the heart and lungs, but more importantly, for what it does for the mind.

Duration

I believe duration is where most people get cardio wrong, believing more time equals more results or benefits. Similar to nutrition, quality trumps quantity when it comes to exercise. When training for a marathon or triathlon, we have to put in the time. However, if our goal is to get in better cardiovascular shape, 10-25 minutes of moderate to high-intensity cardio on a regular basis is all we need.

Intensity

Intensity is the level of difficulty to sustain the exercise or movement. A leisurely walk or bike ride is great, but to see adaptations to the cardiovascular system, we must get a little uncomfortable. If the exercise is too hard and can only last a few minutes before we have to stop, the intensity may be too high (redlining). If the intensity is too low, the body will only make minimal adaptations, and we will get fewer benefits from the cardio exercise. Here are a few ways to monitor intensity.

Visual

Body language and postural alignment are great indicators that the intensity is too high. When the intensity is too demanding, the body begins to make compensations, leading to poor posture. If the intensity is too low, it becomes a leisure activity.

Breath—Talk Test

I used to talk to my clients while they did their cardio. If they could easily carry on a conversation, I knew their intensity level was too low to create a training effect. If they could not talk, then the intensity most likely was too high.

Perceived Exertion

Perceived exertion can be measured on a 1-10 scale with 1-2 being easy, 4-6 moderate, and 8-10 extremely difficult. Perceived exertion may vary from person to person but can be an easy way to assess the difficulty of cardio movements. Monitor exertion on a scale of 1-10. Are you working out at a 3, 5 or 8? Or do you vary intensity by doing a few intervals?

Heart Rate

Traditionally, heart rate is the gold standard for monitoring exercise intensity. Heart rate is a great indicator of current fitness level, perceived stress, and is a great way to measure the intensity level of a particular exercise. As fitness levels improve, so does heart rate range. With a resting heart rate of 60 and a maximum heart rate of 160, the heart rate range is 100. As fitness levels increase, the heart rate range increases, leading to greater cardio capacity. Using heart rate to gauge intensity levels is the gold standard for most competitive athletes. For most, however, starting with how we look, feel, and whether we can talk during exercise is enough.

How do you currently monitor your cardio intensity level?

____

____

When starting a movement or exercise program, start slowly and over time begin to challenge yourself. Start with a heart rate around 95-110 beats per minute. For a moderate exerciser, start with 111-140 beats per minutes and for the advanced exerciser or when doing intervals, 125-175 beats per minute.

Remember, these are just guidelines. Monitor your heart rate further with the talk test and by assessing your perceived exertion to see how your heart rate measures up.

One last point. It is always a good idea to consult with your healthcare professional prior to beginning any exercise program. Start slowly and let your body slowly acclimate to your movement plan. Remember, you cannot out-exercise a poor diet!

Cardio Essentials

Big Picture

- Cardio has many wonderful health benefits for the mind and body.
- Oxygen uptake is low in people who do not exercise and high in those who do regular aerobic exercise.
- Lower resting heart rates indicate higher fitness levels.
- Increasing cardiovascular capacity requires both aerobic and anaerobic exercise.
- Aerobic demand meets the supply of oxygen. Anaerobic demand exceeds the supply of oxygen.
- A cardio plan to meet your goals includes what you do (modality), how hard you do it (intensity), how often you do it (frequency), and how long you do it (duration).

Ask Yourself

- How much time are you spending on cardio each week?
- Do you redline too often?
- Is your current cardio plan in line with your goals?
- How can you improve your cardio experience?

Small Steps

- Walk, jog, skip rope, swim, climb, get your heart pumping, and get out of breath on a regular basis.
- Find cardio activities you enjoy.
- Sprinkle some high-intensity intervals into your cardio plan.

27 Strength Training

The fourth MOVE building block and one of my favorites is Strength Training.

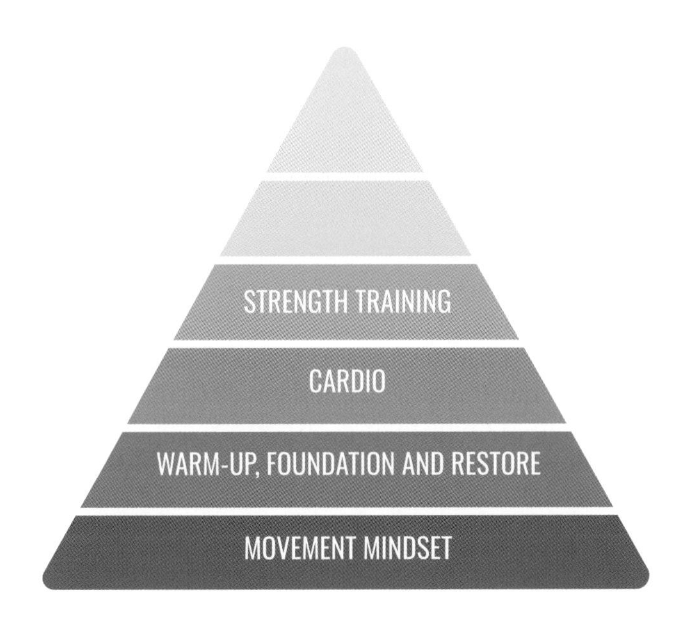

If there is one form of exercise that can turn back the hands of time, it is strength training. Even people in their 80s and 90s can improve their strength, mobility, balance, flexibility, and bone density with strength training. I have witnessed incredible benefits from strength training with my clients, seminar attendees, family, and friends. Strength training can be magical in keeping the body strong and vibrant.

A Gift that Keeps on Giving

For my 11th birthday, I received 110-pound barbell set from my parents. Who gives their kid a barbell set for their 11th birthday? This was over 50 years ago, and I still have some of the original plates. Who would have guessed this would be a lifelong passion of mine? I guess my parents knew what they were doing.

What is Strength Training?

Strength is the ability to exert force in order to overcome resistance. Strength training is a movement or exercise that uses resistance to place demands on the nervous system, hormones, bones, connective tissue, and muscles. Strength training is generally done in short bursts (10-30 seconds) of the strength training phase, which is when the muscle is under tension. For example, when doing a bicep curl, lifting the weight up shortens the muscle. This is the concentric phase of the movement. Lowering the weight back down lengthens the muscle. This is the eccentric phase of the movement. Each exercise is followed by a rest or recovery phase, lasting from 10 seconds to over 5 minutes depending on the desired goals.

With the right intensity, strength training can tax the anaerobic system, leading to a stimulation of youthful building hormones, growth hormone, and testosterone. To my women readers, do not be afraid of "bulking up" with strength training. Men have a great deal more growth hormone and testosterone than women do. It takes a tremendous amount of effort, good nutrition, and the right genetic material to get larger muscles. I have been trying to build bigger muscles for years, and it is difficult to do.

I have been strength training for over 50 years. When I was young my main goal was to build large muscles and enhance my athletic performance. Today at the age of 64, I am still trying to get stronger and build my body, but I also understand that strength training provides so much more than that. Strength training can improve posture, prevent injuries, reduce stress, increase bone density, heighten athletic performance, and improve mobility, flexibility, balance, metabolism, and weight control. Strength training not only improves the way we look, but more importantly, it improves the way we feel.

Strength training can increase our vitality. After I strength train, my mind is clear. My mood is great and I feel energized. Strength training can be done in a variety of methods. We can use our own body weight such as in a push-up, pull-up, or a bodyweight squat. Or we can add resistance using free weights, kettle bells, resistance bands, a Swiss ball, or strength training machines. These are just a sample of strength training methods to choose from.

Strength Training Guidelines

Here are a few simple guidelines to follow when putting a strength training routine in place.

Posture

Good posture is job one when beginning any type of strength training plan. Before starting each exercise or movement, get into great posture and maintain this posture alignment throughout the entire exercise or movement. When posture alignment begins to break down, stop the movement.

Breathing

How we breathe during the day, the night, and when strength training is a big deal. If the breath gets out of rhythm, intensity may be too high. Get in the flow with each breath. Exhale during the exertional or concentric phase of each strength training movement. Inhale during the lowering or eccentric phase.

Focus

Focus on the movement being performed. Concentrate on alignment and form. How does it feel? What muscles are engaged? Is there a connection between the brain and the muscles? This is the neuromuscular system at work. This is the intrinsic motivation I like to teach with strength training. Feel the body with every movement. This takes focus and concentration. The mind becomes one with the body. This is not always easy but is a skill we can all learn.

Technique

Performing a strength training exercise correctly is critical. The correct training technique matters. What surprises me is the mindset many people have when it comes to strength training. Many people think there cannot be much to it. Just pick up a few weights, count the reps, and that is it. They have had no instruction, no guidance. Maybe they picked up these exercises in a magazine or book or saw them on social media. It is, however, the quality of the movements that is critical to success when strength training.

Scapula Retraction

When doing strength training for the upper body, it is important to learn how to use the scapula (the shoulder blades) correctly. Retracting the scapula, pulling them down and in, creates necessary space in the chest, shoulders, and back to improve the function and effectiveness of the exercise and decrease the risk of injury. When doing a push-up, lat pull-down, or standing row, pull the scapula down and in. Hold this position throughout the entire exercise or movement. Scapula retraction is dynamic, requiring both mobility and stability.

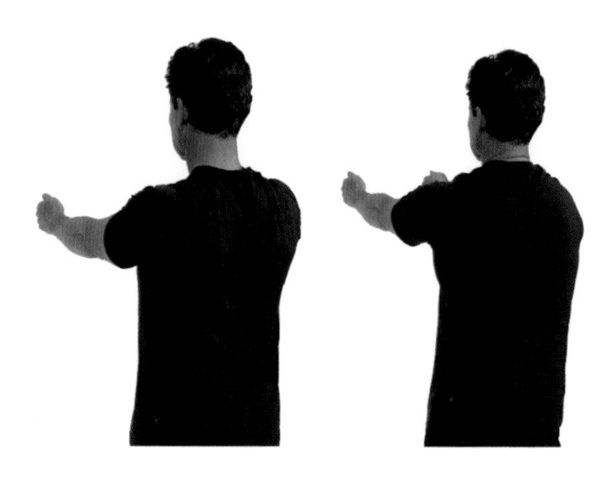

Scapula Retraction

Reps and Sets

Once the strength training movements have been selected, it is time to focus on setting the number of reps and sets.

Reps

Start with 5-13 repetitions (reps) per strength training movement and focus on doing each rep perfectly. Use reps as a guide to measure intensity and progress. More important than the number of reps is maintaining proper posture throughout each strength training movement or exercise. If posture and body alignment begin to break down, stop the exercise regardless of whether the desired reps have been achieved. Losing proper posture and body alignment is how people get injured, develop muscle imbalances, and poor movement patterns.

Sets

A set is taking the specific number of reps and repeating the reps in a set. For example, doing a push-up 8 times (reps) then repeating those 8 reps after a short rest break is 2 sets. When beginning, start with 1-2 sets of each exercise. To advance, move to 3-5 sets per movement or exercise. Each month I like to change the number of reps and sets for each strength training exercise. For example, in the first month, I do 5 sets of 5 reps for each exercise with high resistance. In the second month, it is 4 sets of 8 reps of each exercise with moderate resistance. In the third month, 3 sets of 13 reps with even lower resistance. Changing reps and sets each month, along with a few other strength training variables, will keep a workout fresh, reduce injury, and challenge the mind and body to adapt.

3 Rs of Strength Training

Now that we have a general understanding of reps and sets, let's go a little deeper into developing a strength training plan by learning how to use the "3 Rs." Using the 3 Rs allows endless ways to exercise especially when it comes to strength training.

Range

The first R is **Range**. Increasing the range of motion with each exercise or movement increases the intensity. Imagine doing a bodyweight squat and lowering down just 6 inches versus lowering down 24-30 inches to 90 degrees. It is the same exercise, but with a completely different intensity level and bottom-line results. So, before considering more weight or resistance, expand the range of motion.

Quality versus Quantity

Years ago, I started working with a guy whose goal was to get stronger for downhill skiing without getting injured. He was having knee and hip pain, so I took a look at his current strength workout. I was shocked to learn that he was currently pressing over 300 pounds! There was no way this guy could move this amount of weight with any range of motion. After a few minutes of warming up, I asked him to demonstrate how he used the leg press machine. He loaded it up with 300 pounds, held his breath, and moved the weight maybe 6-8 inches. We then discussed his goals and I suggested we start by going through the 3 Rs, beginning with range. We stripped the leg press down to 100 pounds and worked on his form and range of motion. After just 2 sets of 8 repetitions with 100 pounds and going through a much larger range of motion, he said his legs were smoked. By reducing the weight and increasing the range of motion, his knee and hip pain started to disappear in less than one month. He also felt his legs getting stronger and more conditioned for his upcoming ski trip.

Rate

The second R is **Rate**, how fast or slow each exercise or movement is performed. Imagine doing a simple push-up with a full range of motion and scapula retraction (technique), pausing at the top of the push-up, slowly lowering down, then pausing at the bottom, and slowly coming back up. Now change the rate/speed of the push-up again by slowly coming down, pausing at the bottom, and quickly exploding up, pausing at the top, and repeating this movement again. The change in rate would make a simple push-up exercise extremely challenging and goal specific. An entire strength training workout or multiple workouts can be done entirely by only focusing on rate. It is this awareness of the rate of each exercise or movement that expands our strength and fitness capacity.

Resistance

The third R is **Resistance**. This is the load used in a given rep or set to perform each movement. Resistance can be in the form of our own body weight, such as in a push-up or pull-up. Or we can add resistance with dumbbells, kettlebells, machines, or bands. There are endless ways to add resistance to each movement. Choosing the correct resistance can be challenging at first. The goal with every exercise or movement is to create and maintain good posture and body alignment, range of motion, rate, and then to slowly add resistance. This is what is called progressive overload. As the body is challenged, it will begin to adapt. This includes changes taking place within the nervous and cardiovascular systems, connective tissue, and muscles. This is the "training effect" at work. The general rule is when doing fewer reps, the resistance is higher. When doing more reps, the resistance is lower. Always listen to your body and maintain perfect form. Do not get caught up just pushing weight.

The Importance of Rest and Recovery

It is important to focus on the amount of time for rest and recovery between each strength training movement or exercise. The rest taken between sets allows time for the body to recover. This can be critical for adaptation, growth, and injury prevention, along with keeping the workout fresh and enjoyable. The more intensity and resistance within each exercise set, the more recovery time will be necessary between sets. If the goal is to push it, such as doing a specific number of squats, push-ups or pull-ups, a longer recovery time may be needed, ranging from 1-5 minutes between sets. If the goal is to integrate many exercises with a moderate amount of resistance, then a shorter recovery time is needed, ranging from 10-45 seconds between sets. Rest and recovery time should be adjusted over time to fit a specific training goal.

Stability and Balance

Balance = Strength and Strength = Balance. Once our strength and fitness levels improve, we can start to challenge our stability and balance. It is much easier to strength train when on a stable surface such as sitting in a chest press or lat pull-down machine. It is much more challenging to do a push-up with toes on a Swiss ball or doing a bodyweight pull-up. As you advance in your strength training routine, think about challenging your stability and balance.

Power

Can a person be strong but not powerful? The answer is yes. This takes us back to our training specificity conversation. If our goal is to hit the golf ball farther, strength training can greatly improve the distance the golf ball travels. We must also understand power.

Power is the ability to overcome resistance in the shortest period of time leading to the ability to produce higher velocities against a given load. This is where rate or speed of strength training movements come in. As our strength training advances, we can improve our power by changing the rate of speed of each strength training movement. As we build our strength base, we can start to experiment with the rate, stability, and balance of each movement. This can translate into more explosive power.

There are so many variables to strength training. That is what makes strength training so interesting. Start with just the basics. Gaining experience and knowledge will expand the vast world of strength training possibilities.

Progressions

Proper progressions are the magic recipe for sustainable success in strength training. Learning how to safely and effectively challenge the body takes time and practice. I see so many people doing the same exact workout day after day, same range of motion, same speed of the movements, same resistance, same reps, and same rest. Many get disappointed in their progress. Learning how to switch up a few variables now and then can make all the difference in a strength training workout in order to achieve the desired results.

Whether you plan to strength train in the gym or at home, I highly recommend getting some professional instruction. Set up a few training sessions with a professional personal trainer to learn proper technique and help create a strength training plan specific for you and your goals.

Strength Training Movements

Here are a variety of strength training movements or exercises to choose from.

STRENGTH TRAINING—UPPER BODY

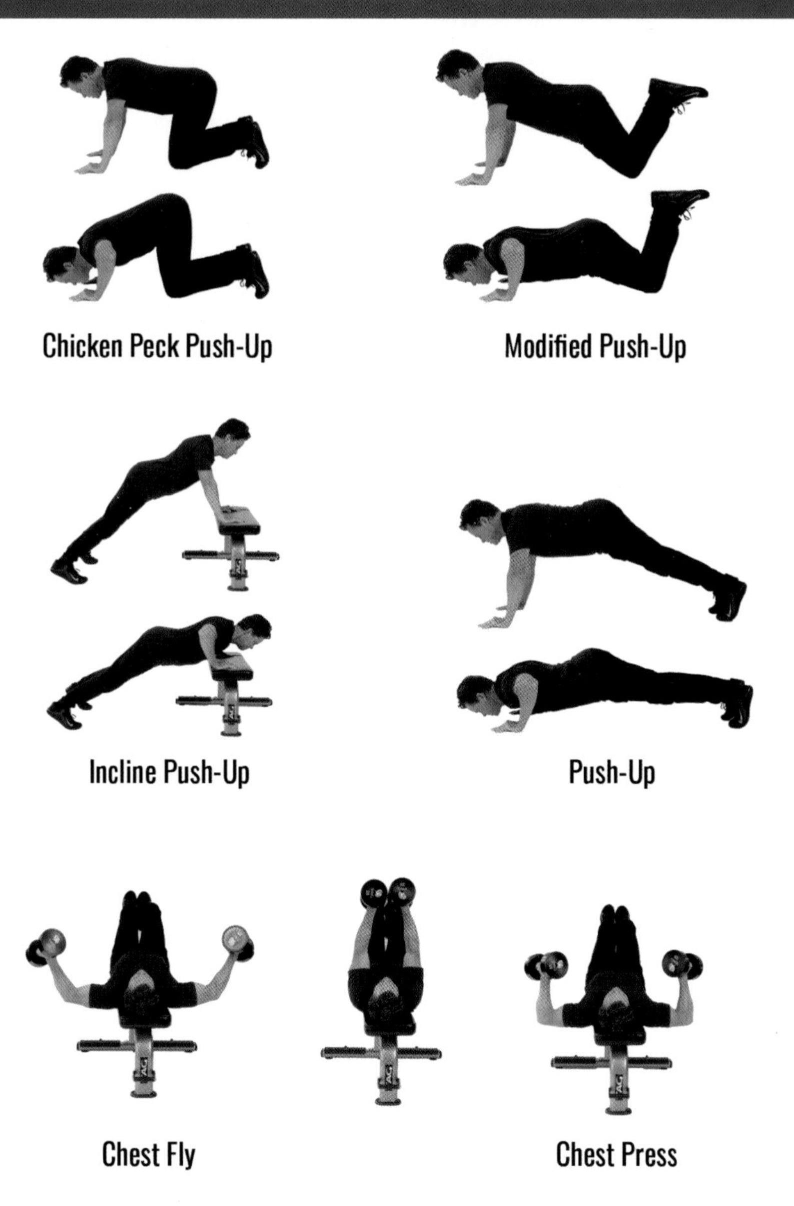

STRENGTH TRAINING—UPPER BODY

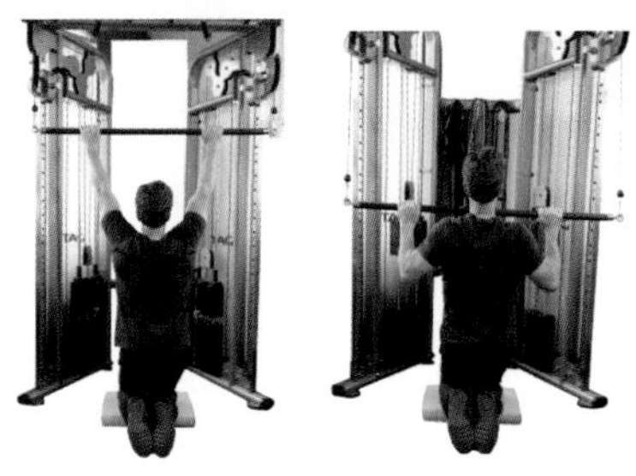

Lat Pull-Down

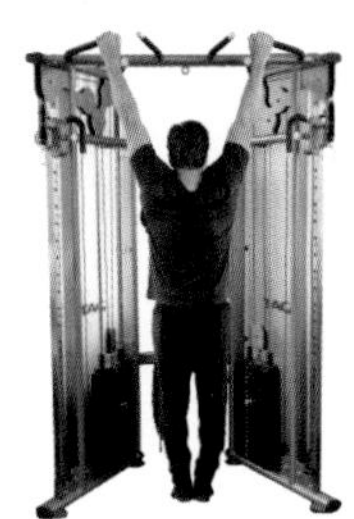

Pull-Up

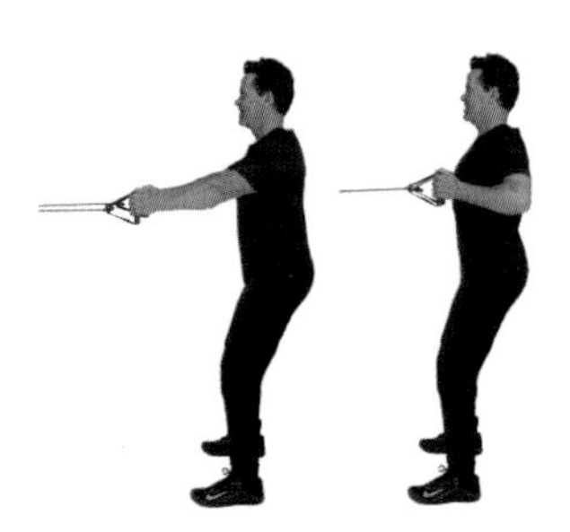

Row with Bands

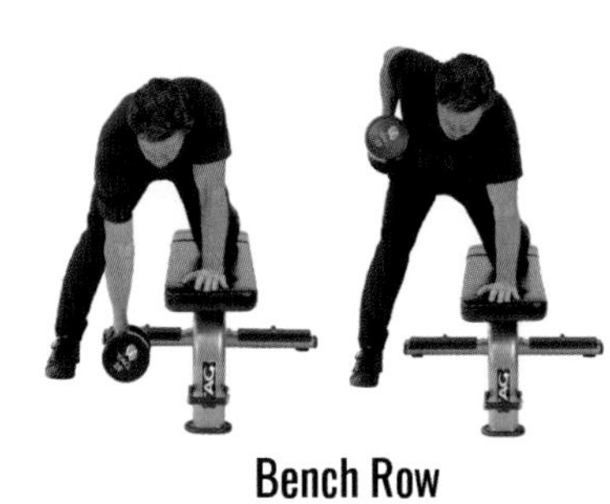

Bench Row

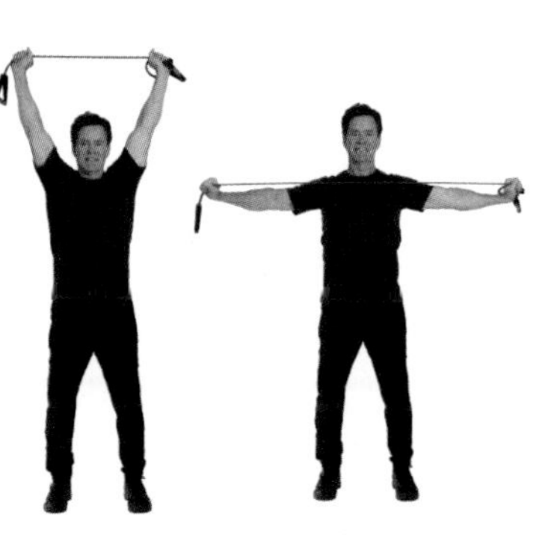

Standing Pull-Over

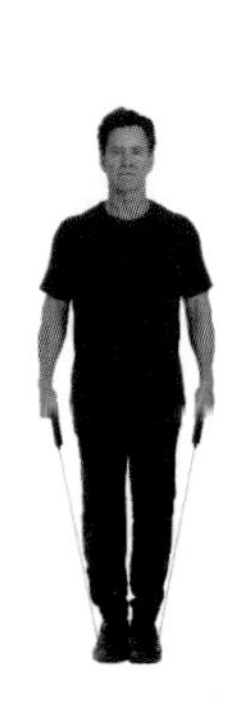

Overhead Thoracic Extension

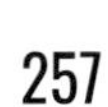

STRENGTH TRAINING—UPPER BODY

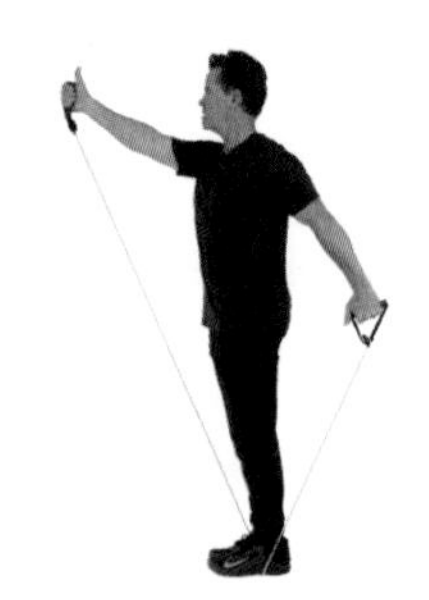

Toy Soldier

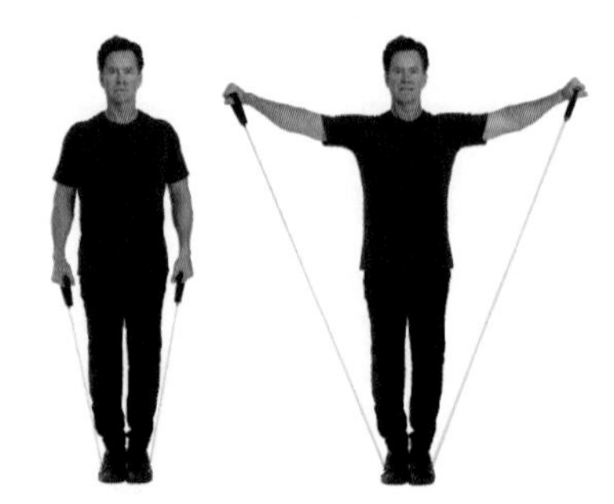

Side Raise

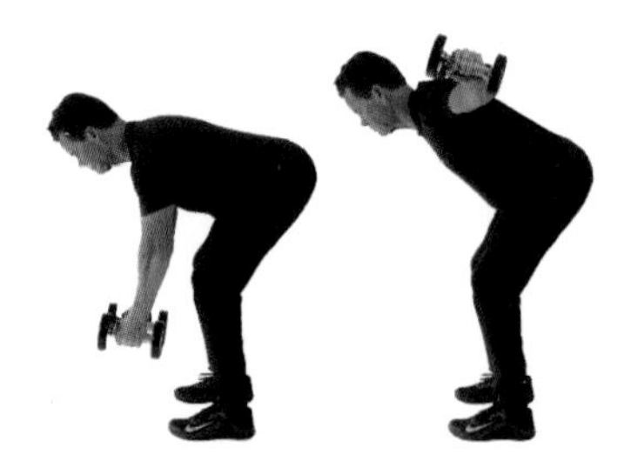

Reverse Fly

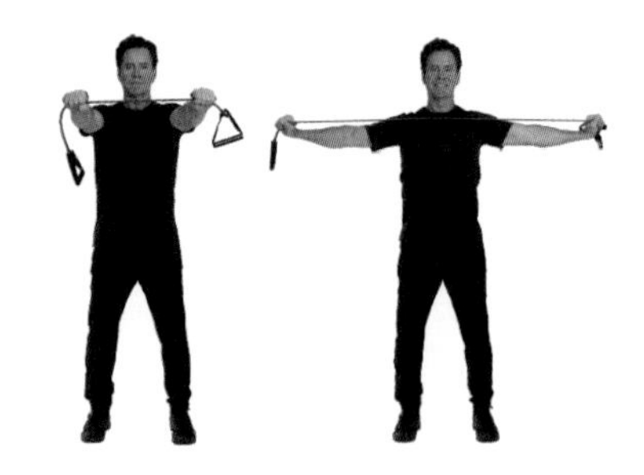

Wide Pull

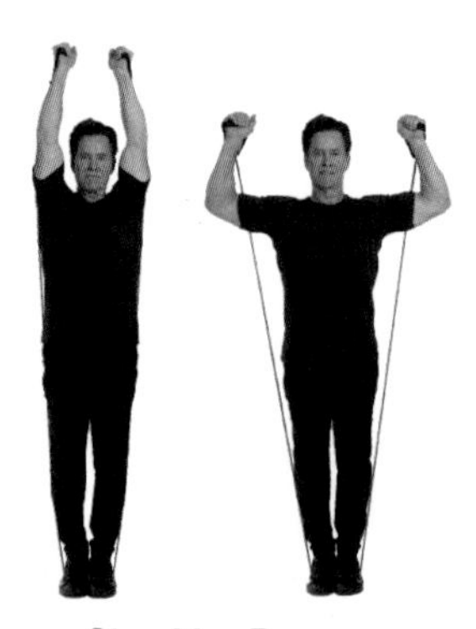

Shoulder Press

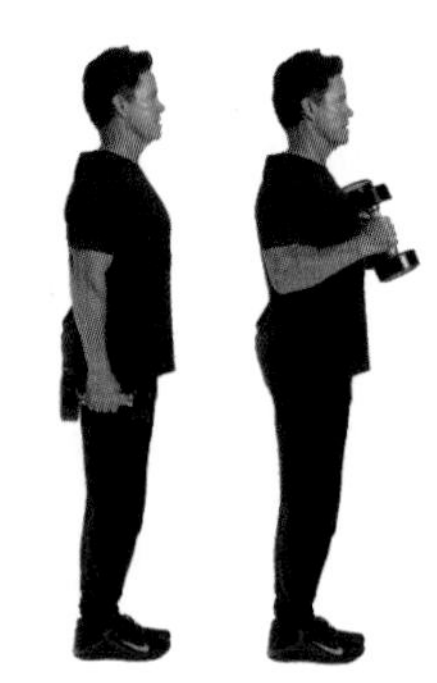

Biceps/Hammer Curl

STRENGTH TRAINING—UPPER BODY

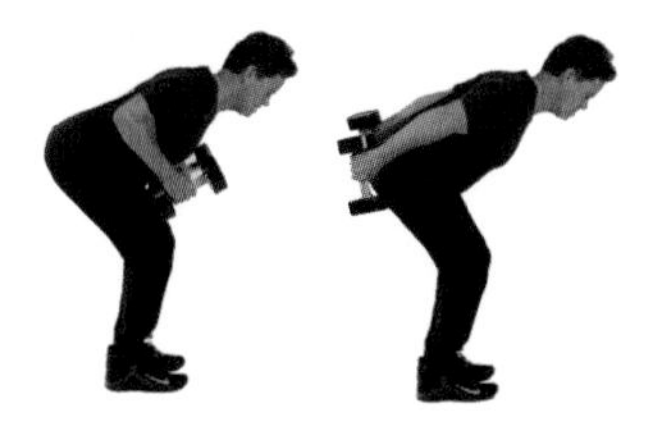

Triceps Kick-Back

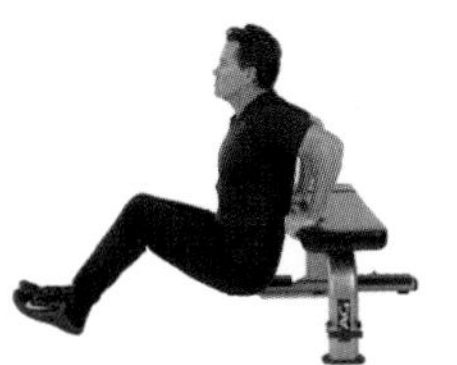

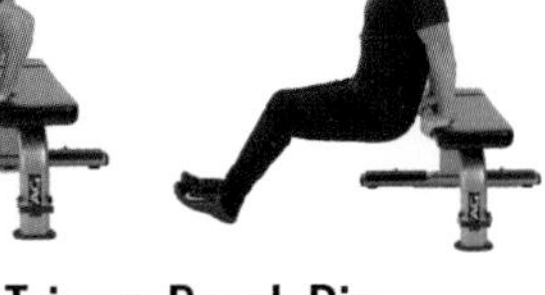

Triceps Bench Dip

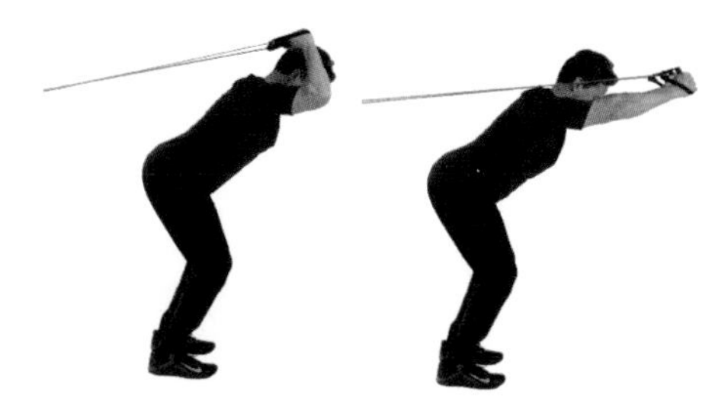

Triceps Extension

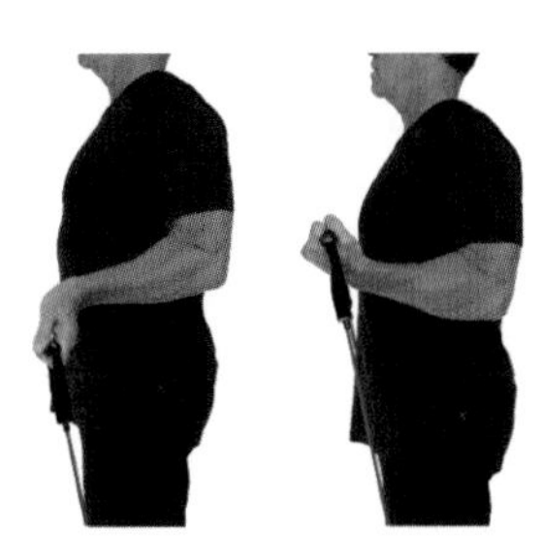

Forearms Flexion

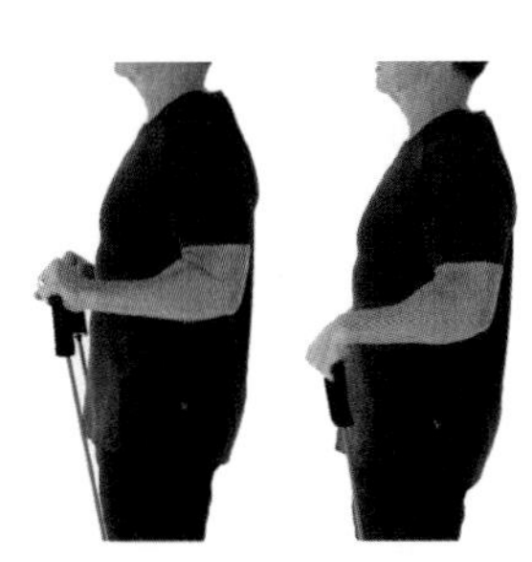

Forearms Extension

STRENGTH TRAINING—LOWER BODY

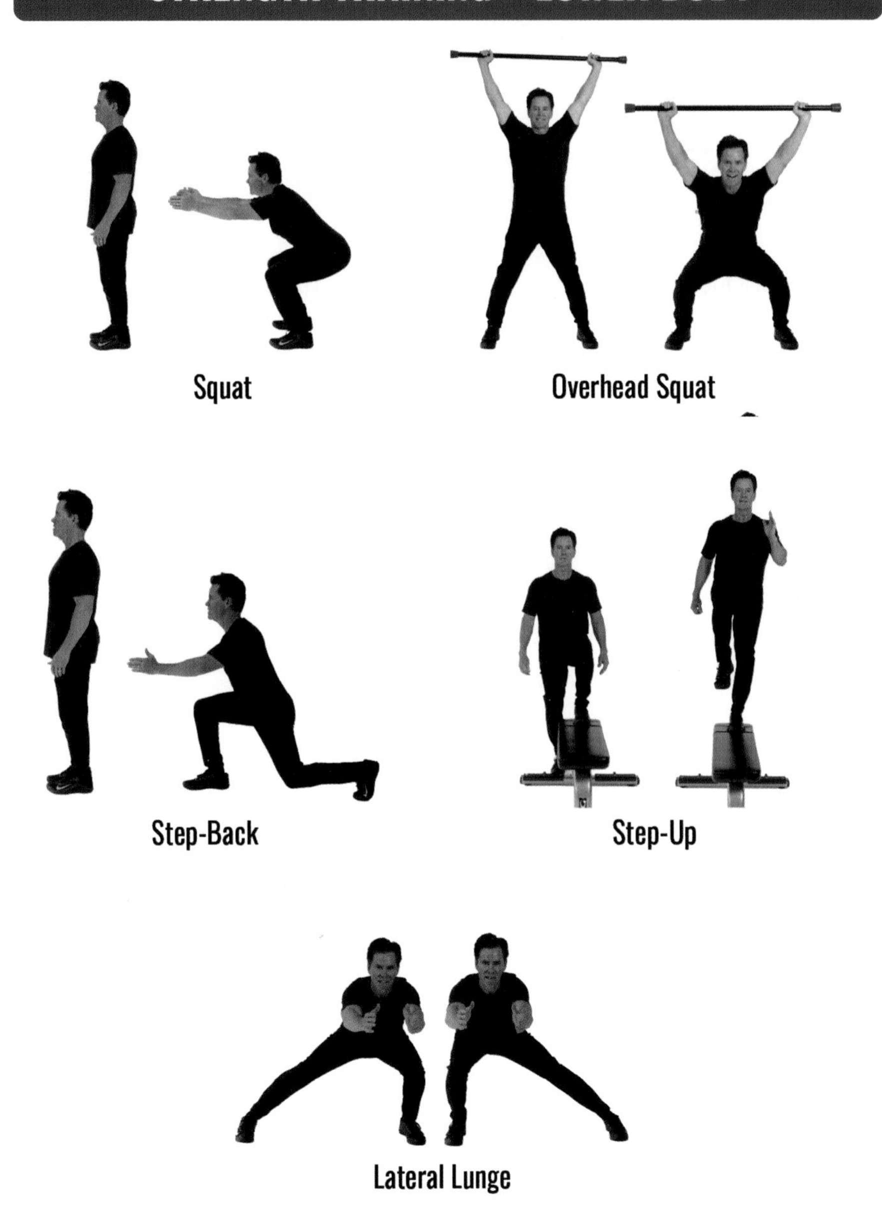

Squat

Overhead Squat

Step-Back

Step-Up

Lateral Lunge

STRENGTH TRAINING—LOWER BODY

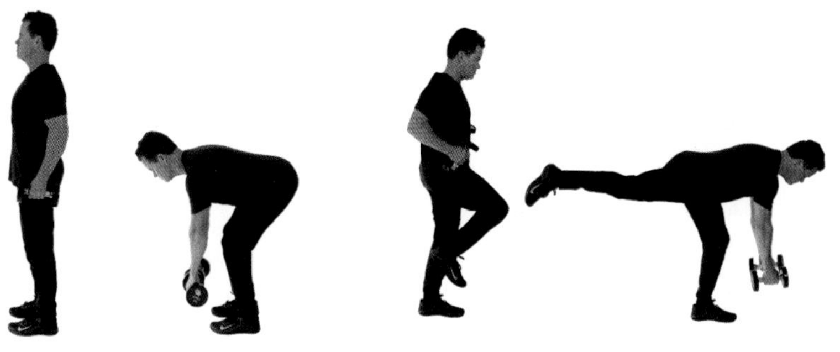

Bent Over Hamstrings

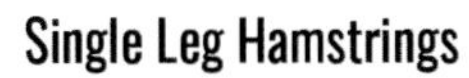

Single Leg Hamstrings

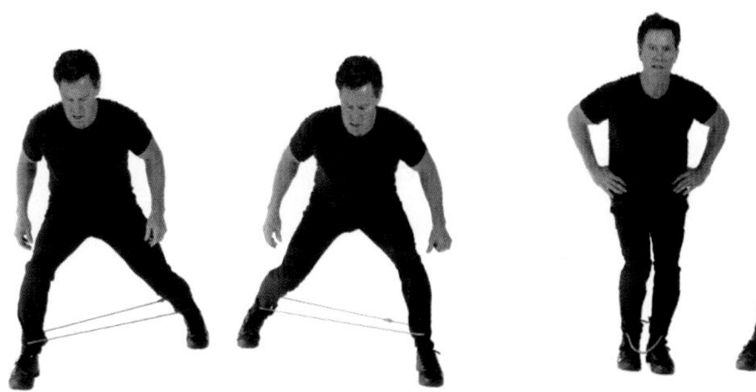

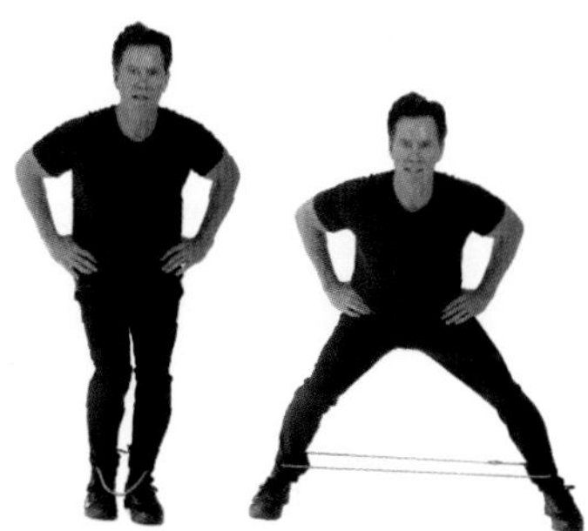

Tubing Monster Walk

Tubing Side Step

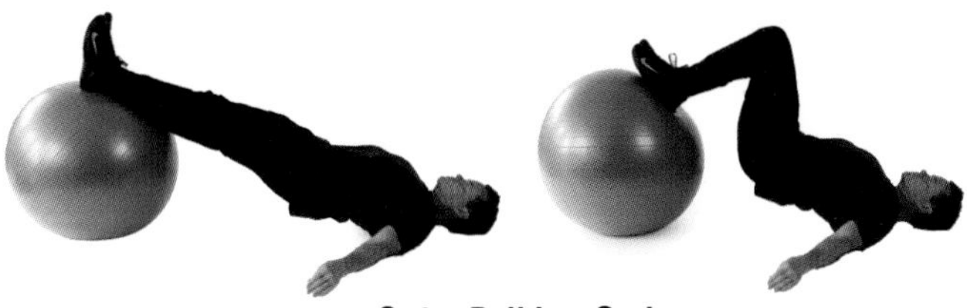

Swiss Ball Leg Curl

STRENGTH TRAINING—LOWER BODY

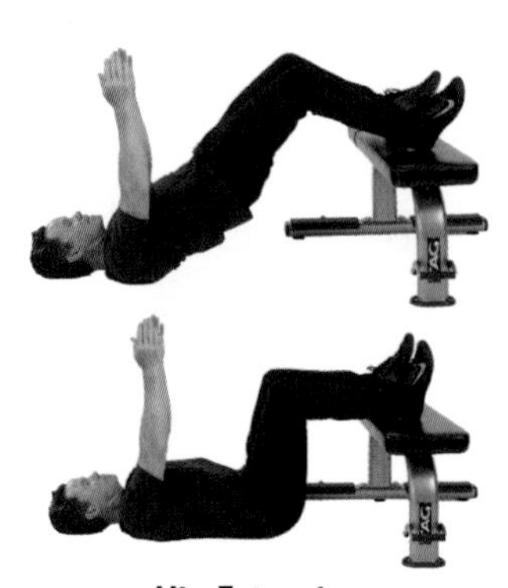

Hip Extension

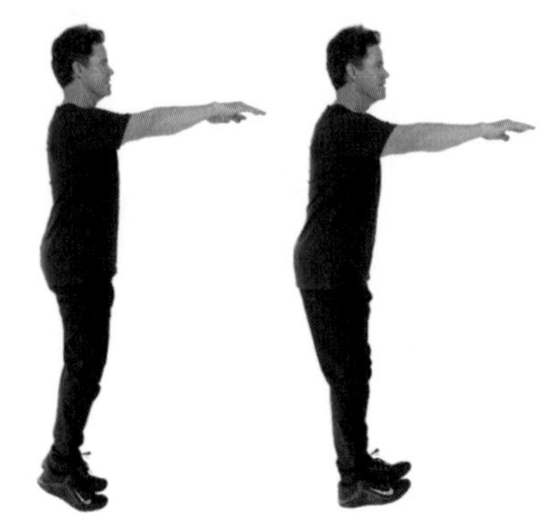

Calf Raise

STRENGTH TRAINING—CORE

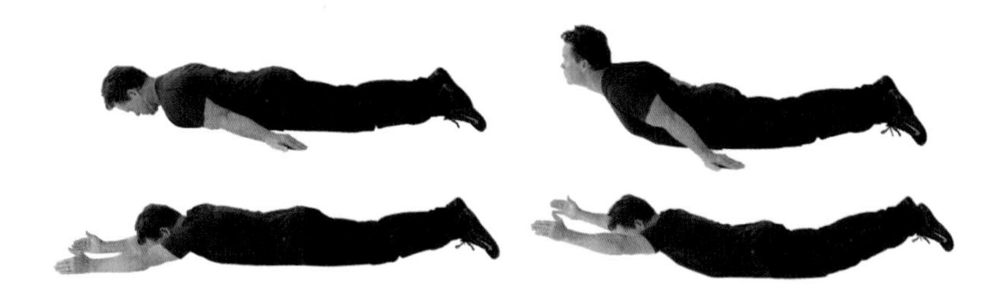

Back Extension

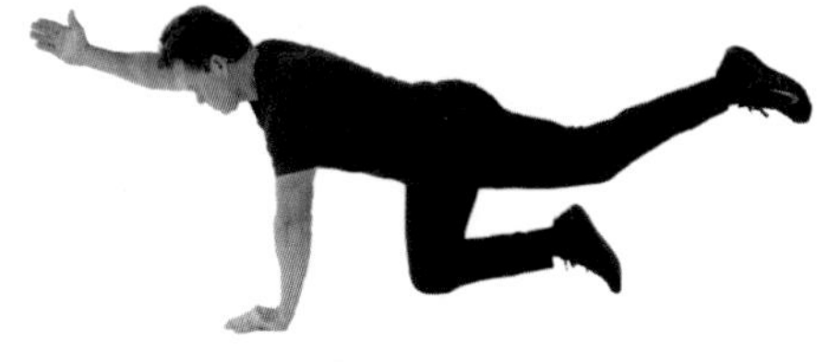

Spinal Balance

STRENGTH TRAINING—CORE

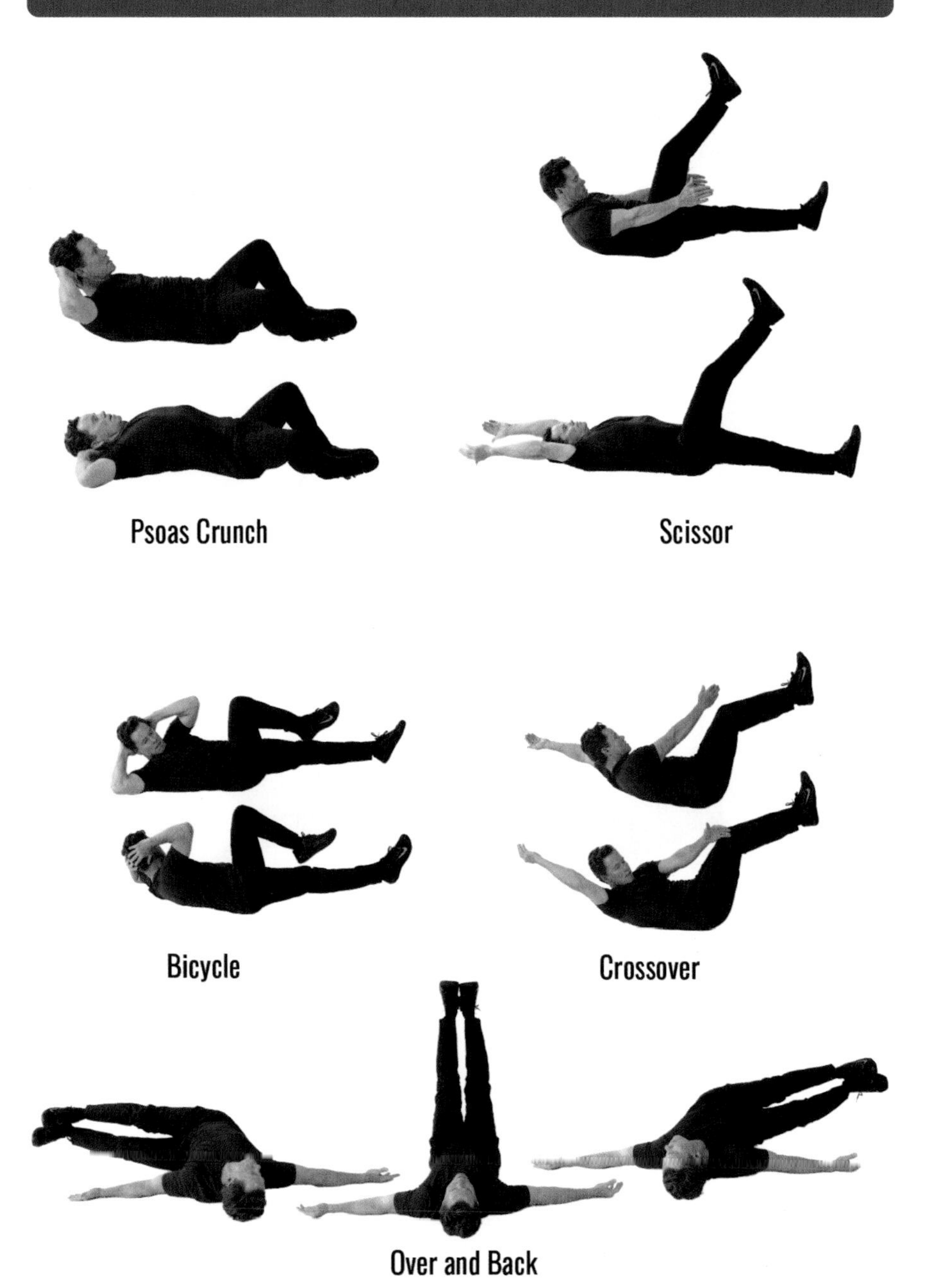

STRENGTH TRAINING—CORE

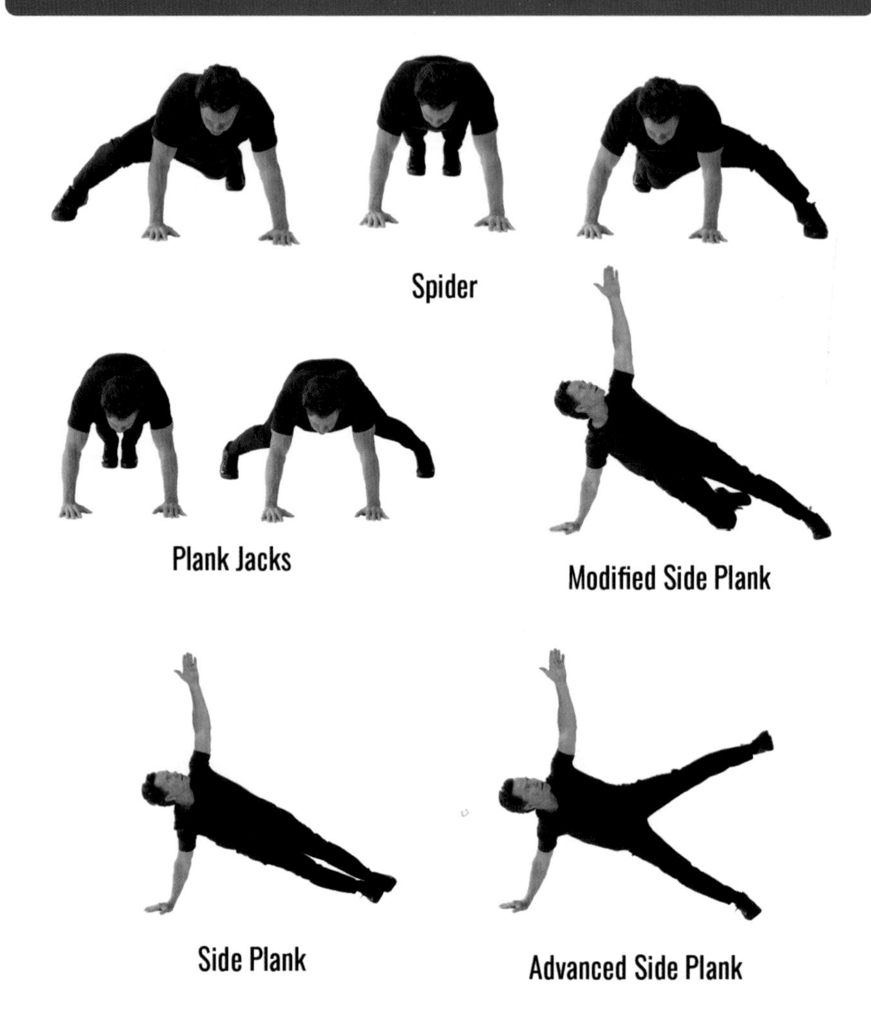

Spider

Plank Jacks

Modified Side Plank

Side Plank

Advanced Side Plank

STRENGTH TRAINING—CORE

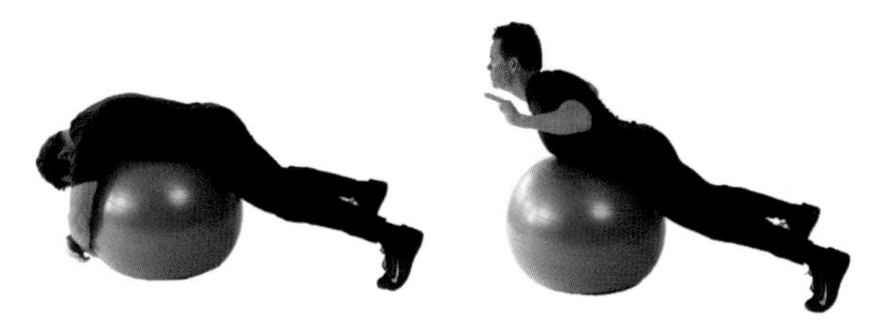

Swiss Ball Back Extension

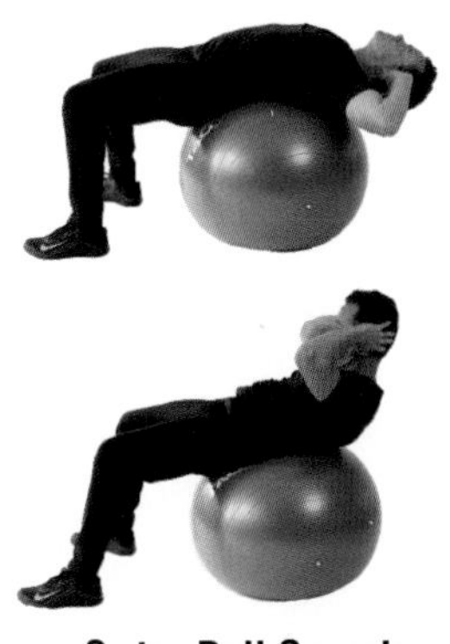

Swiss Ball Crunch

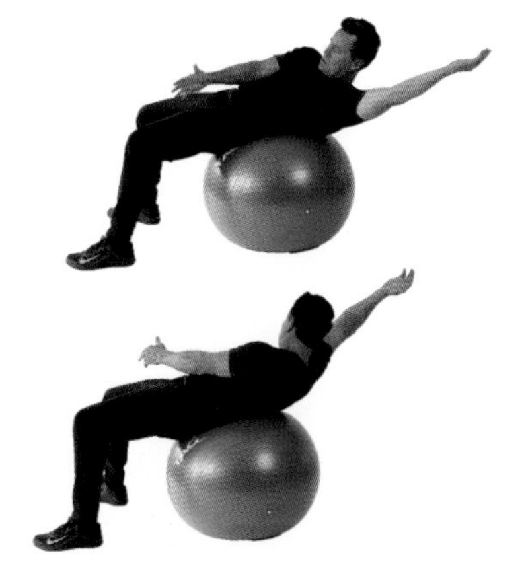

Swiss Ball Crossover

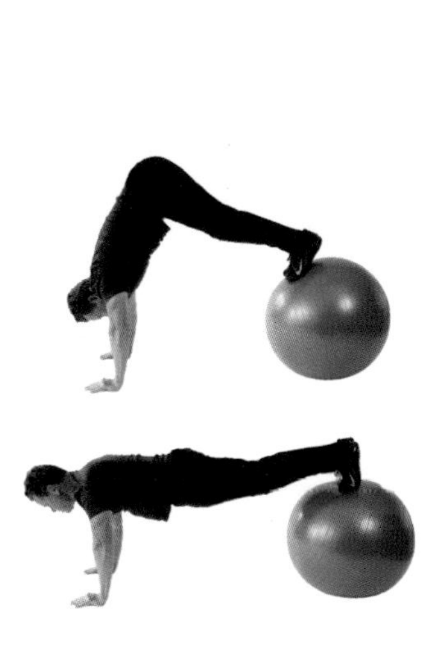

Swiss Ball Pike

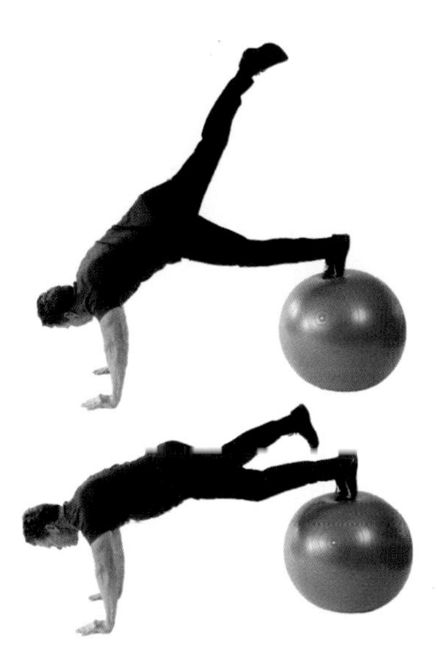

Swiss Ball Pommel Horse

Designing a Strength Training Program

Full-Body Strength Training Routine

A full-body strength training routine is a great option if you do not plan to strength train every day or if you are new to strength training. Work the entire body by doing 4-6 movements. As you progress add a few more strength training movements.

Here is a sample full-body strength training workout of six movements. All of these exercises can be performed in the gym or at home.

- Squat
- Step-Up
- Push-Up
- Standing Row
- Psoas Crunch
- Spinal Balance

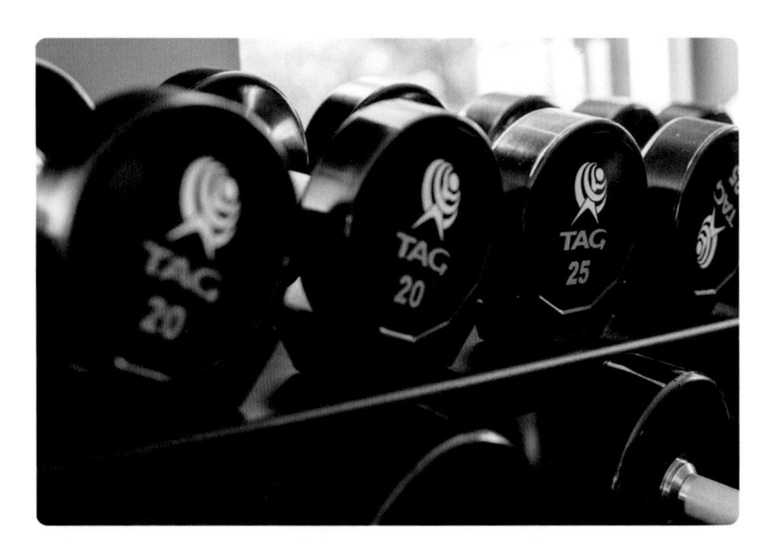

3-Day Split Strength Training Routine

As your strength training needs advance, add a few more movements or divide the routine into splits, such as upper body on one day and lower body on the next. I personally do a 3-day split strength training routine. Day one is chest/back/core. Day two is shoulders/arms core. Day three is lower body/core. It is quick, focused, efficient, effective, and I enjoy the workouts.

Here is a sample 3-day split strength training routine. All of these strength training movements can be performed in the gym or at home.

Day One: Chest/Back/Core

- Dumbbell Chest Press
- Lat Pull-Down or Pull-Up
- Cable, Band or Dumbbell Fly
- Standing Row
- Push-Up
- Standing Pull-Over
- Spinal Balance
- Back Extension

Day Two: Shoulders/Arms/Core

- Side Raise
- Thoracic Overhead Extension
- Reverse Fly or Wide Pull
- Biceps Curl
- Triceps Push-Down or Bench Dips
- Hammer Curls
- Triceps Extension
- Forearms - Flexion/Extension
- Spider
- Plank Jacks

Day Three: Lower Body/Core

- Squat
- Step-Up or Step-Back
- Lateral Lunge
- Supine Hip Extension or Swiss Ball Leg Curl
- Tubing Side Steps and Monster Walks
- Calf Raise - Flexion/Extension
- Floor Core Sequence
    - Psoas Crunch
    - Crossover
    - Over and Back

Before beginning a strength training program, ask yourself a few simple questions.

How would you rate your current fitness level on a 1-10 scale?

____

Are you new to strength training or are you looking to take your game up a notch or two? ______________________________

____

Have you ever used a professional personal trainer? Yes or No

What specific goals do you have in mind?

____

____

What injuries or challenges do you need to address prior to beginning your strength training plan?

____

____

How much time do you want to invest in your strength training plan to fit your needs or goals? ______________________________

____

Home Gym Equipment

Here are a few recommendations on how to set up a home gym.

- Determine the type of strength training you enjoy.
- Consider safety.
- Set a budget.
- Equipment options:
    - o Resistance Bands
    - o Dumbbells
    - o Padded Barbells
    - o Pull-Up Bar
    - o Swiss Ball
    - o Medicine Ball
    - o Multi-Station Strength Machine
    - o Mini Trampoline
    - o Portable Bench

Periodization Training

Years ago, my friend and colleague Matthew Cross first introduced me to a periodization training program to help me reach peak performance on demand. Matthew Cross is an international speaker and the founder and president of Leadership Alliance, a dynamic learning and training organization. Matthew has written multiple books. Two of my favorites are the *Divine Code* and *The Hoshin Success Compass*. As a thought leader, he works with some of the largest organizations in the world helping to guide them with his premier strategic alignment process.

Matthew is also an elite runner. Matthew knew I had competed in bodybuilding contests in the past. He wanted to share with me some of his thoughts on training using Fibonacci numbers and a specific book titled *Consistent Winning* written by Ronald Sandler and Dennis Lobstein. *Consistent Winning* explains the science behind periodization. Periodization refers to structured training periods built into an exercise training routine. Whether you are training for your first 5K, to climb Mt. Kilimanjaro, or to get in the best shape of your life, *Consistent Winning* is a great resource for taking your training to the next level.

89-Day Periodization Training Program

I have put together a sample 89-day training program that I follow a few times each year using the *Consistent Winning* process to bring more focus and energy to my training program. I start by taking some time to set the specific goals and metrics I want to accomplish. Then I follow it up by adopting targeted habits and a training plan. This plan is challenging. As I have learned over the years, the journey is where all the good stuff takes place.

Step 1: Set up Goals and Metrics

- Breaths per minute: 5
- Resting Heart Rate: 45
- Resting Blood Pressure: 110/70
- Body Weight: 170-175 lbs
- 10 Pull-Ups and 40 Push-Ups
- DB Chest Press: 90 lbs x 5 reps
- Diamond Handstand
- Improve Strength, Flexibility, Balance and Mobility
- Know My Numbers (blood work)
- Vibrant Health

Step 2: Set up Daily/Weekly/Monthly Habits

- Breath Work: 5-10 minutes/day
- Sleep: 8 hours
- Water: 80 ounces with lemons/oranges
- Fasting: 12-14 hour overnight fast
- Superfoods: wheatgrass, spirulina/chlorella, flax, hemp, chia, coconut, ginger, beets, greens
- 80/20 Rule
- 3-day Split Strength Training Routine
- Flexibility/Restorative Movements: 15-30 minutes daily
- Yoga: 30-45 minutes 1-2 x week
- Foam Roller: 5 minutes daily
- Epsom Salt Bath: 2 x week
- Massage: 2 x month

Step 3: Set up the Training Program

Dynamic Warm-up: 2-3 minutes daily

Foundation Movements: 5-6 minutes daily

Restorative Movements: 5-10-minutes daily

Cardio: 10-25 minutes 3-6 x week

Strength Training: 3-Day Split Strength Routine **(see pages 266-277)**

Reps/Sets/3 Rs: Begin each exercise with an easy warm-up set. As you flow through each set you will quickly get a feel for the amount of resistance needed for each movement or exercise and set. Also, there will be a few strength training movements where the resistance may change a little.

Active Rest: At the end of each week or month take a few days off to rest and recover. One way to help the mind and body recover is to participate in some form of active rest. Active rest activities are easy and relaxing. Here are a few of my favorite active rest activities: restorative movements, light stretching, a walk in the woods, an easy swim, or a fun game of ping pong.

Complete Rest: We all need to shut it down from time to time. Every week take a day off to rest. At the end of each month take 2 full days of complete rest. This allows your mind and body to heal and recover. Work on your breathing or meditate. Take an Epsom salt bath or get a massage. Take a nap. Give your mind and body the necessary time to rest and rejuvenate!

Sample Strength Training Monthly Progressions

Month One Training: (5 reps/5 sets)
Rest: 2 days of Active Rest
2 days of Complete Rest

Month Two Training: (8 reps/4 sets)
Rest: 2 days of Active Rest
2 days of Complete Rest

Month Three Training: (13 reps/3 sets)
Rest: 2 days of Active Rest
2 days of Complete Rest

Training Tips: Focus on posture, technique, range of motion, rate of movement, number of reps and sets, and resistance. Don't forget to sprinkle in some valuable rest and recovery.

There is no greater exercise to turn back the hands of time than strength training!

Videos of these strength training movements can be found on our ***app*** at ***ontargetliving.com***.

Strength Training Essentials

Big Picture

- Proper posture alignment is essential for injury prevention and greater performance.
- Learn how to strength train from an experienced professional.
- Breath is a great indicator if the intensity of the strength movement is too high.
- Reps = the number of repetitions per exercise or movement.
- Sets = the number of times you repeat the movement.
- The "3 Rs" are Range, Rate, and Resistance.
- Rest and recovery play an important role in your health and fitness plan.
- Every strength training movement has a progression.
- Training Specificity—Exercise with a specific goal in mind.

Ask Yourself

- How would you rate your current fitness level?
- Have you ever done any form of strength training before?
- Where did you learn how to strength train?
- What are some of the goals you want to accomplish through strength training?

Small Steps

- Start with 4-6 simple strength training exercises that may be done at home or in the gym.
- Hire a professional personal trainer for 2-5 sessions to help you develop your strength training plan.
- Posture! Posture! Posture! Maintaining good posture is essential for greater results and staying free of injury when strength training.
- Enjoy the incredible benefits strength training can bring to your life
- To fully engage, download our ***app*** at ***ontargetliving.com***.

28 Perfecting the Ordinary

I wanted to introduce a variety of small but powerful nuggets that are rarely discussed. This is what I like to call "Perfecting the Ordinary."

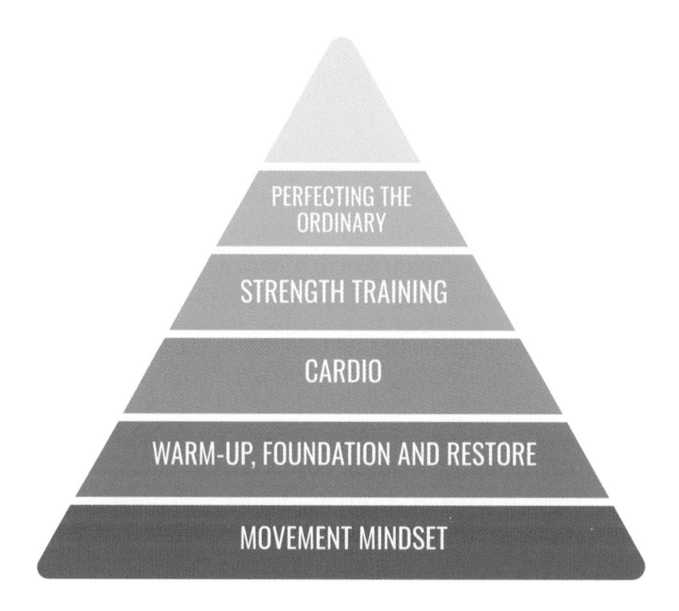

Much of the wisdom in this chapter comes from spending thousands of hours in the gym personally and professionally. Sometimes what we learn does not come from a textbook, a certification, or taking another class. It comes from doing, from trial and error, from colleagues and clients, and it comes from the love, passion, and the precious time we put into our craft. No shortcuts, no hacking. It comes from time. Therefore, I am highlighting some of the most important things to focus on and practice so they can be perfected and adopted as habits and rituals.

Learning From Others

I have been given an incredible gift over my 30-plus year career. I have been able to be inspired by and work with some of the best and brightest friends, healthcare professionals, and personal trainers in the world! Friends and colleagues such as Tab, Dennie, Marty, John, Phil, Matthew, Todd, Tracy, Beth, Jason, Justin, Gabe, Stacey, Damian, Brian, Jeremy, Jen, Gay, and Ann.

One personal trainer I want to highlight is my friend and colleague Walt Reynolds. Walt and I have been friends for over 30 years, and Walt is the guy I go to see for my training. To set the table, Walt was an Olympic-caliber high jumper back in his days at the University of Oregon, jumping over 7 feet. This guy has some hops! Today at the age of 57, Walt is a co-owner of The Trainers Studio, a very successful private training studio located in our community. I describe Walt this way, "Walt is a freak show." Standing 6 feet tall, Walt is lean, strong, and extremely flexible. Some of the movements Walt can still do today are hard to believe. When I think I am doing pretty good and sitting high in the saddle, I go see Walt and he opens up my eyes to what is possible.

Walt's knowledge in the exercise and training space is off the charts. Not only is Walt a great thinker, but I believe one of Walt's greatest attributes is his kindness. He is one of the kindest people you will ever meet.

When Walt and I get in a room together our conversations around health, fitness, and life can go on for hours. I hope you enjoy some of these Health & Fitness movement nuggets, and that they will help you Perfect the Ordinary!

Compound Interest

One of the hardest things in helping others change their lifestyle is to get people to embrace the concept of compound interest. Understanding that even the smallest improvements in lifestyle, applied on a daily basis, will pay off greatly in the future. This is the power of compound interest. We all know that when we make deposits, large or small, day in and day out into our bank account, our money continues to grow and grow and grow. The same is true when it comes our "health and fitness" bank account. Consistent deposits each day will reap great rewards to our lifestyle in the future.

- Drink that extra 8 ounces of water each day.
- Take 1 tablespoon of cod liver oil each morning.
- Walk for 10 minutes every morning.
- Do 1-2 sets of 8-10 repetitions of push-ups or squats.
- Eat a big salad 3-5 times each week.
- Get that extra 30 minutes of sleep.
- Take an Epsom salt bath prior to bed.
- Practice breathing exercises for 1-2 minutes a day.

It is the small stuff that adds up to huge changes over time. As Warren Buffet says, "Patterns Matter."

Posture Awareness and Practice

As was mentioned in chapter 24, posture is a big deal. We are all fighting a battle with gravity as we age. We all can recognize great posture when we watch someone walk into a room with their chest up, shoulders down, and head held high. Good posture is a look of health and vitality.

During your day, be aware of your posture when you are sitting, standing, walking, playing, and exercising. Good posture can be learned and must be practiced daily. Here are the five key checkpoints for ideal posture. When they all line up the body sings. (See page 219)

- Ear
- Shoulder
- Hip
- Knee
- Ankle

One Perfect Rep

When exercising or moving our body, whether it is some form of strength training, stretching, walking, jogging, running, or swimming laps, try to focus on doing one perfect rep. What would a perfect push-up, a perfect pull-up, or perfect squat look like? What would it feel like? As we strive to perfect each movement or exercise, we not only train our muscles and connective tissue, we also train our nervous system. Our nervous system tells our mind and body how to move in space. This is why it is so important to learn how to do a specific movement or exercise correctly right from the beginning. Try the "One Perfect Rep" training method when performing a push-up, pull-up, standing row, bodyweight squat, handstand, or when training to swim or run more efficiently.

Whatever type of training or movement plan you currently follow, step back and ask yourself how you can make each movement better or each individual rep better. If you can do one perfect push-up or one perfect bodyweight squat when you hit 90 years old, not only will you have the capacity to move better, you will also look like you can move. Remember, form follows function.

Find Your Edge

Imagine standing on the edge of a cliff with solid and secure footing. What would happen if you moved a few feet closer or stepped off the edge? One of the challenges when exercising or moving is finding our edge. The greatest gains take place at the edge. Maybe running a 7-mph pace is no problem, but how would taking it to 8 mph feel? How would our hamstrings and lungs respond? Maybe a handstand with the hands positioned 18 inches from the wall is attainable but moving the hands 6 inches closer to the wall would be more challenging for the shoulders.

The next time you work out, pick one or two exercises, and try to find your edge. It could be a simple bodyweight squat and your edge is limited due to a lack of flexibility stemming from your ankles or knees. Finding your edge allows you to make the greatest gains without getting injured in the process.

Gain a New Perspective

The huge value when working with a personal trainer is not always the Xs and Os. It can be picking their brain on how they think. When do they fit their daily exercise in or what do their sleep habits look like? How do they plan their recovery, sleep, morning rituals, meals, workouts, or goals?

Anytime I discuss nutrition, training, or anything related to health and fitness with a client, friend, family member, or colleague, I ask them what they have learned.

When on a diet what is going on in your mind? How do you feel? What does your self-talk look like? What have you learned? How can you apply this knowledge to your future success?

How you THINK is...........How you MOVE is.............How you LIVE!

Changing the narrative on how you think is priceless!

Never Stop Learning

I love to learn new things or new ways to tackle a problem or challenge. Developing new lifestyle habits that fit into a daily routine may take some time and additional learning along the way.

Lifelong Learning

While in graduate school at Michigan State University I had the privilege to study under some incredible professors including Dr. Wayne Van Huss. Dr. Van Huss was the director of the Human Energy Research Laboratory and professor in the Department of Kinesiology. Dr. Van Huss along with Dr. William Heusner were also involved in helping NASA astronauts deal with the effects of space on human organs. Both of these men where legends in the field of exercise physiology.

Because I was working full-time while in school, I had a commitment that would not allow me to take the final exam on the designated date. I asked

Dr. Van Huss if I could take the exam at another time. He said that was no problem. A few days later, I met Dr. Van Huss to take my exam. He walked downstairs with me to an empty classroom and handed me the exam. As he was about to close the door he said, "Chris, I am heading home for the day. When you are done with your exam, slide it under the door."

A few days later I met with Dr. Van Huss to go over my test results. After we discussed the exam, I inquired of Dr. Van Huss, "You put me in a room, shut the door, and told me to put the exam under the door when it was completed. I had a backpack full of books and notes. Didn't you worry about me cheating?" I will never forget what he said. "Chris, you are here to learn. You are not here to get a score. Life is not about the score, but the learning that takes place along the way." Dr. Wayne Van Huss believed that the character of a person, rather than their achievements, mattered the most.

The Magic Dust is in the Journey

I recently listened to a podcast which debated the different methods of training to reap maximal benefits. The discussion included one scientific study after another. What was missing in the debate were the hundreds of other intangibles that take place when moving the body.

One day I posed a question to one of my favorite personal clients Bob Cornwell. If I could give him a pill to help get in the best shape of his life, would he take it? Without hesitation Bob said no. Bob quickly pointed out, "The Magic Dust is in the journey. Why would I want to take a pill and lose out on all the special experiences that take place during my journey? The magic dust is how it affects my mind, my emotions, how it helps me relieve stress and gain patience, perseverance, grit, and confidence. It is the journey that makes it special!"

Learning how to find enjoyment in your lifestyle journey is often overlooked. Finding physical activities that you enjoy is a powerful way to stay intrinsically motivated and moving for life! Get into your body. Be still and take out the earbuds.

What does your mind and body say to you when you are moving?

____

____

Do you enjoy the process of strength training, walking, jogging, playing tennis or pickleball, or going for a swim? Yes or No

How can you enjoy moving your body?

____

____

What are some new movement activities you would like to try?

____

____

How do you feel after you have moved your body?

____

____

What have you learned about yourself?

____

____

Perfecting the Ordinary Essentials

Big Picture

- Compound interest is a powerful lifestyle ingredient.
- One perfect rep is foundational to optimal results.
- Find your edge.
- Stay curious.
- Never stop learning.
- Remember, the magic dust takes place during the journey.

Ask Yourself

- What do you think about when you are moving your body?
- How can you enjoy the process of exercise or moving your body?
- What have you learned from dieting?
- What can you learn from working with a trainer?
- Have you ever tried to do one perfect rep?
- How can you perfect the ordinary?

Small Steps

- Apply compound interest to your movement plan.
- The next time you exercise, apply the perfect rep principle to your entire workout.
- Take one or two exercises and find your edge.
- Try new activities.
- Think about what you have learned during your movement journey.
- Find Your Magic Dust!

29 Time to Play

What would a world with no play look like, feel like, or sound like? What if there was no running, no jumping, no climbing, no skipping, or no games? It is hard to imagine. Let's take a journey back in time and examine the world of play and how play impacts the health of our mind and the health of our body from birth to the end of life. Play completes the MOVE pyramid.

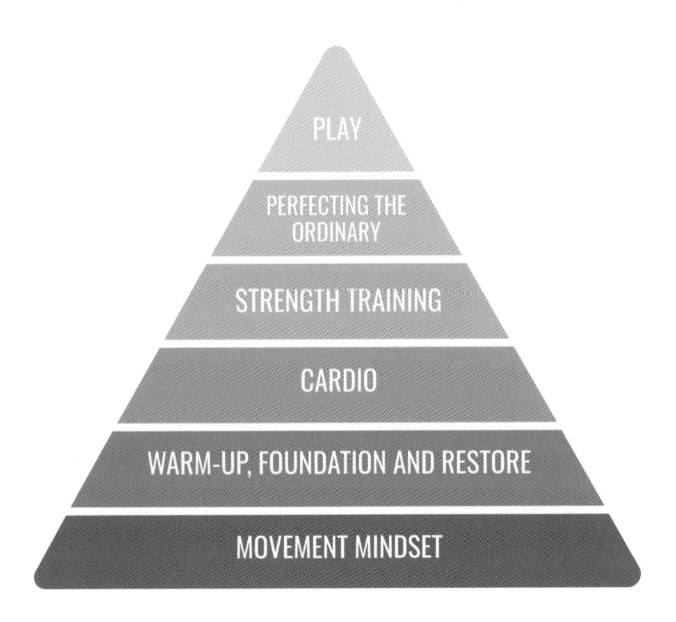

Definition of Play

A survey of 100 people on their definition of play would most likely result in 100 different answers. Wikipedia defines play as "a range of intrinsically motivated activities done for recreational pleasure and enjoyment." Play is commonly associated with children, but play occurs at any life stage, and among higher-functioning animals as well, most notably mammals and birds. My big takeaway from this definition comes from two words—"intrinsically motivated"—motivation that is driven from within. There are so many interpretations and definitions of play. Here are just a few.

- Body Play: Jumping up and down or wiggling around
- Object Play: Molding a piece of clay or a snowball with our hands
- Rough and Tumble Play: Always one of my favorite ways to play
- Solo Play: Building a sandcastle at the beach

- Group Play: Pick-up games of baseball, basketball, or football with the kids in the neighborhood
- Imagination Play: Hitting a home run in the bottom of the 9th or walking on the moon
- Verbal and Non-Verbal Play: Joking, teasing, flirting

Play may be difficult to define, but I believe most people recognize play when they see or hear it. Take a moment to observe and listen to a playground full of kids. They are climbing on the monkey bars, swinging on the swing set, running around playing tag, throwing a ball, or playing a game. What can be seen and heard is energy, laughter, fun, joy, excitement, and engagement. I think we all know what play looks, sounds, and feels like, and we like what play brings to our children.

Benefits of Play

The benefits of play are incredibly powerful. Play allows children to use their creativity while developing their physical, cognitive, and emotional strengths. Play is important to brain development. It helps children conquer their fears, explore, learn empathy and compassion, and interact with the world around them. Undirected play allows children to work together in groups, to share, negotiate, resolve conflicts, develop trust, and learn how to speak up for themselves.

Physically, play builds muscles and bones, improves coordination and dexterity, enhances body awareness, contributes to hormonal development, and burns calories. The more often a child plays, the more likely they will play as an adult. Play leads to a lifetime of movement.

What does play do for the brain? Nothing fires up the brain more than play. The cerebellum, frontal lobe, and the entire brain come alive during play. Play enhances memory and is essential for mental health.

As kids, when my older brother Nick and I started fighting, it drove our parents crazy. My mom would tell us to go outside and play. Most of the time that play would help us settle our differences by calming our minds and relaxing our bodies. How did mom know that going outside to play would work? Moms are so smart.

I believe one of the greatest benefits of play is the emotional impact it brings. The opposite of play is not work. The opposite of play is depression. If we do not play, we do not develop a fully functioning brain.

How do you feel when you are playing? How do you feel after you have played? Play brings joy to our hearts and souls.

Power of Play

I have been fascinated by play my entire life. Mom used to say, "All that boy likes to do is play." Even as an adult and now a grandpa, I love to play. I think my play gene came from my dad. He loved to play cards, croquet, golf, basketball, football, and games, as well as wrestle, tease, and joke. Dad was always in a playful mood. I loved this about him.

I became more interested in the topic of play after listening to an interview conducted by Guy Raz, the host of the Ted Radio Hour. Guy interviewed Dr. Stuart Brown, one of the leading authorities on the world of play. Dr. Brown's research shows that play is not just joyful and energizing. It is deeply involved with human development and intelligence. As the founder of the National Institute for Play, Dr. Brown is focused on the effect and importance of play in our lives. His research indicates that play is as basic a natural phenomenon as sleep, and, like sleep, many of us are not getting enough of it. A life devoid of play faces major health risks, such as depression, a compromised immune system, and many stress-related diseases including heart disease and cancer. On a larger scale, a culture devoid of play may even experience higher rates of violence and crime.

During the interview I learned that Dr. Brown was thrown into the world of play almost by accident. As a psychiatry student at Baylor in the 1960s, Dr. Brown was asked to interview mass murderer Charles Whitman to learn why he killed 16 people and wounded 31 others. Dr. Brown uncovered that as a child, little Charles was rarely seen outside playing in his yard. If Charles was found playing, his father severely punished him. Charles grew up in a household of violence and with little or no play.

The following year Dr. Brown took a trip to the Huntsville Prison in Texas to interview 26 convicted murderers in his quest to learn more about aggression, violence, empathy, and most importantly, to find a common thread among them. After interviewing all 26 convicted murderers, he found one common thread. All 26 men grew up without play! This discovery led Dr. Brown to understand that missing out on childhood play could lead to many physical and emotional problems. For the past 50 years Dr. Brown has been sharing the Power of Play with the world.

We Need to Play More

Unfortunately, many people, including parents, teachers, school systems, and organizations view play as frivolous, having little purpose or no value. This type of thinking has to change. What would happen if we walked into our next meeting with a beach ball and tossed it into the crowd? People would start laughing and smiling as they tossed the ball around. The energy in the room would ignite. We all need a better understanding how play impacts life, from beginning to end. Play is essential for optimal health and happiness throughout our entire life. Despite the incredible benefits derived from play, time for free play has been markedly reduced for both children and adults.

Kindergartners with No Play

When I was in kindergarten class at North Elementary School, my teacher, Mrs. Pick, who I loved, would take away recess if she got behind or the class was acting up. This left a mark on me to this day. How could Mrs. Pick take away the most valuable 40-minutes of our day? If you compared two different kindergarten classrooms, one that got recess and the other that did not, which group do you think would show better performance? The children who had an opportunity to go outside, run around, climb on the monkey bars, swing on the swing set, or play tag? Or the group of children who were stuck twitching in their seats with an incredible amount of pent-up energy?

A 1989 survey taken by the National Association of Elementary School Principals found that 96 percent of surveyed school systems had at least one recess period each day. A decade later the same survey found that only 70 percent of kindergarten classrooms had a recess period.

Play is a dying pastime, but in order for the mind and body to work together in harmony we all need some play. Our electronic devices and television can be engaging, but neither one connects the body to the mind like play does. Have you ever watched a dog play with another dog, or kids playing with other kids or adults? When we play, time seems to disappear. Sometimes our lives get out of sync. Life gets busy, and we may forget about the benefits and joys of play.

When was the last time you just played a basketball game, ran around the house chasing your kids or grandkids, swung on a swing set, jumped rope, went ice skating or sledding, skipped stones on the lake, climbed on the monkey bars, or played hide and seek, hopscotch, a game of tennis, ping pong, or croquet, or a joined a pickup game of baseball, football, or basketball?

Did you grow up playing as a child? Yes or no

What were a few of your favorite play activities as a child?

____

____

How do you feel when you are playing?

____

____

How do you feel after you have played?

____

____

On a 1-10 scale how important is play to you? ______________

How much time do you currently spend playing each week? ________

If you are currently not playing on a regular basis what may be holding you back?

____

____

What is your current favorite play activity?

____

What new play activity you would like to try?

____

Time to Play

To bring more play into our world it is essential to understand that play is more than just fun. Play has a powerful positive impact on our mind and body. Play makes us healthy and happy. What is your play history? Go back in time to some of your fondest memories of play. Maybe it was building a snow fort in the winter or a tree house in the summer. Maybe it was fishing with your grandmother and trying to catch minnows. Maybe it was swimming or water skiing at the lake. Maybe it was exploring in the woods or snow skiing.

Maybe it was racing your mom in the back yard or playing cards with your grandfather. Maybe it was joining a pick-up game of basketball with your neighborhood friends. Explore the past and revisit some of the powerful emotions surrounding play.

Infuse play into your daily life. Keep the activity unstructured with few or no guidelines or rules. Let it be just pure play. Find play activities that you enjoy. Experiment and try new ways to play. There is no right or wrong way to play. Now is the time for all of us to bring back some of that misspent youth. From infancy to the end of life, here's to more PLAY!

The Joy of Play

Growing up in Michigan all we did was play! Football on our knees, basketball without a hoop, and baseball in the basement with a Wiffle ball and a plastic bat were some of our favorite ways to play during long Michigan winters.

As we grew a little older it was baseball in the summer, playing two-on-two with Jeff, Rex, Marty, and me. Right field was closed, pitchers' hand, one ghost runner, four gloves, one or two bats, and one precious ball.

In the fall it was three-on-three or four-on-four football at the field with Paul, Marty, Jeff, Greg, Rock, Rick, John, Bruce, Danny, Fredder, and me. The play calls were simple—hook and pitch right, the bomb, the chair, double reverse, or Fredder's favorite, run straight up the middle.

For basketball in the winter, Don, Mike, Marty, and I shoveled off the neighbor's driveway. We ran the basketball under hot water so it would bounce and played for hours at a time.

Maybe this was a little too much misspent youth, but I would not trade one play date. The memories even today are priceless.

Play Essentials

Big Picture

- Play is a critical component for a healthy mind and body from birth to the end of life.
- Play is a range of intrinsically motivated activities done for recreational pleasure and enjoyment.
- Unfortunately many people, including parents, teachers, school systems, and organizations, view play as frivolous, having little purpose or value. This type of thinking has to change.
- The benefits of play are incredible.

Ask Yourself

- What were some of your favorite play activities growing up?
- How important is play to you now?
- How much time do you spend playing each week?
- What is your favorite play activity?
- How can you bring more play into your life and those around you?

Small Steps

- Understand the value of play and how it can impact your health and happiness.
- Find play activities you enjoy.
- Infuse play into your daily life.
- Plan your play time.
- Let's all bring more play into our world!

SECTION

6

YOUR HEALTH KEEPS SCORE

30 Decoding Your Health

Section 6 contains a variety of content that will help in your lifetime pursuit of greater health and feeling your best. Learning how to listen to your body, learning how to understand your numbers and improve them, and learning what you put in and on your body all play a large role in taking ownership of your health.

Is a headache the sign of an ibuprofen deficiency? Of course not! But for many, that is the first thing they try. Instead, maybe they need some water, some rest, or some food. How do we get so numb to our mind and body that we ignore the signs? When a plant starts to wilt, what do we do? We give it water, sunlight, and food. Sounds simple, but somewhere along the way, many people lose touch with their bodies and the curiosity of asking better questions.

Ask Better Questions

Years ago, while speaking at a large convention in Orlando, Florida, a member of the audience asked a question about atrial fibrillation, the fluttering of the heart. Many men get atrial fibrillation in their 50s, and many women get it in their 60s. Atrial fibrillation has become very common in the United States, but it is not normal and may be the beginning of more severe heart problems.

Six weeks after this conference I received a phone call from a woman who had been in the audience with her husband. She heard my talk about atrial fibrillation but said she had not really grasped everything I covered. She asked for my help for her husband. Help begins with asking good questions.

How old is your husband? Fifty-four years old. How long has your husband had atrial fibrillation? Two years. What medications is he on? An atrial fib medication along with a beta blocker.

I asked, "You have lost your husband, haven't you?" She said it was true, that her husband had little interest in his career and very little interest in her. He was tired all the time and had little energy and no vitality. She stated, "He is not the same guy I married."

Of course, he was not the same guy. He was taking a high dose beta blocker. Beta blockers are very powerful medications that slow everything down, including the heart, blood pressure, and brain waves. Beta blockers put the body in a protective state. One of their main side effects is how they deplete energy.

The questions continued. Is your husband taking any other medications, like pain medications such as Tylenol, Aleve, or Advil? She reported he had been taking Aleve for more than 10 years.

I told her I thought that might be his problem. When we take these powerful pain medications over a long period of time, they can damage gut health and leach out many valuable minerals. If we get a bee sting or toothache, taking these types of pain medications on an occasional basis in most cases is not a problem. However, taking them day in and day out for many years can be a problem. Daily use of pain-relieving medications may cause the body to leach out precious minerals like magnesium. Magnesium is the mineral of relaxation. It helps with headaches, helps you stay asleep, improves your blood pressure, and is essential for the contraction of the heart. I told her I believed her husband was deficient in magnesium and gave her these suggestions along encouraging him to work closely with his doctor.

First, have him stop taking the Aleve and replace it with cod liver oil and ground flaxseeds. Both are natural anti-inflammatory foods.

Second, work with his doctor and do not change any of his medications.

Third, have him start adding more magnesium into his body. He should take an Epsom salt bath twice a week. Put two cups of Epsom salt in a warm bath and soak for 10-15 minutes. Epsom salt is high in magnesium and is absorbed through the skin.

Fourth, bring on foods high in magnesium such as bananas, raisins, dried mangos and figs, cacao nibs, coconut, oatmeal, greens, nuts and many seeds, and frozen wheatgrass.

One year later her husband no longer had atrial fibrillation and was off all of his medications. Now she has her husband back!

Your Body is Always Talking. You Need to Listen!

Imagine driving down the highway and the engine light in the car comes on. Should we ignore it and hope the light goes off or take it to a mechanic?

Similar to the engine light, our body is always talking to us and giving us signs. But are we listening? For many, the thought of learning how to listen to our body may be completely new. That is okay. Self-awareness is the first step in making any change. We know our body better than anyone else, so it is imperative that we take ownership of our personal health.

This chapter is all about helping you understand what your body is telling you and how to listen. One thing I have learned and am still so passionate about after 30 years in this business is this—the magic is in all of us if we would listen and take care.

Our body will try to heal and self-correct if we just give it a chance. There are multiple ways our body talks to us.

- Eyes
- Teeth and Gums
- Breath
- Sleep
- Digestion and Elimination
- Energy
- Muscles, Tendons, and Ligaments
- Bones
- Skin, Hair, and Nails
- Body Weight

Eyes

In my mid 50s I had my first eye exam with one of my close friends, Dr. Ed Peters. Dr. Peters ran me through a battery of tests, took a few pictures of my eyes, and then we sat down to discuss what he had found. He showed me a few sample photos of the eye. We looked at eyes with macular degeneration, type 2 diabetes, high blood pressure, inflammation, along with a photo of a pair of healthy eyes. I was like a kid in the candy store. It was fascinating for me to see the eye and how it revealed so much. He explained how the tiny vessels inside the eyes can become damaged by type 2 diabetes or high blood pressure. In most cases, these conditions show up much earlier in eyes than through a traditional blood test. I never realized how important getting our eyes examined could be. We all need to get a regular eye exam so that changes over time can be detected.

Teeth and Gums

Another way our body talks is through the teeth and gums. Seniors who have great teeth and gums always fascinate me. How many people do you know over the age of 80 who have healthy teeth and gums? How many 80-, 90-, or 100-year-olds have all their original teeth? Healthy teeth and gums tell a great deal about the quality of our health. A dentist or dental hygienist can instantly recognize healthy teeth and gums as soon as we open our mouth.

Growing up, I was always told that if I ate too much sugar, I would get cavities. I did not want cavities, but I really liked sugar. It never dawned on me that what I ate and drank made a difference in the health of my teeth and gums. I figured that if I just brushed my teeth and flossed, I would be okay. Today, I have a much greater appreciation of the health of the teeth and gums and how powerful a role quality nutrition plays in keeping them healthy for life.

Dr. Weston Price, a dentist from Cleveland, Ohio, wrote a book back in 1939 titled *Nutrition and Physical Degeneration*. In it he describes fieldwork he did in the 1920s and 1930s in various world cultures. His book contains numerous photos of people he studied and includes comparison photos of the teeth and gums of people who lived on a traditional diet and people who had adopted or grew up on an industrial or processed food diet.

Dr. Price's research and photos are powerful reminders of how much a healthy lifestyle impacts the teeth and gums. Having regular dental checkups, daily brushing and flossing, keeping pH in balance, eating high-quality foods and beverages, and daily movement, along with proper rest and rejuvenation all play a role in keeping teeth and gums healthy for life.

Breath

As we discussed in Section 3, our breath is a key component to good health. In addition to the mechanics of how we breathe, our breath is an amazing sign of what is going on inside our body. Do you have chronic bad breath? Occasional bad breath is to be expected. When it becomes more chronic, it could be a sign of other health problems.

Years ago, my wife Paula mentioned that my breath smelled funny again. This was usually after working a 14-15-hour day for Butternut Bread and getting less than five hours of sleep. I now realize I had acetone breath due to metabolic acidosis. What causes acetone breath? In most cases it comes from metabolic acidosis, which is a condition that occurs when the body produces too much acid or when the kidneys are not removing enough acid from the body. Too much acid in the body causes it to go into ketosis. While in ketosis, the breath may smell like nail polish. That is why it is referred to as acetone breath. It is a little more complicated than this, but for simplicity's sake, this is the big picture. If left unchecked over time, metabolic acidosis can lead to severe health problems including death.

What causes this excess acid in the body? It could be linked to working long hours without enough rest, too much stress, not getting enough sleep, going too long without eating, dehydration, a high protein or low carbohydrate diet, too much coffee, energy drinks, too much aspirin and anti-inflammatories, over-training in the gym, or not getting enough proper nutrients in our diet.

Acetone breath is not normal. It is another way our body is talking to us. Scientists are now developing tests to diagnose a growing list of diseases based on breath, such as asthma, diabetes, lung cancer, kidney and liver disease, IBS, and lactose intolerance, to name a few. Scientists are identifying thousands of chemical compounds that create these distinct odors. This type of noninvasive technology is exciting for the future.

Sleep

When life starts getting out of balance, sleep may begin to suffer, leading to a drop in energy, a compromised immune system, and a foggy brain. The answer to a better night of sleep is not found in a sleep aid, but in learning how to listen to our body. Review Section 3 to learn more about the power of sleep.

Digestion and Elimination

Much was said about digestion and elimination in Section 4. Remember that the health of the human body begins in the gut. It is not only what we put into the body that makes the difference in our health, but also how our body breaks down, absorbs, and eliminates the nutrients we eat and drink. If we are not having a regular bowel movement or it does not look like a soft banana, the body is talking and telling us something is not right.

When the body is dehydrated, urine will look too dark. If we pinch the skin on our hand and it does not bounce back, we may be dehydrated. When skin does not look healthy, poor digestion or elimination can be the root cause.

Energy

Another way our body is talking to us is our energy. Energy is our most precious commodity, but very few of us have been taught how to recognize ways to build and protect our energy. Energy is critical for optimal health and performance.

When I am on the road, I know it is essential for me to eat right, consume my superfoods, stay well-hydrated, stretch, move my body, take hot and cold showers, do my breath work, and get plenty of sleep. Without these, I will not feel and be my best.

It is not a shock that today many people are constantly complaining about their lack of energy. I had to laugh when I did an internet search for the word, "energy." The first thing that popped up on the screen was an advertisement for low testosterone. Not one word was mentioned about lack of sleep, poor nutrition, or too much stress. I believe that we could all use more energy now and then. But the answer cannot be found by consuming more caffeine or energy drinks.

The conversation begins with where and how we get our energy. Our main source of energy comes from the foods and beverages we consume, followed by a good night of sleep, sunlight, space, daily movement, and controlling stress.

If we lack energy, could it be due to some poor lifestyle habits? Could low energy be due to some of the medications we currently take? If our energy is not what we think it should be, we need to begin with the basics and build energy habits and strategies into each day to help maintain great energy throughout the day.

How would you rate your energy level on a 1-10 scale, with 10 having great energy most of the time? ______________________________

Do you feel fatigued more than you think you should? Yes or No

Do you need caffeine or some type of stimulant to get through your day? Yes or No

How do you feel on a regular basis? ______________________________

____

Muscles, Tendons, and Ligaments

One of the areas that many people recognize, but may be confused by, is why their muscles, tendons, and ligaments ache.

Do you feel stiff on a daily basis? Yes or No

Have you lost flexibility? Yes or No

Do your muscles ache more than you think they should? Yes or No

Has your strength slowly declined? Yes or No

What do you believe may be contributing to your stiffness, lack of flexibility, or aching muscles?

____

____

The answer is not more anti-inflammatories or pain medications. The answer lies within us. Too much acid may lead to inflammation and joint pain.

Is your pH out of balance and you are too acidic? Yes or No

Does your diet need some improvement? Yes or No

Is your diet deficient in valuable nutrients such as B vitamins, zinc, magnesium, or omega-3 fats? Yes or No

Do you get a good night of sleep on a regular basis? Yes or No

Are your stress levels out of control? Yes or No

Do you move your body on a daily basis? Yes or No

Is strength training part of your current exercise program? Yes or No

There are several ways to keep muscles and connective tissue strong and flexible and keep pain and discomfort under control without using anti-inflammatories. One big strategy is to consume more high-quality foods and beverages. These include white figs, dried mangos, bananas, raisins, berries, greens, cacao nibs, coconut, macadamia nuts, frozen wheatgrass, spirulina/chlorella, cod liver oil, ground flaxseeds, and water with lemon or ginger. Add in regular strength training, dynamic warm-up, foundation, and restorative movements. Use a foam roller and get massages twice a month. Take Epsom salt baths and plan downtime. All can play a major role in keeping muscles and connective tissue strong with less pain.

The Solution Does Not Come in a Pill

One day as I was getting dressed at my local health club, a guy a few lockers away asked me if I had a Motrin for his headache. I did not have a Motrin or any other type of headache medicine. I wondered whether I should let this conversation go or should I go a little deeper and ask a few more questions about his headache? In most cases, I try not to be the food or exercise police, but sometimes I cannot help myself. So, I began asking him a few questions. How much water are you drinking? Are you consuming any type of omega-3 fats? How is your sleep? Do you breathe with your chest or belly? Do you consume foods high in magnesium or vitamin D3?

You should have seen this guy scrambling to get out of the locker room. I think he set a land speed record for getting dressed. What started as a simple request for a Motrin led to a battery of questions.

Bone Health and Calcium

We receive many questions from people asking about calcium supplements or specific medications to improve bone health. Why do we have such poor bone health in the United States, when in fact we have the highest intake of calcium in the world? In America, calcium in the diet is often synonymous with the use of dairy products.

I rarely recommend taking calcium supplements or consuming dairy products to improve bone health. Most calcium supplements are difficult for the body to absorb leading to high levels of calcium in the bloodstream and increased calcification in our vessels. Second, dairy is a poor source of calcium. Over 32 percent of available calcium is destroyed when food is heated above 150 degrees Fahrenheit. This makes pasteurized milk a poor source of calcium.

In Petaluma, California, known as the egg capital of the world, egg farmers know that if they want to produce eggshells hard enough not to break, they feed kale, spinach, and foods high in chlorophyll, not dairy, to the hens. For a list of foods high in calcium, magnesium, and iodine. See Section 2.

Other Contributors to Bone Health

Decreasing the consumption of processed sugar, soda pop, alcohol, and processed foods improves pH balance. A more alkaline gut protects and preserves calcium and magnesium, two powerful minerals for healthy bones. Magnesium is essential for calcium absorption. Lowering stress can prevent leaching this and other valuable minerals from the body.

Vitamin D is also necessary for greater bone health. Get outside into some natural sunlight and take a dose of cod liver oil every day. Both are essential to improving vitamin D3 levels.

Of course, we must not forget the role that movement, especially strength training, plays in bone health. Bones are alive and they adapt when added stress is applied. Regular weight bearing exercises, along with strength training, stress the bones and connective tissue and make them adapt and become stronger.

Skin, Hair, and Nails

The body also talks to us through our skin, hair, and nails. Skin rashes, cracked or discolored nails, psoriasis, brittle or thinning hair, or dandruff mean that there is some imbalance in the body, and it is time to take notice.

The first signs of poor digestion, poor elimination, and deficiencies in vitamins, minerals, and healthy carbohydrates, proteins, or fats may show up in skin, hair, and nails. When beginning our journey to a healthier lifestyle, most people will see results first in their skin, hair, and nails. Skin will look vibrant and healthy. Hair becomes shiny and thicker, and nails begin to grow faster and look healthier. One of the first things we teach our On Target Living health coaches is to check a person's skin, hair, and nails for the ways their body is talking to them.

Body Weight

There has already been a great deal said about body weight throughout this book. Body weight is a powerful indicator of what is happening in the mind and body. Do you have a body weight range you would like to maintain 24/7? Is it realistic? Finding and maintaining a healthy body weight is part of everyone's journey to feeling and being their best.

The human body is truly amazing in its ability to try to self-correct and heal itself if given the proper resources. Learning how to decode our health is a gift that keeps on giving. Slow down and take the time to listen. When feeling out of balance, start by asking better questions.

Your body is always talking to you. Take the time to listen!

Decoding Your Health Essentials

Big Picture

- Decoding your health begins by asking better questions.
- Learn how to listen to your body.
- Nobody knows your body better than you.
- Your body will try to heal and self-correct if you give it a chance.
- There are multiple ways your body is talking back to you, and most have nothing to do with a blood test.

Ask Yourself

- What questions do you need to ask to learn more about your health?
- Do you pay attention to the warning signals your body sends out?
- Do you feel like you have enough space in your life?
- When was the last time you had an eye exam?
- How many hours of sleep do you average per night?
- How often do you have a bowel movement?
- Do you move your body on a daily basis?
- Is strength training part of your regular workout plan?
- Are you a chest or diaphragmatic breather?
- Can you touch your toes easily?
- Are you consuming a minimum of 50 ounces of water a day?
- Do you consume calcium and magnesium-rich foods?
- Do you consume omega-3 fats on a daily basis?

Small Steps

- Step back and listen for signs, signals, and clues your body is telling you.
- Get your eyes examined on a regular basis.
- Give yourself enough space to get eight hours of sleep.
- Work on your posture and flexibility by doing a 60-second micro break—standing wall extension and standing up and down dog stretch.
- Drink more water, consume superfoods, upgrade food choices, and fast 12 hours overnight.
- Don't ignore your body. It is now time to listen!

31 Know and Improve Your Numbers

Over my 30-plus year career, I have acquired a body of knowledge and experience. I have incorporated my expertise in exercise physiology with hospital-based wellness programs and designed exercise and nutrition programs for high-risk patients and clients. I have developed systematic health and fitness programs for a major health club and trained numerous personal trainers, and personal coaches.

What is very clear is that people are unhealthy and over-medicated for many reasons. Understanding those reasons is fundamental to starting the journey to optimal health. Health is about the entire person.

In chapter 30, we discussed decoding our health, being mindful about cues and clues that our body is telling us, and to take the time to step back and listen. A big part of decoding our health is to have a better understanding of our numbers, learning how to interpret them, and understanding our risk. We need to know how to converse with our healthcare professionals and realize what we can do to improve our numbers.

Know Your Numbers

Knowing our numbers and learning how to improve those numbers is essential for optimal health. A blood test will give us and our healthcare professionals meaningful information. A blood test does not keep secrets. If something is not working right inside of us, a blood test may reveal what may be ailing us.

Unfortunately, many people have little knowledge or understanding of what blood test numbers mean. They just hope their numbers fall into the normal range. If our numbers are not in the normal range and the doctor wants to prescribe a medication, we may feel helpless due to our lack of education.

My goal in this chapter is to provide a better understanding of common test numbers, so that you can understand your risk. I will share strategies to help you improve those numbers. I will provide information that will help you have a healthier and more productive conversation with your healthcare professional. A blood test is just one method of evaluation. Our body talks to us in a variety of ways.

Cholesterol

Cholesterol is a hot topic. The cholesterol scare has been rampant for decades. When I take a survey almost everyone reports that they have had their cholesterol checked in the past few years. When I ask the same group if they have had their homocysteine or highly sensitive C-reactive protein checked, just a few raise their hands. Most have never heard of these two blood tests before. Why is this? The short answer is that there are no medications to prescribe if these tests come back out of the norm. However, homocysteine and highly sensitive C-reactive protein are two important blood tests to help predict the risk for heart disease, cancer, and stroke.

Ever thought of cholesterol as being good thing? The latest research suggests that we may actually live longer if we have high cholesterol levels that are in balance. Most people have been led to believe that having high cholesterol is the most important risk factor for having a heart attack or stroke, yet more than 60 percent of all heart attacks occur in people with normal cholesterol levels. Over 25 percent of adults in the United States currently take a statin medication to lower cholesterol. More than $60 billion is spent each year globally on statin medications. Here is the real kicker, the incidence of heart disease is not getting any better.

An unbalanced cholesterol profile may be a risk for having a heart attack or stroke, but there are many other risk factors that need to be addressed. Many people still believe that having low cholesterol is good and having high cholesterol is bad. What if the opposite was true? Let's go deeper and start having a better understanding of cholesterol, so we can have a better conversation with our healthcare professionals and take greater ownership in our personal health.

What Does Cholesterol Do?

I believe most people think of cholesterol as something bad or believe low cholesterol is better. Let's change this thinking right now. Cholesterol is essential for optimal health. Cholesterol makes up every cell membrane in the human body. Cholesterol heals the body, creates our stress hormones and building (sex) hormones, transports vitamins and minerals, and helps absorb Vitamin D. Cholesterol is essential for memory and brain health. Cholesterol is necessary for strength, vitality, and the production of CoQ10, a powerful antioxidant involved in energy production of every cell in the body, and most famously for keeping the heart healthy.

During my daughter-in-law's first pregnancy, her blood work included a test for cholesterol by mistake. Her total cholesterol came back extremely high, but her doctor told her not to worry. During pregnancy cholesterol levels rise dramatically. This is completely normal when making a new life. Cholesterol is amazing, and without it we would not have life.

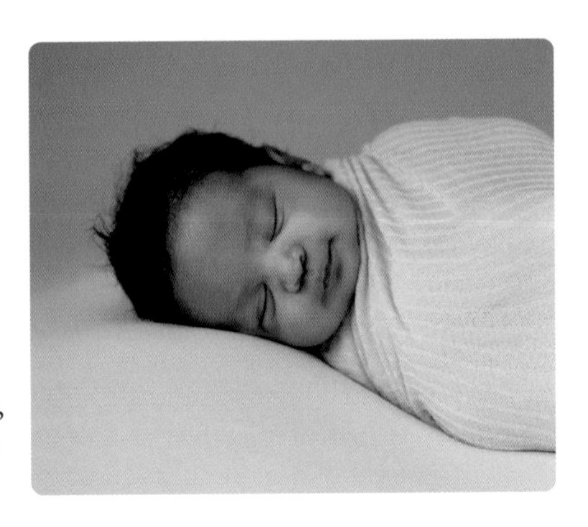

Causes of High or Unbalanced Cholesterol

A balanced cholesterol level is what we should all strive for. If cholesterol is too high or out of balance, we need to ask why. Remember, cholesterol is the raw material that makes hormones and keeps our cells energized and healthy. High levels of stress take a toll on the body, causing high inflammation and sleep issues. Consuming too many processed foods or drinking too much coffee, soda pop, energy drinks, or alcohol cause the body to go into healing mode. In healing mode, the liver begins producing more cholesterol for hormonal balance and repair. Some people may also have a genetic predisposition to produce more cholesterol than the average person. In most of these cases the goal again is to create balance within the cholesterol profile.

Cholesterol is not the risk factor. Unbalanced cholesterol is the risk factor.

Statin Medications

Obviously, I am not your doctor. My intention is to empower you with greater knowledge and understanding so that you can work with your doctor or healthcare professional to make informed decisions about your health. I will share my thoughts and strategies for improving cholesterol profiles and lowering the risk of having a heart attack or stroke as an alternative to using a statin medication.

What is a statin medication? Statin medications have been on the market for over 30 years and are the most prescribed medication around the world to help lower cholesterol. Statins are big business, a multi-billion-dollar business, and one that continues to grow.

The statin class of medications is very effective at reducing cholesterol. They do their work in the liver by suppressing an enzyme called HMG-CoA.

Blocking this enzyme also blocks the production of CoQ10, a powerful antioxidant that protects the heart. A deficiency in CoQ10 can lead to multiple problems, such as leg pain, muscle cramps, erectile dysfunction, depression and memory loss, type 2 diabetes, shortness of breath or fatigue, cardiac palpitations, and liver enzyme abnormalities. Statin medications have many side effects.

Earlier I discussed the role of cholesterol and its importance in healthy hormones. Cholesterol is the raw material for all building (sex) hormones. This means that all healing hormones, growth hormone, testosterone, estrogens, progestins, mineralocorticoids, and glucocorticoids are made from cholesterol. If cholesterol production is blocked by a statin medication, many of these hormones get compromised.

Every week we receive copies of blood work from people wanting to learn more and have a better understanding of their numbers. When I see an extremely low reading of total cholesterol followed by an extremely low reading of testosterone, I know this person most likely is taking a statin medication.

Statins block cholesterol production and compromise the production of building hormones and healing hormones. We must ask why sales of erectile dysfunction medications are skyrocketing. Could one answer to the epidemic levels of erectile dysfunction be from the overconsumption of statin medications?

Another concern is the epidemic increases in brain and nerve diseases such as Alzheimer's, Parkinson's, and multiple sclerosis. All of these diseases are based on the breakdown of the myelin sheath, the protective coating that surrounds every nerve in the human body. One of the possible side effects of statin medications is the breakdown of the myelin sheath.

As you can tell, I am not a fan of statin medications due to the vast array of potential side effects. If you want to improve your cholesterol profile, I believe there are safer and much more effective paths to take.

Know Your Risk Factors

We all have to take more ownership in our personal health and become more educated. In today's world of medicine most doctors spend less than 12 minutes per office visit. 12 minutes! How do we expect our healthcare professionals to fix sleep, high blood pressure, type 2 diabetes, or an unbalanced cholesterol profile in less than 12 minutes? In such a short visit, is it possible for the doctor and patient to fully discuss and agree to future lifestyle changes?

Understanding our risk factors is critical to our future health. Here is a snapshot of what we need to know.

Cholesterol/HDL Ratio

The cholesterol/HDL ratio is where we should begin to understand risk. Here is an easy example. Total cholesterol of 210 and an HDL of 70. Divide the total cholesterol by the HDL (210/70 = 3.0).

For women, the cholesterol/HDL ratio should be 3.5 or less.

For men, it should be 4.5 or less.

Triglyceride/HDL Ratio

Another simple cholesterol screen is the triglyceride/HDL ratio. For example, triglycerides of 100 and HDL of 50. Divide the total triglycerides by the HDL (100/50=2.0).

A ratio below 2 indicates a low risk of heart attack or stroke.

Cholesterol Particle Size

Another cholesterol screen is the weight and size of cholesterol particles. It turns out that LDL particles are not all created equal. Smaller, more tightly packed LDL particles have an easier time getting into arteries. Larger fluffier particles have difficulty getting into the arteries, making them less dangerous.

The Goal: Cholesterol particles like beach balls—large and fluffy.

Optimal < 1,000

Fibrinogen

Fibrinogen may be tested alongside other heart measurements and is an indicator of the stickiness of platelets. The lower the fibrinogen, the less likely for clotting to take place, which lowers the risk for a heart attack or stroke.

Normal Fibrinogen Value: 200-400 mg/dL

Calcium Score

Another method to help you understand your overall risk of heart disease or a stroke is to get a calcium score (sometimes called an Agatston score). The calcium score is calculated on the amount of plaque observed in the CT scan. It may be converted to a percentile rank based on your age and gender.

Calcium Score:	**Low Risk: 0-99**
Moderate Risk:	**100-400**
High Risk:	**400 plus**

The lower your calcium score and percentile rank, the less likely you are to have a cardiac event compared to other men or women your age. While the likelihood of having heart disease or a heart attack may correlate with your calcium score, remember that this is just one of many methods to help you evaluate your risk of having heart disease.

> ***What is Your Risk?***
>
> *Recently I received an email from a 52-year-old man. He had seen me speak multiple times over the years and wanted to get my thoughts on what his doctor had told him from his recent blood test.*
>
> *He reported that his doctor only had one concern, his cholesterol reading of 242. He also reported that he had always had high cholesterol, ate a healthy diet, and exercised on a regular basis. He had asked the doctor about lowering cholesterol through some lifestyle improvements, but his doctor told him that 80 percent of cholesterol is hereditary and wanted to put him on a cholesterol-lowering statin medication. He wanted to hear my thoughts about his cholesterol and possible next steps.*
>
> *This is what I told him. First, you need to have a better understanding of your risk. Most likely there was little conversation about other risk factors, such as blood pressure, resting heart rate, breaths per minute, sleep, stress, blood glucose, cholesterol balance, cholesterol particle size, oxidation, and inflammation. How can you put a person on a cholesterol-lowering medication prior to fully understanding their risk factors?*

How to Improve Your Cholesterol Profile

Over the last 30 years I have helped hundreds of people avoid taking statin medications or to work with their healthcare professional to wean them off their statins by taking a few basic steps. Consistent targeted lifestyle changes will help you play offense versus defense with your health.

Step 1: Understand Your Risk

Understand your numbers and talk with your doctor or healthcare professional before heading down the medication path.

Step 2: Get Enough Rest

Getting enough rest is critical for balancing cholesterol and improving overall health. Breathe through the nose and use the diaphragm. Slow breathing down. Sleep 8 hours each night. Create space by taking more micro, medium, and macro breaks.

Step 3: Hydrate

Drink more water—one-half of your body weight in ounces per day or 6-8 ounces per hour.

Step 4: Add Cod Liver Oil to Your Routine

Take 1-2 tablespoons of cod liver oil each morning. This is great for decreasing inflammation, lowering triglycerides, and raising HDL.

Step 5: Consume Flaxseeds or Chia Seeds

Take 1-2 tablespoons of ground flaxseeds or chia seeds 4-7 times per week.

Step 6: Consume Foods High in Vitamin C and Ancient Grains

Berries, lemons, oranges, grapefruit, limes, watermelon, pineapple, apples, broccoli, kale, asparagus, sweet potatoes, oatmeal, teff, and amaranth can all help bring cholesterol levels back into balance.

Step 7: Add Superfoods to Your Routine

Add spirulina/chlorella, frozen wheatgrass, greens, pumpkin seeds, hempseeds, Brazil nuts, apples, walnuts, coconut, cacao nibs, and beans to your diet. Use the Food Target as your guide.

Step 8: Move Your Body Daily

Move the body on a daily basis and play more. Find movement activities you enjoy.

How to Get Off or Lower the Dose of Cholesterol Medications

Step 1: Continue Taking Your Medications

Do not change your medications for the first month or two.

Step 2: Get New Habits in Place

Add cod liver oil, flaxseeds, oatmeal, and citrus to your diet. Cut out low-quality foods and upgrade your food and beverage choices. Move your body on a daily basis, and work on getting a good night of sleep.

Step 3: Make an Appointment with Your Doctor

Make a plan to discuss your intention to slowly get off your cholesterol medications with your doctor or healthcare professional.

Step 4: Get Another Test in Three Months

After three months, get another blood test to monitor your cholesterol profile and other risk factors. If you are seeing your profile start to change, ask your doctor if it is time to start lowering your dose of medications. If you are currently taking 40 milligrams of your cholesterol medication, ask your doctor to cut the dose in half to 20 milligrams and get another blood test in three months.

Step 5: As Your Profile Improves, Continue to Lower Your Dose

Ask your doctor again if it is time to cut your statin dosage in half to 10 milligrams and follow the same protocol until you get off your statin medication.

I am very passionate about helping people get off their cholesterol-lowering medications because I know it is possible and I know what I am sharing with you works. By slowly working with your doctor and improving your lifestyle habits, your need for cholesterol medications can disappear.

You have the power!

Triglycerides

Triglycerides are another fat in the blood similar to cholesterol. Triglycerides are produced in the liver and are extremely sensitive to the foods and beverages we consume. A cholesterol profile may take months to be impacted by new healthy lifestyle habits, but triglycerides are impacted almost immediately. Triglycerides are a great indicator of current lifestyle, good or bad. It is like looking into a mirror. The mirror does not lie. When people tell me they are eating healthy and their triglyceride levels are elevated, I know they are not giving me the full picture.

Causes of High Triglycerides

Why are triglyceride levels too high? In most cases they become elevated due to too many processed foods, fast food, and beverages such as soda pop, energy drinks and alcohol. Stress and a sedentary lifestyle can also contribute to high triglyceride levels.

A target triglyceride reading should be under 100.

How to Improve Triglycerides

Step 1: Consume Foods High in Omega-3 Fats

One of the fastest ways to reduce triglycerides is by consuming omega-3 fats such as cod liver oil, ground flaxseeds, and chia seeds.

Step 2: Consume Foods High in Chlorophyll

Consume foods high in chlorophyll. Greens such as spirulina/chlorella, frozen wheatgrass, broccoli, kale, and spinach all help improve triglycerides.

Step 3: Cut back on Processed Carbohydrates

These are found in sweets, alcohol, soda pop, energy drinks, and processed foods.

Step 4: Add Helpful Foods

Eat hempseeds, pumpkin seeds, walnuts, and colorful fruits and vegetables.

Step 5: Hydrate

Diabetes

In 1960, **1 in 4,000** people had type 2 diabetes in the United States. Today that number is **1 in 10**, and trending to 1 in 4. What is wrong with this picture? If we stay on this rapid pace, we may have over 100 million type 2 diabetics in the United States over the next 8-10 years, costing upwards of $450 billion in healthcare costs and even more importantly costing millions of lives!

Type 2 diabetes is no longer a problem facing just the United States. Type 2 diabetes has now turned into a global problem.

What is Diabetes?

When we consume foods or beverages that contain calories, glucose is absorbed into the intestines and distributed by the blood to all cells in the body. To maintain a constant blood glucose level, the pancreas produces two opposing hormones, insulin and glucagon. The major role of insulin is to open the cell for glucose to enter the cell. As a review, go to back to Section 2 for a full explanation of the cell and how it works.

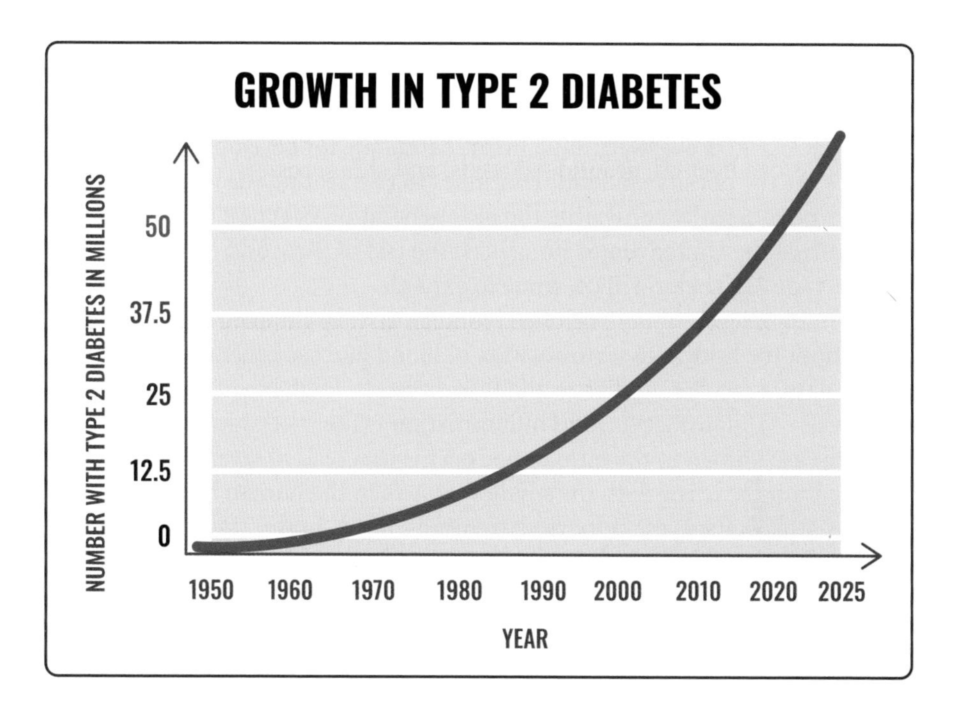

After a meal, blood glucose begins to rise. The pancreas then releases insulin which opens the membrane of the cell allowing glucose to enter and feed the cell. Without insulin, glucose cannot enter the cell. Glucagon, on the other hand, is the opposing hormone to insulin. Glucagon is released by the pancreas when blood glucose begins to drop, almost as a safety net for maintaining a steady flow of glucose to the cells. Glucagon does this by releasing stored reserves of glucose, called glycogen.

There are two types of diabetes, type 1 and type 2. For type 1 diabetics the pancreas does not produce insulin. For type 2 diabetics insulin is produced but has a difficult time opening the cell.

For type 1 diabetes, insulin must be taken because the pancreas does not produce insulin. Most type 1 diabetics are born with this condition. However, today we are also seeing a major rise in the number of type 1 diabetics due to unhealthy lifestyles that lead to a vast increase in autoimmune diseases that may damage and breakdown the pancreas.

Type 2 diabetes, on the other hand, is a lifestyle disease in which the cell membrane becomes stiff and rigid over time. When the cell membrane becomes stiff and rigid, it is extremely difficult for insulin to open membrane of the cell for glucose to enter, like a rusty lock on a door. Today, approximately 90-95 percent of all diabetics around the world are type 2.

Type 2 Diabetes Damages the Body

Obesity and type 2 diabetes often occur together. A person who is over the age of 35 and is overweight is a prime candidate for developing type 2 diabetes. As the obesity epidemic continues to rise around the world, it is as if we are purposefully cultivating the next generation of type 2 diabetics. As the health of the United States along with the rest of the world continues to decline, type 2 diabetes will continue to explode.

When high levels of uncontrolled blood glucose begin to circulate throughout the body, the accumulation of blood glucose generates free-radical damage to the capillaries and blood vessels. High blood glucose creates high levels of inflammation, and inflammation is the root cause of almost every disease known to the human body. This may lead to several health complications, starting with the smallest vessels in the human body. Type 2 diabetes attacks the eyes, kidneys, extremities, heart, brain, and may cause impotency. Type 2 diabetes is a wrecking crew that slowly destroys the mind and the body.

Diagnosing Type 2 Diabetes

Developing type 2 diabetes does not happen overnight. Type 2 diabetes takes time to develop and may show up in a variety of symptoms, such as increased urination, extreme thirst or hunger, fatigue, sleep apnea, eczema or psoriasis, dry mouth, headaches, blurred vision, or cuts and bruises that are slow to heal, along with tingling, pain, or numbness in the hands or feet.

There are two screening blood test measurements for diabetes. First is a blood glucose test. Second, is the blood test, hemoglobin A1C. This test measures glucose over a period of time. The test for blood glucose levels is like checking the stock market for a day. The hemoglobin A1C test looks at the stock market over a 6–12-week period and is used in conjunction with blood glucose monitoring.

A normal blood glucose level should be less than 100 mg/dL. If blood glucose measures closer to that 100 marker, a hemoglobin A1C should be checked.

Hemoglobin A1C results are expressed as the percentage of hemoglobin molecules that have glucose molecules bound to them. If there is not enough insulin for the amount of glucose, the level of hemoglobin A1C will rise.

A normal hemoglobin A1C test is between 4 and 5.6 percent. Hemoglobin A1C levels between 5.7 and 6.4 percent indicate increased risk of diabetes, and levels 6.5 percent or higher indicate diabetes.

Causes of High Blood Glucose or Hemoglobin A1C

Most people believe that type 2 diabetes is caused by eating too many carbohydrates. Type 2 diabetes is not a disease of carbohydrates and sugars. It is a disease of the cell. The problem is an unhealthy cell. Type 2 diabetes begins at the cellular level. As the cell membrane becomes stiff and rigid like an M & M candy shell, insulin has a difficult time opening the cell.

Most type 2 diabetics have been told to cut back on the consumption of carbohydrates. What is truly important is to consider the source of the carbohydrates. Are they real food, such as fruits, vegetables, ancient grains or starchy carbohydrates close to the source? Dehydration, nutritional deficiencies especially omega-3 fats, medications, stress, poor breathing, and lack of sleep also contribute to the skyrocketing increase of type 2 diabetes around the world.

How to Prevent or Reverse Type 2 Diabetes

It is possible to reverse type 2 diabetes. For over 30 years I have worked with hundreds of type 2 diabetics. My first conversation always begins with questions about their beliefs. If we do not address their beliefs, they are not going to get the outcome they most desire—improved health.

One of the first questions is whether they know that type 2 diabetes is preventable and most importantly reversible. Most have been told that type 2 diabetes is not reversible, but manageable, if they create a healthier lifestyle, eat better, and move more. Almost everyone says that they have been told to increase protein and cut out carbohydrates, to avoid all foods that contain sugar including most fruits, potatoes, and ancient grains. This is a disaster in the making, leading to high levels of acid, inflammation, and an unhealthy cell to boot. Type 2 diabetes certainly can be improved, managed, and reversed through an improved lifestyle.

The human body has an incredible ability to heal and self-correct if given the proper tools. The first step is getting the cell membrane soft and permeable. As the cell membrane becomes healthier, it allows insulin to easily open the cell door for glucose to enter. As the health of cells improves so does the improvement of overall health. Blood glucose levels slowly begin to come back into balance.

Preventing and reversing type 2 diabetes begins with the three foundational pillars for optimal health: how we **REST**, how we **EAT**, and how we **MOVE**!

Step 1: Develop Good Breathing Habits

- Increase breath awareness. Stay in tune with the breath.
- Breathe through the nose. The nose is the switchboard to calm the mind and relax the body.
- Use the diaphragm. The diaphragm is powerful muscle at the base of the lungs that needs to be exercised to maintain lung capacity, allowing the cells to absorb more oxygen.
- Practice slow breathing. Inhale for 5 seconds and exhale for 5 seconds. Do this for 2-5 minutes every day.

Step 2: Improve Sleep

- Value sleep.
- Plan sleep.
- Create a healthy sleep environment—dark, cool, and quiet.
- Consume magnesium-rich foods that help to relax the body.
- Move daily.
- Limit screen time.

Step 3: Hydrate

- Stay properly hydrated to keep the cells healthy, soft, and permeable.
- Drink 8 ounces of water first thing in the morning.
- Drink half your body weight in ounces of water each day.
- Add lemon, lime, or ginger slices to a glass of water.

Step 4: Consume Foods High in Omega-3 Fats

- Over 95 percent of Americans are deficient in omega-3 essential fatty acids.
- Omega-3 fats are essential in making and keeping the cell soft and permeable.
- Add cod liver oil, flaxseeds, and chia seeds to your nutrition plan.

Step 5: Add Superfoods to Your Routine

- Foods high in chlorophyll are like scrubbing bubbles, cleaning the cell membrane.
- Bring on the Superfoods. Spirulina/chlorella and frozen wheatgrass are the two oldest and most powerful superfoods, highest in chlorophyll, nucleic acid, and minerals, and fantastic for cellular health.
- Include broccoli, kale, spinach, asparagus, and any food dark green in color to your diet.

Step 6: Add Magnesium through Foods and Baths

- Magnesium is the mineral of relaxation and also increases cellular sensitivity.
- Foods rich in magnesium include avocados, oatmeal, coconut, cacao nibs, greens, dates, figs, raisins, prunes, bananas, mangos, ginger, walnuts, chia seeds, beans, and beets.
- Epsom salt is high in magnesium, Add 2 cups of Epsom salt to a warm bath. Soak for 15-minutes, 1-2 times a week.

Step 7: Consume Foods Good for Gut Health

- Cellular health begins with a healthy gut.
- Apples, strawberries, berries, cherries, celery, sauerkraut, pickles, mushrooms, onions, bok choy, garlic, apple cider vinegar, sea vegetables, root vegetables, potatoes, squash, teff, amaranth, buckwheat, salmon, beans, nuts, seeds, cinnamon, and turmeric all provide healthy nutrients for the gut and the cells.

Step 8: Add Vitamin D through Foods and Sunshine

- Vitamin D is a powerful healer and improves cellular sensitivity.
- Sunshine: Get at least 30 minutes of sunshine daily.
- Cod liver oil is high in vitamin D3. Take 1-2 tablespoons every day.

Step 9: Cut Out Low-Quality Foods and Beverages

- Slowly begin to upgrade foods and beverages to give the cells a chance to heal and repair.
- Avoid trans fats, fast food, and processed foods and beverages which make the cell stiff and rigid, making it extremely difficult for insulin to open it up.
- Use the Food Target to make upgrades.

Step 10: Move Daily

- One of the greatest ways to improve the sensitivity of our cells is to move the body on a daily basis.
- Create a new mindset around moving the body every day. Start with 10 minutes or more per day.
- Find enjoyable physical activities.
- Don't forget the healing power of play.

Homocysteine

We have been discussing blood tests that are very common and familiar to all of us. One test that is relatively unknown but provides valuable insight is homocysteine. Homocysteine is an amino acid that can be measured in a simple blood test that measures oxidation. What is oxidation? Oxidation occurs when rain hits metal and it begins to rust, or when we bite into an apple and it immediately begins to turn brown. Homocysteine that is not cleared in the blood and left intact begins attacking blood vessel walls, creating havoc throughout the entire body. Homocysteine is now considered the new cholesterol and a powerful risk factor for heart disease and stroke.

With all the research on heart disease, we have recently learned that approximately 60-70 percent of all heart attacks occur in people with normal cholesterol levels. The mere presence of cholesterol does not cause heart disease. Oxidation and inflammation also must occur for a heart attack or stroke. Therefore, it is important to look at all risk factors, including homocysteine, before taking a statin medication to lower cholesterol.

So why have most people not had this test if it is such a powerful risk factor for heart disease and stroke? For one thing, not all healthcare professionals know much about homocysteine. Second, there are no medications for lowering homocysteine.

Homocysteine levels above 13 are a risk fact for heart disease, stroke, inflammation, cancer, Alzheimer's, and Parkinson's diseases, to name a few.

Causes of High Homocysteine

For most people, an essential amino acid found in meat is an indirect source of homocysteine. There are many circumstances when homocysteine may become deadly if not broken down and cleared from the bloodstream. A lack of B vitamins may impair homocysteine metabolism, as can high levels of acid in the diet from eating too much animal protein, processed foods and acidic beverages. An extremely low carbohydrate diet, along with lack of sleep, and too much stress may also increase homocysteine levels.

A Recipe for High Levels of Homocysteine

Many years ago, while interviewing a new personal training client, the subject of cholesterol came up. My new client, a woman in her early 50s and in great physical shape, stated that she was concerned about heart disease due to her mother and sister both having a history of heart problems. She felt good because her cholesterol levels were already low, and she exercised daily. I asked her if she knew what her homocysteine level was. She had no idea what homocysteine was or why she needed it to be checked. Her doctor had never mentioned it. I explained that it was a blood test that measured oxidation, a risk factor for heart disease and stroke. I recommended she request it be tested the next time she got a blood test. Her annual physical was coming up in the next few weeks, so she agreed to do it. I also asked her to do a three-day sleep, nutrition, and exercise log.

A few weeks later, she returned with her blood test results and her log. I was shocked to see her homocysteine level at 39—three times the norm! I told her homocysteine level should be between 5 and 13. When I looked at her food log, she had been on an extremely high protein, low carbohydrate diet for over a year. She was eating lots of meat and cheese, and little to no fruit, ancient grains, or starchy carbohydrates. She was drinking four cups of coffee along with artificially sweetened beverages throughout the day. Her entire diet was extremely deficient in many vitamins and minerals, along with being highly acidic. Her hair was brittle, her skin was dry, and her breath had the smell of acetone. She was very lean, and it was her goal to stay lean. After our second session, she never came back. I do not think she wanted to hear what I had to say. Unfortunately, two years later she had a heart attack. Thank goodness she survived her heart attack. Could her heart attack have been prevented by changing her diet and lowering her homocysteine level?

How to Improve Homocysteine

Step 1: Ask for a Homocysteine Blood Test

The amount of oxidation in the body is a risk fact for heart disease, stroke, cancer, type 2 diabetes, arthritis, and an aging body.

Step 2: Eat Foods High in Folate—Vitamin B9

Folate plays an extremely important role in clearing homocysteine from the body. Foods high in folate include leafy greens, asparagus, broccoli, cucumbers, beets, sweet potatoes, squash, strawberries, flaxseeds, spirulina/chlorella, and frozen wheatgrass. When taking folate in a supplement form, take folate, not folic acid. Folic acid is a synthetic form of folate.

Step 3: Eat Foods High in Pyridoxine - Vitamin B6

Vitamin B6 is involved in the metabolism of proteins and carbohydrates. Low levels of B6 allow homocysteine to increase. Foods high in B6 include beans, nuts, bananas, cabbage, cauliflower, potatoes, and whole grains such as oatmeal, amaranth, teff, and millet.

Step 4: Eat foods High in Methylcobalamin - Vitamin B12

Vitamin B12 is also essential during the metabolism of protein, carbohydrates, and fats. As with folate and B6, vitamin B12 must be present to rid the body of harmful amounts of homocysteine. Foods high in B12 include Brussels sprouts, kale, parsley, whole grains, nuts, seeds, sea vegetables, spirulina/chlorella, and fish.

Step 5: Bring on the Choline

Choline is another B vitamin and is a building block for fats necessary for building cell membranes. Choline is important for brain function and memory. A few foods high in choline include nuts, peas, lentils, broccoli, cauliflower, eggs, and fish.

Step 6: Eat More Antioxidant Foods

Antioxidant foods decrease oxidation. Consume more omega-3 fats along with colorful fruits and vegetables.

Highly Sensitive C-Reactive Protein (HS-CRP)

Another blood test that most people are not familiar with is called Highly Sensitive C-Reactive Protein (HS-CRP). A high level of HS-CRP in the blood is a marker of inflammation. It can be caused by a wide variety of conditions from infection to cancer. HS-CRP levels can also indicate that there is inflammation in the arteries of the heart. This can mean a higher risk of heart attack or stroke.

It was not until the year 2000 that the role of inflammation and heart disease started to gain momentum. Dr. Paul Ridker of Harvard Medical School developed this blood test and reported in the *New England Journal of Medicine* that women with elevated HS-CRP levels were four times more likely to suffer heart attack compared to women who had normal HS-CRP levels.

The American Heart Association and U.S. Centers for Disease Control and Prevention have defined HS-CRP risk groups as follows:

Low risk: Less than 1.0 mg/L
Average risk: 1.0 to 3.0 mg/L
High risk: Above 3.0 mg/L

Causes of HS-CRP

There are many factors that contribute to high levels of inflammation throughout the body. First and foremost is a high level of acid or a pH imbalance. Remember, high acid levels raise inflammation throughout the body. This can be caused by consumption of too many processed foods, fast foods, and processed omega-6 fats, such as corn or soybean oil, as well as too much alcohol, soda pop, energy drinks, animal protein, and trans fats. High levels of stress, dehydration, lack of essential nutrients, and poor sleep can all add up to high levels of inflammation.

How to Lower HS-CRP

Step 1: Ask for a Highly Sensitive C-Reactive Protein Test

As with homocysteine, step one is to get a HS-CRP test. The amount of inflammation in the body contributes to risk factors for heart disease, cancer, type 2 diabetes, arthritis, poor bone health, pain, and a compromised immune system.

Step 2: Adopt an Anti-Inflammatory Diet

Start by cutting out processed, acidic, highly inflammatory foods and beverages. Foods and beverages in the red area of the food target are highly processed, acidic, and extremely inflammatory.

Step 3: Bring on the Healthy Fats

Omega-3 fats such as cod liver oil, ground flaxseeds, and chia seeds are extremely anti-inflammatory, as are healthy fats such as extra virgin coconut oil, extra virgin olive oil, avocados, almonds, macadamia nuts, pumpkin seeds, Brazil nuts, and hempseeds. Most raw nuts and seeds are also anti-inflammatory. Cut out all the processed oils such as corn, soy, and canola.

Step 4: Eat from the Green Area of the Food Target

Foods in the green area are more alkaline and nutrient-dense, and lower inflammation.

Step 5: Add Super Greens to the Diet

Spirulina/chlorella, frozen wheatgrass, kale, spinach, bok choy, broccoli, and asparagus are all high in chlorophyll, extremely alkaline, and lower inflammation.

Step 6: Hydrate

Staying well hydrated is essential for almost anything related to having a healthy body and is extremely important in decreasing inflammation.

Step 7: Make Space for Rest and Rejuvenation

I have had clients who have healthy diets, but their stress levels are out of control. When their HS-CRP levels come back high, they are very confused as to why. Too much stress and a lack of rest can contribute to an imbalanced pH and create a great deal of inflammation throughout the body. Some people have a hard time believing that how they think can make them sick. As I have pointed out multiple times throughout this book, stress coupled with a lack of rest and rejuvenation can be linked to most of diseases around the world. Getting enough rest and rejuvenation is key for lowering inflammation.

Prostate-Specific Antigen (PSA)

Prostate cancer is now one of the most common cancers in men in the United States with over 250,000 new cases of prostate cancer and 35,000 deaths each year. Prostate-specific antigen (PSA) is a protein produced by cells of the prostate gland. The PSA test, a screening for prostate cancer, measures the level of PSA in a man's blood. Prostate cancer screening can help identify cancer early on when treatment is most effective. A normal PSA test combined with a rectal exam can provide reassurance about the risk of prostate cancer.

Professional organizations vary in their recommendations about who should and who should not get a PSA screening test. Most agree to encourage the screening in men between the ages of 40-80, and in men with an increased risk of prostate cancer. Whether to have a PSA test is something you should decide after discussing it with your doctor and considering your risk.

A normal PSA reading is 00. to 4.00ng/ml.

Causes of High PSA

Consuming processed foods and beverages, too much alcohol, smoking, high levels of stress, and a sedentary lifestyle all contribute to increased cancer risk, including prostate cancer. Being deficient in nutrients such as iodine and zinc may also contribute to an increase in prostate cancer.

How to Improve Prostate Health

Step 1: Get Regular Check Ups

All men over the age of 50 should have their prostate physically checked on a yearly basis, especially when there is a family history of prostate problems.

Step 2: Consume Foods High in Gamma-Linolenic Acid (GLA)

GLA is an omega-6 fat that helps boost the immune system protecting the body from cancer. Foods high in GLA include pumpkin seeds, Brazil nuts, hempseeds, evening primrose oil, black currant seed oil, and spirulina/ chlorella.

Step 3: Consume Sea Vegetables

Sea vegetables such as sushi nori, kelp, dulse, and kombu, and many others are very cooling and help reduce tumors and unwanted growths. Sea vegetables are also high in iodine, which helps to support the prostate gland.

Step 4: Consume Cereal Grasses

Cereal grasses such as wheatgrass are high in minerals and chlorophyll and contain anti-inflammatory properties that help protect the prostate.

Step 5: Bring on the Trace Mineral Zinc

Zinc is tied directly to the immune system. For many people zinc levels quickly decline with age. Foods high in zinc include chicken, lamb, spinach, beef, squash, broccoli, asparagus, greens, oatmeal, teff, amaranth, millet, pumpkin seeds, spirulina/chlorella, and many beans.

Step 6: Understand How Medications Deplete Zinc

Many prescriptions and over-the-counter medications deplete the valuable mineral zinc. Ibuprofen, aspirin, antacids, and medications for acid reflux, blood pressure, cholesterol, and hormonal replacement therapy all have a leaching effect on zinc and should be used in moderation or avoided.

Thyroid-Stimulating Hormone (TSH-Ultra Sensitive)

Thyroid problems are on the rise, especially in women. The thyroid stimulating hormone is often the test of choice for evaluating thyroid function. There are two common conditions of imbalance in the thyroid. In hyperthyroidism, the thyroid is speeded up beyond normal function and uses iodine rapidly. In hypothyroidism, the thyroid functions below normal, often because of lack of iodine. The hyperthyroid person moves faster than a speeding bullet, while the hypothyroid person moves like a turtle with sore feet.

A normal reading for TSH is 0.35 to 5.5.

Causes of Thyroid Imbalance

The body needs iodine to make the thyroid hormone, so a lack of iodine can cause havoc in the body and lead to a host of problems, such as compromised immune system, breast cancer, prostate cancer, diabetes, heart arrhythmias, diabetes, low energy, little or no sex drive, depression, and weight gain. A nutrient-deficient diet, a high-acid diet, too much stress, and lack of sleep, along with a host of medications that may rob the body of valuable minerals including iodine, can easily put the body out of balance.

How to Balance the Thyroid Gland

A balanced pH is critical for bringing the thyroid back into balance. Planned recovery coupled with daily movement and high-quality nutrition all play a role in having a healthy thyroid.

Step 1: Get Your Rest

I believe one reason we are having an epidemic increase in thyroid problems is due to stress and not getting enough rest and rejuvenation. Adrenal exhaustion has become widespread with millions suffering from stress diseases. Many people believe having a rest and rejuvenation strategy plugged in their life is a luxury. I cannot tell you how many times I have talked with men and women with thyroid problems who want some advice on how to improve their thyroid. When I ask them about their current rest and rejuvenation strategies, they often look at me like I have a third eye. The best way to improve thyroid hormone function is to get restful sleep, breathe with the diaphragm, use a foam roller, get regular massages, play soft music, and create more space in life. These simple strategies can truly make a difference.

Step 2: Consume Foods High in Iodine

The body needs iodine to make the thyroid hormone. Foods high in iodine include asparagus, Brussels sprouts, carrots, coconut, fish, kale, oats, green onions, sweet potatoes, squash, strawberries, tomatoes, watermelon, spirulina/chlorella, and sea vegetables.

Step 3: Consume Foods High in Zinc

Zinc is not only essential for prostate health but also for a healthy thyroid. Low levels of zinc may cause the development of hypothyroidism that could lead to hair loss, weight gain, fatigue, a feeling of being cold, depression, low sex drive, insomnia, dry skin, and brittle nails. Foods high in zinc include chicken, lamb, spinach, beef, squash, broccoli, asparagus, greens, oats, teff, amaranth, pumpkin seeds, and most beans.

Step 4: Keep Your Liver Healthy

A clean liver equals a healthy thyroid. If the liver is stagnant and sluggish due to too much processed food, alcohol, and dehydration, the thyroid may also become sluggish. Proper hydration, foods high in chlorophyll, and daily movement all contribute to keeping the liver clean and functioning at its best.

Step 5: Get Good Sleep

Sleep is critical for thyroid gland health. Breathe with your diaphragm. Get outside and move daily. Eat right and drink less alcohol. Plan your sleep.

25-Hydroxyvitamin D Total

The 25-hydroxyvitamin D Total is a blood test to determine if bone weakness, bone malformation, or abnormal metabolism of calcium is occurring because of a vitamin D deficiency. Once ingested, vitamin D turns into a powerful hormone that helps build strong bones and muscles, lowers cancer risk by increasing immune function, and lowers the risk of type 2 diabetes by improving insulin sensitivity. Vitamin D is necessary to help absorb important minerals such as calcium and phosphorus, both necessary for healthy bones. Vitamin D is powerful, yet today more and more people around the world are becoming vitamin D deficient.

A normal 25-hydroxyvitamin D total is 25.0-80.0 ng/mL.

Causes of Vitamin D Deficiency

Lack of sunlight is one of the greatest reasons for being vitamin D deficient. Lack of consuming wild cold-water fish along with taking medications that leach out vitamin D also contribute to deficiency.

How to Improve Vitamin D Levels

Step 1: Get Out into The Sun

Just 30 minutes of sunshine daily will provide approximately 10,000 to 20,000 IU of vitamin D.

Step 2: Consume Cod Liver Oil

Our On Target Living cod liver oil, harvested in Dutch Harbor, Alaska, has the highest source of vitamin D3 (cholecalciferol) of any food source in the world. The livers of the cod are processed on the boat immediately after harvest to preserve the naturally occurring D3. Taking 1-2 tablespoons of cod liver oil on a daily basis provides approximately 600-1200 IU of vitamin D3 each day or 4200-8400 IU of vitamin D3 per week.

Step 3: Consume Foods High in Chlorophyll

All plants touched by sunlight contain chlorophyll. Green plants contain the highest amount of chlorophyll. Fortunately, chlorophyll foods act as a form of stored sunshine, performing like vitamin D in the body to regulate calcium. Foods such as frozen wheatgrass, spirulina/chlorella, spinach, kale, broccoli, asparagus, collard greens, romaine lettuce, and sea vegetables all contain high levels of chlorophyll.

Step 4: Limit Medications

Many medications rob the body of valuable nutrients including vitamin D. Limiting medications as much as possible can help maintain Vitamin D levels in the body.

Testosterone

Testosterone is one of the greatest indicators of how well we are aging. I like to call the testosterone test the vitality blood test.

We have all heard the term Low-T and the products touted to address it such as Ageless Male or AndroGel. There are a growing number of prescription pills, gels, and patches all aimed at boosting testosterone levels in men struggling with growing older and symptoms, such as decreased sex drive, erectile dysfunction, increased belly fat, loss of lean muscle, hair loss, poor sleep, depression, and fatigue. Advertising targeting testosterone is everywhere. Today testosterone supplements and medications have turned into a multi-billion dollar industry.

Do we really believe a pill, gel, or patch is going to fix the problem overnight? Let's first ask some better questions.

- Why do testosterone levels drop?
- Could it be linked to stress, lack of sleep, little or no space, poor diet, and a lack of exercise?
- Is it possible to move the testosterone needle by improving many of lifestyle habits first?

It may surprise many people that men do not have a monopoly on testosterone. Testosterone belongs to a class of hormones called androgens, but women also produce testosterone. Testosterone is a powerful hormone that keeps the body young and is involved in many processes in the body, such as growth, repair, energy, mood, sex drive, weight control, and muscle, bone, skin, hair, and nail health. As we age, testosterone levels slowly begin to drop. This may lead to a host of problems, such as loss of muscle, weakened bones, dry skin and hair, brittle nails, low energy, depression, low sex drive, erectile dysfunction, and weight gain.

A baseline testosterone blood test for both men and women can be very helpful in monitoring the aging process. These are the normal testosterone ranges for both men and women from the National Institutes of Health.

Women:	**25-95 ng/dL**
Men:	**300-1200 ng/dL**

While total testosterone levels of 30 ng/dL for women and 300 ng/dL for men are considered in the normal range, these numbers do not indicate thriving health by any means. Total testosterone levels greater than 35 ng/dL for women and greater than 500 ng/dL for men move people in the thriving category. Total testosterone levels also vary with age.

Not Enough Recovery

At the age of 56, my blood test came back with a drop in testosterone of almost 200 points in just over one year. I felt like I was doing all the right things: taking my superfoods, drinking water, strength training, and eating well.

When discussing this with my son, he speculated that my drop in testosterone must be due to my crazy work schedule. During the prior year, I had conducted more than 100 speaking events all around the world. He reminded me that the number one way to build and protect testosterone and health is to get enough rest and rejuvenation. I wasn't taking my own advice and needed this wake-up call.

We then discussed a new plan to improve my testosterone. For every four days on the road, I needed at least three days at home to recharge my batteries. I also needed to focus on getting enough sleep, practicing my breathing, taking Epsom salt baths, getting regular massages, consuming superfoods, and strength training. Eighteen months later my testosterone level bounced back to the original level. I just needed more REST and REJUVENATION!

Causes of Low or Imbalanced Testosterone

We frequently get calls about hormone replacement therapy (HRT) from men who had their testosterone checked and it came back low. For many, the doctor had suggested HRT. HRT may be an option, but let's begin by asking some better questions. Let's first try to uncover the why behind the problem before we head down the HRT path.

On a scale of 1-10, how do you rate your stress? ____________________

Are you getting a good night of sleep? Yes or No

Remember cholesterol is the raw material that makes testosterone. Are you on a statin medication? Yes or No

Are you drinking too much alcohol? Yes or No

Is your diet too acidic? Yes or No

Are you deficient in omega-3 fats, selenium, or zinc? Yes or No

Are you doing any strength training exercises? Yes or No

How to Improve Testosterone Levels

Step 1: Reduce Stress

Too much stress can produce too much of the stress hormone, cortisol, which can steal from your building (sex) hormones, and that includes testosterone.

Step 2: Get Good Sleep

A good night of sleep is essential for hormonal balance and healthy testosterone production. Testosterone is produced when we sleep. Taking a sleep medication is not the remedy for improving your testosterone levels. A daily rest and rejuvenation strategy is essential for healthy testosterone levels.

Step 3: Consume Foods High in Omega-3 Fats

Omega-3 fats are the raw material to make healthy hormones, including testosterone. Cod liver oil, flaxseeds, and chia seeds are a must for hormonal harmony.

Step 4: Consume Foods High in Selenium and Zinc

Selenium and zinc are two more raw materials for building testosterone. Brazil nuts, pumpkin seeds, hempseeds, broccoli, asparagus, greens, beans, oats, millet, amaranth, chicken, eggs, lamb, and beef are all foods high in selenium and zinc.

Step 5: Add Strength Training to Your Routine

I am a huge fan of strength training for both men and women. I like to call strength training the Fountain of Youth. Strength training stimulates testosterone and growth hormone production. If you are not currently strength training, start slowly with a few exercises like a bodyweight squat or a push-up.

If you are currently strength training and feel like you are doing the same old thing, change your rep ranges up each month. For example, one month choose five reps, with higher resistance and greater intensity. During month two, go to eight reps with a little less resistance. At month three, go to 13 reps and even less resistance. Maintain your body alignment and posture with each exercise. At the end of each month, take a few days off for recovery.

Step 6: Avoid Statin Medications

Statin medications block the production of cholesterol, the backbone for building steroidal hormones including testosterone. When you block the production of cholesterol, you compromise hormonal balance, including testosterone.

It is extremely important to get your testosterone measured on an annual basis as a great indicator of how you are aging.

Glomerular Filtration Rate (GFR)

Glomerular filtration rate (GFR) is a blood test that checks how well the kidneys are working. It is one of several ways to measure kidney function. The kidneys have tiny filters called glomeruli. These filters help remove waste and excess fluid from the blood. A GFR test estimates how much blood passes through these filters each minute.

A normal GFR is 60-120.

Causes of Low GFR

There are many lifestyle factors that may contribute to low GFR reading. Dehydration, processed foods, alcohol, soda pop, energy drinks, excessive protein, protein powders, acidic diet, stress, lack of sleep, lack of movement, high blood pressure, and type 2 diabetes all can play a role in putting excessive stress on the kidneys and a drop in GFR.

How to Improve GFR

Step 1: Hydrate

Staying properly hydrated is essential for healthy kidneys.

Step 2: Consume Foods High in Chlorophyll

Foods high in chlorophyll are natural detoxifiers for the kidneys. Green foods such as spirulina/chlorella, wheatgrass, kale, spinach, collard greens, broccoli, bok choy, and many more help the kidneys function at high levels.

Step 3: Consume Detoxifying Fruits and Vegetables

Berries, bananas, oranges, watermelon, strawberries, lemons, limes, ginger, beets, and sweet potatoes are excellent foods for kidney health.

Step 4: Cut Out Low-Quality Foods and Beverages

It is not about being perfect, but consuming less alcohol, coffee, soda pop, energy drinks, protein powders, and processed foods all play a role in improving kidney health.

Step 5: Upgrade Your Lifestyle.

Breathing practices, sleep, space, stress management, and daily movement all play a role in having a healthy GFR.

Breaths Per Minute

Breaths per minute is a great indicator of whether the nervous system is in or out of balance. The fewer breaths taken each day, the healthier we will be. It is that simple. We have become a society of overbreathers (or hyperventilators), averaging up to 18 breaths per minute, equating to over 25,000 breaths per day. That is a lot of inhalations and exhalations each day. Overbreathing puts an enormous amount of physical stress on the entire body, especially the heart and lungs. Alternatively, taking slow, diaphragmatic breaths through the nose creates efficiency and balance throughout the entire body. Breathe better by taking 10 breaths or less per minute, equating to 9,000 to 14,000 breaths per day. This change can affect our health, energy, and our mind. I think your mind and body would love the new you!

When breathing at a normal rate, our lungs can absorb about a quarter of the available oxygen from the outside air. The majority of oxygen is exhaled right back out. By taking longer slower breaths, we allow the lungs to soak up more oxygen in fewer breaths. When we slow down our breathing, we train the lungs to be more efficient. By taking fewer breaths we do not decrease oxygen, we are actually increasing oxygen due to greater absorption. For a deeper dive on breathing, go back and review Section 3.

How many breaths do you take per minute? ____________

Resting Heart Rate

One of the best indicators of improved fitness and health is a low resting heart rate. As fitness levels improve, resting heart rate begins to slow down. This is due to increased efficiency in the cardiovascular system, specifically an increase in stroke volume. Stroke volume is the strength of the contraction of the heart. As we become more fit, each beat of the heart can push out more blood due to an increase in stroke volume. One of the greatest indicators of overall health and fitness level is a low resting heart rate.

For most healthy adults, the resting heart rate should be under 60 beats per minute.

Low Fitness Level:	**Above 72 beats/minute**
Moderate Fitness Level:	**60-72 beats/minute**
High Fitness Level:	**Under 55 beats/minute**

How to Calculate Resting Heart Rate

To get an accurate resting heart rate, find the pulse in your wrist.

Take your pulse for 10 seconds and multiply it by 6 to calculate beats per minute.

Do this first thing in the morning before you get out of bed.

What is your resting heart rate? __________

Causes of High Resting Heart Rate

When stress levels are high, or we lack sleep, eat and drink too many unhealthy foods and beverages, and get little movement in our day, our resting heart rate will begin to rise. Resting heart rate is a great example of how the body is talking to us.

How to Lower the Resting Heart Rate

Step 1: Move Your Body Daily

Step 2: Practice Diaphragmatic Breathing

Step 3: Create More Space in Your Life

Step 4: Get More Restful Sleep

Step 5: Eat and Drink High-Quality Foods and Beverages

Blood Pressure

High blood pressure can be extremely debilitating to good health. Many people are not aware they have high blood pressure. That is why high blood pressure is sometimes called the "Silent Killer." High blood pressure stresses the arterial walls, which may then lead to stroke or damaged arteries. It also puts more demand on the heart muscle, creating a thicker heart. As the heart thickens stroke volume declines leading to a drop in cardiac output.

Monitor blood pressure on a regular basis. Also, measure blood pressure at different times during the day to detect differences from morning to evening. There are many home blood pressure kits that are easy to use and very effective.

What is your blood pressure? ____________

Causes of High Blood Pressure

There are multiple reasons for high blood pressure. These include obesity, poor nutrition, stress, lack of sleep, poor fitness, lack of exercise, pH imbalance, mineral deficiencies (such as lack of magnesium), dehydration, and medication side effects to name a few.

How to Lower Blood Pressure

Step 1: Breathe with the Diaphragm

Diaphragmatic breathing stimulates the vagus nerve, which in turn stimulates the parasympathetic nervous system, which slows everything down, including heart rate, brainwaves, and blood pressure.

Step 2: Consume High-Quality Foods and Beverages

The consumption of high-quality foods and beverages including avocados, macadamia nuts, cod liver oil, flaxseeds, chia seeds, and healthy fats such as extra-virgin olive oil may help lower blood pressure.

Step 3: Consume Foods High in Magnesium

Foods rich in magnesium include avocados, oatmeal, coconut, cacao nibs, greens, dates, figs, raisins, prunes, bananas, mangos, ginger, walnuts, chia seeds, beans, and beets.

Step 4: Take an Epsom Salt Bath Regularly

Epsom salt is high in magnesium. Add 2 cups of Epsom salt to a warm bath. Soak for 15-minutes, 1-2 times a week.

Step 4: Get Enough Rest and Rejuvenation

Know Your Numbers Handout

I want to make this crystal clear. I am not your doctor, but for over 30 years I have helped thousands of people understand and improve their numbers. A copy of our "Know Your Numbers" handout is included on the next page and is also available at ***ontargetliving.com***. Take it with you to the doctor. It provides the basics to help you have a greater understanding of your risk and take ownership in your own health.

Work with your doctor, understand your risk factors, and ask better questions. And always remember, the human body was designed to heal and self-correct. The magic is in you!

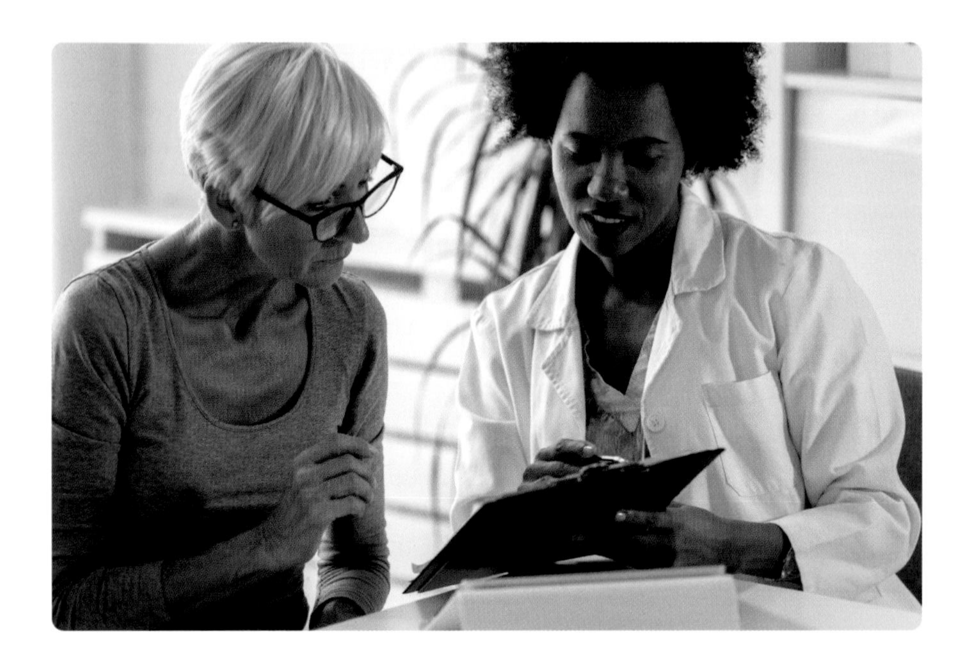

On Target Living®

KNOW YOUR NUMBERS

TEST	RESULTS	DATE	NORMS	GOAL
Cholesterol			150-250 mg/dl	
HDL Cholesterol			45-90 mg/dl	
LDL Cholesterol			60-130 mg/dl	
Cholesterol/HDL Ratio			<3.5 f / <4.5 m	
Triglycerides			<110 mg/dl	
Triglycerides/HDL Ratio			2.0 or less	
Glucose			65-99 mg/dl	
Hemoglobin A1C			4%-5.6%	
Homocysteine			4-13 mcmol/L	
High Sensitive C-Reactive Protein			low risk < 1.0 mg/L avg. risk < 1.0-3.0 mg/L high risk > 3.0 mg/L	
Prostate-Sensitive Antigen Screening (PSA)			0-4 ng/ml	
Thyroid Stimulating Hormone (TSH Ultra-Sensitive)			35 -5.50 mU/L or mcU/ml	
T3			27%-47%	
T4			4-12 mcg/dl	
25-Hydroxy Vitamin D Total			25.0-80.0 ng/dl	
Total Testosterone			30-95 ng.dl for women 400-1000 ng/dl for men	
Free Testosterone			49.0>185 pg/ml	
Glomerular Filtration Rate (GFR)			60-120	
Body Weight				
THE BIG 3: Breaths per Minute			5-12	
THE BIG 3: Resting Heart Rate (RHR)			<65 bpm	
THE BIG 3: Resting Blood Pressure			<120/80	

This handout can be downloaded at ***ontargetliving.com.***

Know Your Numbers Essentials

Big Picture

- Blood tests give you and your doctor or healthcare professional a meaningful look into your health.
- A big part of decoding your health is a better understanding of your numbers, learning how to interpret your numbers, and understanding your risk. This will help you have a better conversation with your doctor or healthcare professional on how to set a strategy to improve your numbers.
- Of all heart attacks, 60-70 percent occur in people with normal cholesterol levels.
- In 1960, 1 in 4,000 people in the United States had type 2 diabetes. Today that number is 1 in 10 and trending to 1 in 4!
- Nobody knows your body better than YOU!

Ask Yourself

- Do you know your risk factors?
- How many hours of sleep do you normally get per night?
- Do you drink at least 50 ounces of water each day?
- Is movement part of your daily plan?
- When was the last time you had your blood tested? Did you have your homocysteine, highly sensitive C-reactive protein, and total testosterone levels checked?
- How many breaths do you take per minute?
- What is your resting heart rate?
- Do you monitor your blood pressure on a regular basis?

Small Steps

- Get your blood tested yearly and track your progress with the Know Your Numbers handout.
- Prior to going to your doctor, take a little time to prepare and educate yourself on your numbers.
- Take ownership in your personal health. Work with your doctor or healthcare professional. Ask better questions and take the necessary steps to better understand your numbers.
- Most importantly, improve those numbers!

32 Body Care

What we expose our bodies to can make a huge difference in our health, energy, and performance in all aspects of life.

Bathtub of Health

My sister Paula Johnson has always said, "Your health is like a bathtub." Paula is a registered occupational therapist and has been in practice for over 30 years. She is also a certified naturopathic practitioner and the author of the book, *Nature's Child, Healing Children from the Inside Out*. Paula likes to say, "Imagine filling up your bathtub with water. The water is analogous to your health. Then slowly start letting the water out, but do not put any water back in. We keep making withdrawals but make few deposits. Over time we begin to squander our health!"

If we continue to expose our bodies to chemicals and toxins, over time our health will be affected. From the air we breathe, to our environment, what we put on our skin, and the household cleaning supplies we use, everything that encounters the human body can either improve our health or may cause it to become extremely toxic and break down.

As we improve our health by getting more rest, eating better, and moving daily we will also want to take it up a notch by improving our body care. As we build healthier habits, body care upgrades are extremely important for our future health.

Identify the body care and cleaning products you use the most.

____

____

Check the ingredients on some of the body care and cleaning products you use. Are you surprised at what you find? Yes or No.

What products do you want to start upgrading?

____

____

The Endocrine System

Let's begin our body care conversation with a little background on our endocrine system, our hormones. The glands in the endocrine system that produce hormones include the thyroid, pituitary, adrenals, pancreas, thymus, ovaries, and testes to name just a few. It is our endocrine system that releases carefully measured hormones into our bloodstream. Hormones are chemical messengers that travel throughout the entire body, controlling and adjusting almost every function in the body. Think of our hormonal system as an orchestra. Each instrument has a specific job to do and staying in balance is critical to making beautiful music.

Our endocrine system is a very sophisticated communication network for the entire body, talking back and forth, and sending messages and signals at warp speed. The endocrine system helps repair vital functions such as growth and repair, stress response, intelligence, metabolism, behavior, sexual development, reproduction, immune function, and insulin production, along with how we age. Hormones play an extremely important role in the health and performance of the human body.

Endocrine Disruptors

Endocrine disruptors are ingredients in many body care products that can cause estrogen dominance in both men and women. They do this by mimicking natural hormones. Endocrine disruptors cause hormonal imbalances that may lead to an overabundance of estrogen in the body. This can be linked to early onset of puberty and menstruation in young girls, uterine fibroids, ovarian cysts, greater menopausal challenges, thyroid problems, and breast cancer in women. For men, it may cause hormonal imbalances with testosterone leading to poor energy, increased belly fat, low sperm count, and poor sperm health. Not only can these endocrine disruptors mimic our natural hormones, but they can also block other hormones from binding to receptor sites.

How to Avoid Endocrine Disruptors

Here are a few of these endocrine disruptors that are found in many body care products and should be avoided. Awareness is the first step in avoiding many of these endocrine disruptors. The second step is learning how to slowly upgrade body care and cleaning products.

Parabens

Parabens are chemicals used as preservatives, which is one reason why they are found in so many products. Parabens can be commonly found in many soaps, moisturizers, shampoos, deodorants, lipsticks, and toothpaste.

Phylates

Phylates are used in many plastics and liquid soaps.

Formaldehyde

Formaldehyde is found in nail products, hair dyes, some shampoos, and maybe even some brands of decaffeinated coffee.

Plastics

Avoid these common plastics:
#3 Polyvinyl chloride (PVCs)
#6 Polystyrene (PSs)
#7 Bisphenol A (BPAs), Polycarbonate (PCs) and Polylactic Acid (PLAs)

Dioxin

Dioxin is found in foods such as milk, eggs, meat, fish, and butter.

Lead

Lead is found in many eyeliners, lipsticks, and cosmetics.

Mercury

Mercury may be found in eye drops, many skincare products, and some seafoods. This is one reason why I recommend wild caught salmon and tungal tuna.

Glycol

Glycol may be found in many paint and cleaning supplies.

Arsenic

Arsenic may be found in our drinking water. This is a great reason to look into installing a water filtration system. I personally use a water ionizer with a filtration system.

Pesticides

Pesticides are used in the food production industry can be found in our food. This is one reason buying organic is the best way to avoid them. Start with the "Dirty Dozen." These are fruits and vegetables that have the highest pesticide levels on average.

THE DIRTY DOZEN		
• Apples	• Cherries	• Peaches
• Bell peppers	• Grapes	• Pears
• Carrots	• Lettuce	• Spinach
• Celery	• Nectarines	• Strawberries

The Lymphatic System

As was mentioned in Section 4, a healthy lymphatic system is one of the keys to health, especially important to the health of our eyes and skin. The lymphatic system is the body's built-in sanitation system, the plumbing that carries away and filters out carcinogens and toxins from every cell, tissue, and organ in the human body.

The lymphatic system also plays an extremely important role in a strong immune system. Think of the lymphatic system as a street cleaner and garbage collector for the human body. Unlike the heart, which pumps blood throughout the entire body, the lymphatic system has no pump, so it needs help in moving fluid throughout the body.

The lymphatic system is made up of lymphatic vessels that carry waste out through sweat, urine, and bowels. Lymphocytes, a type of white blood cell, are the primary cells of the lymphatic system. There are two classes of lymphocytes: T cells that kill invaders and B cells that protect the body. The thymus, the gland underneath the breastbone, produces white blood cells. The spleen is connected to the lymph system and produces lymphocytes. Bone marrow is where lymphocytes are born.

Lymph nodes are filtering stations that are found in the armpit and pubic area of the body. This is one reason why it is important to never block these lymph nodes with odor blocking agents. Tonsils, adenoids, and the appendix all play a large role in a vibrant and healthy immune system. There is a lot going on inside the lymphatic system. Here is the point. A congested lymphatic system is a major contributor to an increase of inflammation and disease.

Causes of a Congested and Sluggish Lymphatic System

- Lack of movement
- Dehydration
- Stress
- Constipation or diarrhea
- Processed foods
- Unhealthy skincare products
- Exposure to toxins and carcinogens

How to Improve the Lymphatic System

Step 1: Practice Better Breathing

Breathe through the nose, use the diaphragm, and take slow rhythmic breaths.

Step 2: Hydrate

Staying properly hydrated is essential for a healthy lymphatic system.

Step 3: Move Your Body Daily

Any activity, such as walking, stretching, or mini trampoline, gets the body moving. That is essential for a healthy, vibrant lymphatic system.

Step 4: Dry Brush Skin Before Showering

Dry brushing allows the skin to breathe better.

Step 5: Massage Your Body

The foam roller is my daily massage. Try to get a real massage once or twice a month.

Step 6: Use an Infrared Sauna

If you have access, this is a fantastic way to detox a few times each week.

Step 7: Wear Loose Breathable Clothing

Step 8: Use Healthy Skincare Products

Step 9: Eat More Whole Foods, Especially Fruits and Vegetables

Step 10: Consume Foods High in Chlorophyll

Chlorophyll is a natural detoxifier and cleanser. Kale, spinach, broccoli, and asparagus are high in chlorophyll. The highest sources are found in spirulina/chlorella and frozen wheatgrass.

Step 11: Consume Herbal Teas

My favorites are ginger, turmeric and cinnamon.

The goal is to keep the lymphatic system running smoothly so it can help rejuvenate and build a vibrant immune system!

Healthy Skin

Did you know that skin is an organ? In fact, our skin is the largest organ in the human body spanning over 20 square feet and containing over 16 percent of our body weight. Our skin is a living organism. It has many jobs to do to keep the human body healthy. Our skin protects the body from microbes and invaders, regulates body temperature, and creates sensations of touch, hot, and cold. Another important role of the skin is elimination. Many toxins are eliminated from our body through our skin.

I think we all recognize healthy skin when we see it. It is that healthy glow. If we do not have this healthy glow, our body may be overloaded with toxins. I learned many years ago that skin heals from the inside out. As you may recall, I had major skin problems for almost 10 years of my life. Doctors gave me oral medications and topical creams, but nothing seemed to work. I was told I just had "sensitive skin." I did not have sensitive skin. I was a poor eater. When I changed my diet, my skin became healthier almost overnight.

We have been sold a very misguided version of healthy skin maintenance. Powerful soaps promise to peel off grease, kill bacteria on contact, and smell like a springtime rain. What kind of sales job was that? It must have worked because this was the only soap my mom ever bought. Imagine the ingredients that were in this soap or in shaving creams that foam, deodorants that block body odor, or antiperspirants that block any sign of moisture. Sunblock, shampoo, and cosmetics can impact our health. It is time to step back and analyze what are we putting on our precious, beautiful skin.

Upgrade the Body Care Products Used Daily

We begin by slowly upgrading the body care products used daily. For Christmas one year I gave out healthy body care products to all my family members. They loved it and it has now become an annual ritual.

Here are a few body care products to begin upgrading: toothpaste, deodorant, soap, shampoo, conditioner, skin moisturizer, sunscreen, cosmetics, bath salts, laundry soap, and cleaning supplies. Remember, what goes on our skin can slowly make its way into our body. This is one reason I like to use almond, macadamia nut, or coconut oil as a skin moisturizer. They work great and are extremely healthy for the entire body.

Essential Oils

Here is a little history on essential oils. Essential oils have been used medicinally for hundreds of years to help enhance physical, mental, emotional, and spiritual health. Essential oils are derived from distilling parts of a plant, flower, or tree to make a concentrated oil. For example, to make a small bottle of rose oil, it takes many, many pounds of rose petals. Many of these concentrated oils are extremely strong and when used topically should be mixed with a carrier oil such as almond or jojoba oil. Just a few drops of essential oil mixed with a carrier oil is all that is needed.

The choice of essential oil depends on the purpose. Calming essential oils such as lavender or lemon bring calmness and serenity to the day. Peppermint is an energizing essential oil. To provide healing or soothe a burn or itch, try frankincense oil. There are multiple essential oil options available to meet many specific needs.

How to Use an Essential Oil

Essential oils enter the body primarily in three ways: applied to the skin, inhaled, or ingested. Within each of these, there are many different types of application methods. The application method to choose depends on the desired effect of the essential oil selected.

Topical Application

Most skincare involves topical applications. For example, essential oils can be applied topically with a compress, as a spray, massaged into the skin or in the bath. Other essential oils are irritating to the skin and are better used by inhalation or aromatherapy.

Aromatherapy

Mood effects are most often addressed through inhalation or aromatherapy. I have a diffuser in my office. I add a few drops of my preferred essential oil to the water, such as lavender, orange, or cypress if I want to chill. If I am looking for something more energizing, I use ginger root, bergamot, or peppermint.

To learn more about therapeutic benefits of using essential oils, I would highly recommend reading *Reference Guide to Essential Oils* by Connie and Alan Higley. I would also recommend contacting a highly qualified aromatherapist or naturopath with expertise in essential oils.

Upgrading your body care products can make a huge impact on your health. Start slowly by upgrading what you currently use each and every day, such as toothpaste, deodorant, soap, shampoo, and skin moisturizers. I am sure that you will truly enjoy the health benefits that high-quality body care products can bring your overall health and feeling your best.

Remember, what you put on your body goes into your body. Let's get healthy and beautiful inside and out.

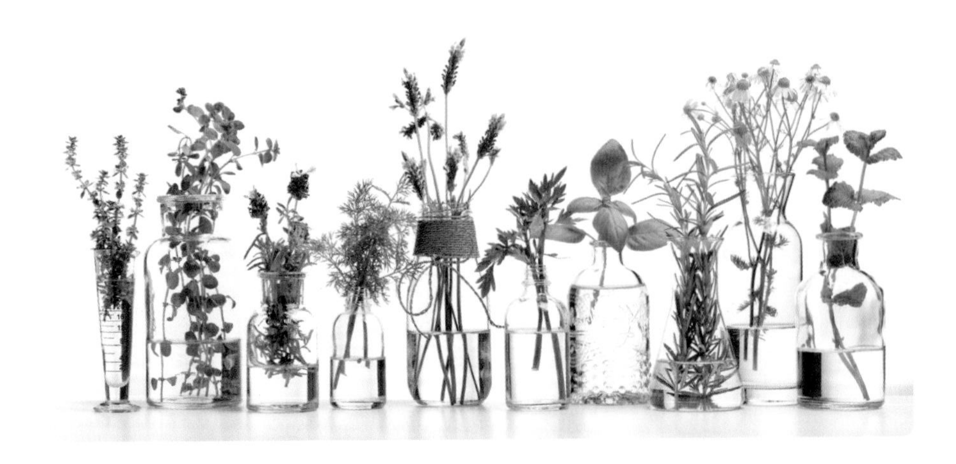

Body Care Essentials

Big Picture

- What we expose our bodies to can make a huge difference in our health, our energy, and our performance in all aspects of life.
- Everything that comes in contact with the human body—the air we breathe, our environment, what we put on our skin, and household cleaning supplies—can either improve our health or may cause the body to be extremely toxic and break down.
- Estrogen disruptors are ingredients in many body care products that can cause estrogen dominance in both men and women.
- The lymphatic system is the street cleaner and garbage collector for the human body. Keeping the lymphatic system running smoothly is essential for greater health.
- What you put on your skin slowly makes its way into the body. The body heals from the inside out.
- Essential oils have been used medicinally for hundreds of years to help enhance physical, mental, emotional, and spiritual health.

Ask Yourself

- Do you check the ingredient list of your body care products?
- What kind of body care and cleaning products do you use on a daily basis that you are willing to upgrade?
- How healthy is your skin?
- What indications do you have that lymphatic system needs improvement?
- What body care products do you need to upgrade or change?

Small Steps

- Read the ingredient list on the back of your body care products. If you cannot read it, do not use it!
- Upgrade 2-3 of your body care products starting today.
- Experiment with a variety of body care products to find products that you love.
- Buy a diffuser and use some essential oils. Experience the power of aromatherapy.

SECTION

7

HAPPINESS IS IN THE PURSUIT

33 You Have the Power

Over the years I have talked to thousands of people who say they aspire to have more energy, lose weight, have a better night of sleep, become medication free, become healthier, and get the juice back in their life.

Unfortunately, many feel like they have Mount Everest staring them in the face, and the task at hand seems too overwhelming. Many also believe they may not have the necessary tools, motivation, or willpower to be successful. I encourage them not to give up hope. Change is possible. I have witnessed many incredible transformations over the 30-plus years that I have been in this business. Success is possible. Lasting change is a process, and in most cases happens in small increments.

How do we stay motivated? How do we build habits that last and keep the momentum going? As we approach the final chapters of this book, it may be clear that this is not the end of the journey. There really is no end to the process of creating a healthy lifestyle. It is a journey with many wonderful stops along the way. It is a lifestyle that is healthy, fun, flavorful, repeatable, and one that gets better over time.

Zero to One

Changing behavior can be extremely challenging especially when it comes to making lifestyle changes. A powerful philosophy to embrace is going from Zero to One. The greatest change occurs when we go from doing nothing to doing something. This point was hit hard in Section 5 during our discussion on movement. Moving forward, try to embrace the thought of getting started rather than focusing on perfection or doing it all at once. Pick a few things in the list below and focus on a few small steps.

REST

- Breathe through your nose and with your diaphragm for 1-2 minutes each day.
- Sleep an additional 30 minutes each night.
- Plan a 2-minute stretch break every afternoon.
- Use a foam roller for 1-2 minutes a day to improve your posture.
- Get a massage 1-2 times each month.
- Take an Epsom salt bath once a week.
- Stop using electronics in bed.

- Block off one morning each month just for YOU.
- Take a vacation day from work to do whatever you want.

EAT

- Drink 6-8 ounces of water when you first wake up.
- Take one tablespoon of cod liver oil every morning.
- Eat an apple 3 times per week.
- Eat a big salad twice a week.
- Fast for 12 hours overnight.

MOVE

- Walk for 5-10 minutes three times a week.
- Do 5 push-ups twice a week.
- Find a new activity you enjoy.
- Play once a week.

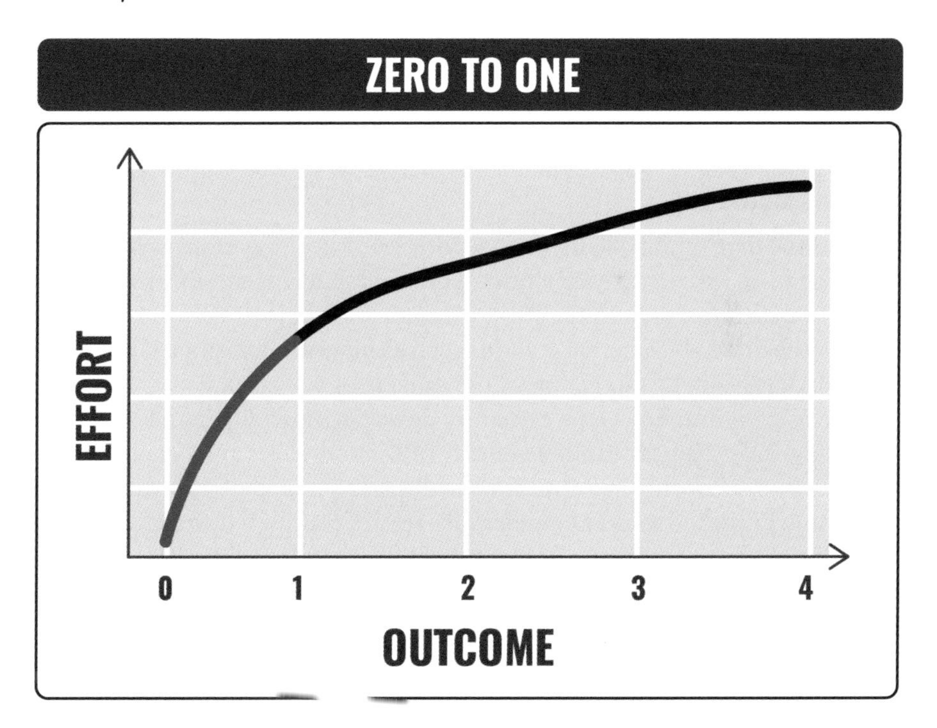

Don't get stuck thinking you have to do it all. There is incredible power when going from Zero to One!

Motivation

Why do we do the things we do? What drives our behaviors? How many times have we said these things to ourselves?

- I have so many great ideas, if only I could get motivated.
- I know that exercise is good for me, but I just cannot seem to find the motivation to get started.
- I want to lose weight but have a hard time staying on a plan without supervision.
- I want to ________________, but I just cannot seem to find the motivation to get started.

The statements all have one thing in common—the need to find motivation. One of the skills successful people have is their ability to motivate themselves.

What is Motivation?

A question we receive on a regular basis is, "How do I get or stay motivated?" Let's begin with a greater understanding of what motivation is and how motivation works. There are two types of motivation: extrinsic or external motivation, and intrinsic or internal motivation.

Extrinsic Motivation

Extrinsic motivation occurs when we are motivated to perform a behavior or engage in an activity to earn a reward or avoid punishment. Extrinsic motivation is the carrot and the stick. Extrinsic motivation refers to behavior that may be driven by external rewards such as money, fame, grades, or praise. Extrinsic motivation comes from **outside** of ourselves.

Extrinsic motivation can be extremely powerful especially in the beginning. Take a job for example. It may offer good wages and benefits in a pleasant work environment. Over time, will this be enough to stay motivated? Do we find joy in the work? Do we feel like we are making a difference?

It is no different than when trying to make a lifestyle change. We may begin working out or eating healthier because we want to lose some weight, decrease inflammation, improve blood pressure, or get off a medication or two. We may be all fired up in the beginning, but slowly the motivation starts slipping away.

As mentioned earlier, the weight loss industry is a $60 billion a year business with over a 90 percent failure rate. Why? Because most people focus on the extrinsic side of motivation versus learning how to enjoy the process, which is the intrinsic side of motivation. Extrinsic motivation may be extremely powerful for simple tasks and in the right situations, but over time extrinsic motivation often loses its power.

We all can benefit from regular doses of extrinsic motivation.

Intrinsic Motivation

Intrinsic motivation involves engaging in a behavior because it is personally rewarding. It is performing an activity for its own sake rather than the desire for some external reward. Intrinsic motivation is doing something because we want to, not because we should or have to. Intrinsic motivation comes from **within**. Here are a few examples of intrinsic motivation.

- Eating healthy because you enjoy the taste and like how eating healthy makes you feel
- Moving your body for the pure joy of it
- Listening to music you find enjoyable
- Solving a puzzle because you find it extremely gratifying
- Taking a hike in the woods because you love to spend time in nature
- Playing

How to Bring More Intrinsic Motivation into Your World

Learning how to stay motivated can be challenging for almost everyone but is a skill that can be learned by all. Here are a few simple tips on how to bring more intrinsic motivation into your world.

- **Connect to Your Values.** Match up your aspirations with your values.
- **Find Your WHY.** Find your driver, your purpose. Your WHY is your jet fuel for change. Anytime your WHY comes from outside of you, this is where the real power lives.
- **Remember the Feeling.** When you do not feel like moving your body, tell yourself that in just a few short minutes you will love the outcome.
- **Take Action.** Sometimes we need show up even when we may not want to.
- **Break Tasks Down into Small Steps.** Habits are formed by taking one tiny step at a time. Floss one day at a time, or write a book one page at a time. Compete in gymnastics one cartwheel at a time, or climb a mountain one step at a time.
- **Create a Sense of Progress.** It is important to measure your progress to help you stay motivated.
- **Ask a Better Question.** How can you lose weight and enjoy the process?
- **Make It a Choice.** Choosing to do something is much more powerful than saying I have to, must do, or should do it. You get to choose.

- **Impress Yourself First.** Small wins can be extremely motivating. There is great power in learning how to amaze and please yourself first.
- **Find a Routine.** Experiment and develop your routines. Maybe it is a new superfood and oatmeal routine in the morning or a 3-minute stretch break in the afternoon. Develop routines you can learn to enjoy.
- **Embrace Getting a Little Uncomfortable.** To truly change we all have to get a little uncomfortable at times.
- **Play to Your Strengths.** Keep striving to grow. Self-mastery is an extremely powerful motivator.

One of my favorite sayings from our seminars and training is this—Your WHY must be bigger than your BUT!

Habits

One of the keys to building a healthier lifestyle is learning how to develop new behaviors that lead to new habits. I am always intrigued by how we develop our own personal habits. Some habits may be healthy and others not so much. How we brush our teeth, take a shower, put on our clothes, drive to work, exercise or not, grocery shop, make the bed, eat breakfast or not—we all have daily personal habits that require little thought or planning.

A habit is a behavior that starts as a choice but over time becomes a subconscious pattern or habit. Seventy to ninety percent of our human behaviors fall into the habit bucket. Imagine if we had to consciously think about every little activity or task throughout our day. We would be exhausted by noon.

In Charles Duhigg's book, *The Power of Habit*, he discusses how habits are formed. He coins it, "The Habit Loop." The Habit Loop is a three-step process that begins with a **cue** or **trigger** that tells the brain to go into automatic mode and which habit or habits to use. Second step is the **routine**. A routine can be physical, emotional, or mental. Finally, there is the **reward** or **benefit**. This helps the brain determine if this specific habit is worth remembering for the future.

THE HABIT LOOP

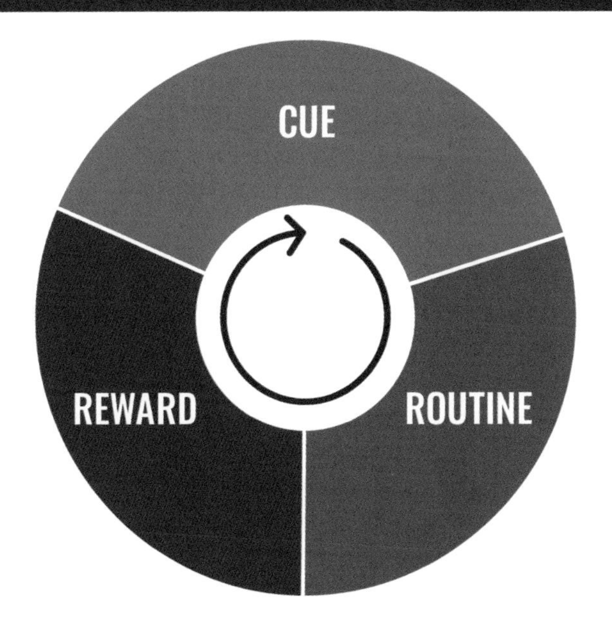

Here are two myths that most people believe about building habits. First, it has to be hard and painful. This is not true. Habit formation is not that hard if we break down each behavior into small actions. Second, most people believe it takes a lot of time to build a new habit. In BJ Fogg's book, *Tiny Habits*, his research reveals that we can build a habit in as little as five days, especially if we reinforce or celebrate our small successes.

Coffee is a habit that more than 70 percent of adults around the world partake in. In the United States alone we consume over 400 million cups of coffee each day or 146 billion cups per year. These numbers continue to rise each year. I am fascinated by how the habit of drinking coffee began for many folks. If you drink coffee, consider how it was first introduced to you. At what age? Were the rewards and benefits of drinking coffee strong right from the start, or did they grow over time? Most would agree that the cues, routine, and rewards all grew over time. Drinking a morning cup of coffee is now ingrained in many people's DNA, and they love it.

When doing research for a recent diabetes presentation, I learned that the country of Norway has very little type 2 diabetes among its people. What does Norway do that most countries around the world do not? One not so surprising fact is that most Norwegians take a shot of cod liver oil as one of their morning habits. Cod liver oil is served in airports, hotels, and restaurants. It is very similar to the American habit of drinking coffee.

As was covered in Section 4, one of the great benefits of taking cod liver oil is that it helps the cell membrane become soft and permeable. As the cell membrane becomes soft and permeable, type 2 diabetes begins to disappear. Is the secret to Norwegian health due to their habit of taking cod liver oil or is there more to the story? Maybe it is that when they feel better, they have less desire for unhealthy processed foods. Or maybe increased energy promotes a more active lifestyle. Whatever it is, I believe a large part of the Norwegian secret is their habit of taking cod liver oil on a daily basis.

Habit of Cod Liver Oil

One of the major healthcare concerns facing our world today is the skyrocketing growth of type 2 diabetes. The United States currently has the highest level of type 2 diabetes followed closely by Mexico. In 1960, approximately 1 in 4,000 people in the United States had type 2 diabetes. Today that number is 1 in 10 trending to 1 in 4, costing billions of dollars each year and even more importantly, costing millions of lives! Could a new habit of cod liver oil help fight this epidemic?

The benefits of cod liver oil are incredible. It is high in DHA, great for brain and heart health, a natural anti-inflammatory, and a powerful raw material for hormonal balance. Cod liver oil is also high in vitamin D3, helping to support the immune system, muscle function, and improve the absorption of calcium. Finally, do not be afraid of the taste. Our On Target Living cod liver oil is flavored with organic lemon for a smooth fresh taste.

Let's dream big. Take a step back and ponder this next question. What would happen to the health of the United States, along with the rest of our planet, if 70 percent of the population started their day by taking one tablespoon of cod liver oil prior to drinking their morning cup of coffee or tea? Is it possible that such a small habit could drastically improve the health of people around the world? I believe so.

So how can we develop the habit of taking cod liver oil?

Build a Habit Loop

Step 1: The Cue or Trigger. Make it as easy as possible. Put the cod liver on the inside of the refrigerator door. When you open the door, it is staring you right in the face.

Step 2: The Routine. Take your cod liver oil first thing in the morning to make it part of your morning ritual. One tablespoon is all you need. This is such a tiny habit that can lead to larger habits down the road.

Step 3: Rewards and Benefits. Make it fun. For our grandkids I call the cod liver oil "Muscle Juice." We have fun with the entire experience. We all change best when we are having fun and feeling our best.

Support Systems

We all need support systems to help us keep the momentum going. There are three support systems that play an integral role in our future success: personal, social, and environmental.

Personal Support Systems

What can we do to support our goals and aspirations? We all need to build and develop personal support systems to support our habits and keep the momentum going.

One of the keys to staying motivated is to learn how to enjoy the process. Many people may not enjoy exercise. What if we could learn a new movement or exercise that we enjoy and may even learn to love?

The same thinking can be also developed around what we eat and drink. I did not start taking cod liver oil or frozen wheatgrass cubes because I liked the taste. My focus was on developing these tiny habits for the benefits and future rewards to my health. In just a short time, I truly looked forward to the habit of taking cod liver oil and wheatgrass. I wanted the results that came with taking them and learned ways to make it work for me.

Do you want to be successful in your aspiration for having a healthier lifestyle? Yes or No

Do you need to change a few of your current beliefs? Yes or No

Is your self-talk positive or is your self-talk holding you back?

____

Do you have the right knowledge, the strategies, tactics, and practices in place? Yes or No

One of the motivating factors for me in writing this book was to help people increase their knowledge and learn strategies and tactics for long-term success. Remember, it is not just knowledge and strategies. It is the practice—the actual doing—that will create the habits and skills.

How to Develop Personal Support Systems

- Find a coach or a friend to meet you at the gym or to go for a walk on a regular basis.
- Listen to motivating music or inspiring podcasts.
- Use the *Target to Table* cookbook for recipes and meal planning.
- Engage with our On Target Living community to help you stay connected with like-minded people to share thoughts, ideas, and practices.

How can you keep yourself motivated and engaged?

____

____

What are you currently doing to support your lifestyle? ____________

____

What personal support system are you going to build into your daily routine?

____

____

Social Support Systems

Who makes up your social network? Are you getting support from your family, friends, and coworkers? Are they accepting and supportive, or is it a constant battle? At times you may feel like you are on an island all by yourself. Sometimes making a shift in your lifestyle may make people around you a little uncomfortable. That is okay. Maybe you will inspire them along the way.

I asked a great friend who happens to be a heart surgeon how often smokers who have had heart surgery quit smoking. He quickly responded, "Hardly ever." I was shocked to hear this. They just had surgery but were not willing to give up their habit of smoking. He went on to say that he always encourages patients after surgery to quit smoking or they may not survive for long. Even though they may want to quit, everyone in their social and support system are smokers, so they do not get the support they need to succeed.

How to Develop a Social Support System

Creating a powerful social support system around us is essential for long-term success. Break the chain. Become a leader for change.

- Graciously invite people in your social circle to get on board with some of your new behaviors and habits.
- Invite 2 or 3 people into your social circle who support your goals.
- Surround yourself with more people who can lift you up.
- Be patient. Building your social support system may take some time.

Is your current social network supportive of your goals? Yes or No

How can you improve your social support system? ________________

____

____

Environmental Support Systems

Creating a healthy environment around us is also critical to our success. Making our behaviors and habits easy to execute is critical for long-term success. For example, I sometimes struggle with drinking enough water. To help me in my desire to drink more water I have water everywhere. I have water at my desk and a water bottle in my car, on the golf course, at the gym, and on my nightstand. If water is not in front of me, I sometimes forget to drink enough of it.

Eating healthier starts with a little pre-planning prior to going to the grocery store. If the refrigerator is packed with high-quality foods, beverages, and maybe a few super foods, it becomes easier to maintain healthy choices going forward.

How to Develop an Environmental Support System

It is easy to get off track when our environment does not support our behavior and habits. Here are few steps to take to set up your environment for success.

- Clean out unhealthy food choices from your pantry and refrigerator.
- Place water in clear view to remind yourself to drink.
- Cut up lemons and limes and keep in the refrigerator for quick access.
- Keep healthy snack options available like fresh fruit, nuts, and dried fruit.
- Pack workout clothes and shoes near the back door to remind you to work out or head to the gym.
- Fill a small cooler with health food and beverages for the day.

At most of our On Target Living corporate events, we work with the meeting planners to create an environment for greater health and performance by offering healthy snacks, meals, superfoods, and beverages. It is always interesting to me that many conferences and training programs offer

SUPPORT SYSTEMS

PERSONAL	SOCIAL	ENVIRONMENTAL
Coach/Training Partner	Family	Meal Prep
Motivating Music	Friends	Travel Planning
On Target Living Community	Coworkers	Clean Out Fridge/Cupboards
Mentor/Friend	Groups	Gym
Positive Self-Talk	Social Media Circles	Dining Out
Strategies/Tactics		Plan Ahead

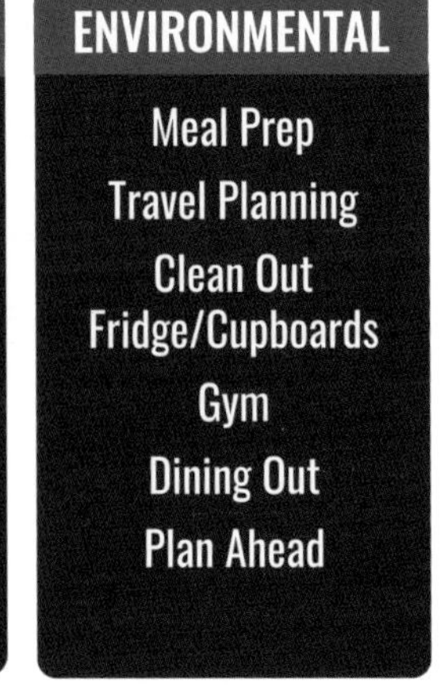

cookies, chips, caffeine, soda pop, and even energy drinks to participants. If people do not have the right fuel, how can they feel and be their best? Imagine feeding a $6 million racehorse a croissant sandwich and coffee for breakfast, or chips, cookies, and a soda pop for a snack. Would the horse perform its best? Take a look at your day. Does your environment support your new behaviors and habits? If not, what do you need to change?

Creating support systems around your new behaviors and habits is essential for your success.

Willpower

How many times have you heard, "If only I had more willpower, I could lose weight . . . get in better shape . . . have greater health . . . save more money . . . Whatever the goal, we could all use a little more willpower. The formal definition of willpower is, "the ability to delay gratification, resisting short-term temptations in order to meet long-term goals. It is the capacity to override an unwanted thought, feeling, or impulse."

Willpower is hard to explain. We cannot touch it or see it, but we all know what it feels like. Willpower is a force or energy that is tied directly to our self-control. The stronger our willpower the more self-control we will have in almost any situation. We have all experienced the temptation to eat ice cream, cookies, or chocolate cake. Many times, we give in even though we have told ourselves multiple times that we do not really need it. We set the alarm to get up early to work out, then turn off the alarm, roll over, and go back to sleep. A major project at work needs to be completed but Netflix sounds better. We have all failed now and then when it comes to self-control. Nobody is perfect in the willpower camp.

On a 1-10 scale how strong is your willpower? ____________________

What causes you to lose your willpower? ____________________

____

____

Here is the good news. We can improve self-control by understanding that willpower is like a muscle that becomes fatigued from overuse but also can be strengthened over the long run through training. In Roy F. Baumeister and John Tierney's book, *WILLPOWER*, they describe the existence of willpower and the power it holds if we can learn how to build and tap into it.

Learning how to build and tap into our own willpower begins with a greater understanding of how willpower works and why it is so fleeting.

First, we rely too much on willpower to get us to the promised land. We set our goals to achieve everything at the start. "I am going to eat in the center of the Food Target for the next three months, exercise 5-7 times each week, get in bed at the right time each night, and meditate daily for 15 minutes." The amount of willpower we have in the tank can be used up very quickly if we try to push too hard. Willpower is like the battery in our phone. If we use the phone too much and never take the time to recharge the battery, the phone will lose its charge and stop working, just like willpower. With all the temptations facing us all, it is extremely easy to use up our precious willpower.

Second, when we put our mind and body in a compromised state, our willpower becomes extremely weak. Stress, broken sleep, unhealthy foods and beverages, and lack of movement may all contribute to a drop in willpower.

The Slippery Slope of Willpower

I remember many years ago on Christmas morning, my wife Paula made her amazing date cookies. As I walked into the kitchen, the date cookies were just coming out of the oven. The smell of warm cookies filled the entire house. So instead of consuming my wheatgrass, cod liver oil, and oatmeal, I said to myself, "I am only going to have one date cookie before I eat my breakfast." I think you know where this story is going.

By eating the date cookie on an empty stomach my blood glucose took off like a rocket. Over the course of the day, I consumed 22 date cookies! My entire family wondered what was wrong with Mr. Positive. Where did my positivity go? I was in a food coma the entire day. My mistake was not eating a date cookie. My mistake was eating a date cookie on an empty stomach. Once my blood glucose got out of balance, my willpower left town!

When we solely rely on willpower to take action, sooner rather than later we are going to fail. When we become stressed, lose space, lack sleep, eat unhealthy foods or beverages, and lack movement, our willpower can easily disappear.

How to Protect and Build Willpower

Some of us start off with more willpower and self-control than others, but willpower can be strengthened with regular practice. We all may run out of willpower now and then, but we can also improve our willpower muscle by paying attention to how we **REST**, **EAT**, and **MOVE**.

Step 1: Build Your Foundation

We all become more resilient when we breathe slowly, get a good night of sleep, fuel our bodies with healthy foods and beverages, and move our body on a regular basis. When our basic physiological needs are not being met, willpower has little chance of survival. It is just a matter of time before our willpower will run out.

Step 2: Use Willpower to Make Gradual Changes

Don't try to do everything at once. Building habits slowly uses less willpower to execute a plan.

Step 3: Set Realistic Goals

Many people use up their willpower by setting unrealistic goals. By setting realistic goals and meeting or exceeding those goals, we build more and more confidence. This leads to strengthened willpower.

Step 4: Develop Strong Support Systems

Building strong support systems makes the process easy to follow and helps protect willpower.

Step 5: Develop Self-Esteem versus Self-Control

As you follow through on your own promises to yourself, your self-esteem will continue to grow. Your confidence and belief in yourself lead to stronger willpower and self-control.

Learn How to Pivot

One of the main reasons why most diets fail is due to the prescriptive approach—being told exactly what to do. A prescriptive approach to almost anything seldom works. You must make mistakes through trial and error and learn how to pivot. If you do not enjoy your current exercise plan or the food you eat, how can you tweak your plan to enjoy the process? This is where pivoting comes in. Pivoting is the ability to make changes depending on our circumstances. When we learn how to pivot, we can make almost any situation better, especially lifestyle changes. If you planned to take a yoga class after work but your day got away from you, how do you fit in 15 minutes to move your body? Or when dining at your favorite restaurant and they are out of your favorite dish, what would be another option that could work for you?

Learning to pivot opens up endless opportunities to develop a lifestyle that works specifically for you!

Keep refining and tweaking the lifestyle you want and deserve.

Momentum

How do we keep the rock rolling down the hill? It is all about building and maintaining momentum. Let's begin with a simple definition of momentum. Momentum is defined as "the amount of motion occurring in something that is moving, or the force that drives something forward to keep it moving."

Law of Momentum P=M x V
P = Momentum
M = Mass
V = Velocity

How do we keep the positive mojo and momentum going? It is not about being on a diet or working out seven days a week. It is about developing a lifestyle that we can sustain and enjoy. In the 80/20 rule, 80 percent of the time we are dialed in and focused on our new lifestyle habits, and the other 20 percent of the time we are taking a few liberties. Nothing fancy, just enough space to live our life the way we want and enjoy. The key is to understand that we can get out of our seat on the bus, but not get off the bus. Think about habits as the seeds to your future. Start planting your seeds today for the future you desire.

If you find yourself struggling to find that needed push, that little nudge, or spark, come back to this chapter over and over. Remember, you are worth it.

All the Energy is Used at Takeoff

My advisor in graduate school, Dr. Kwok Ho, was always coming up with some gold nugget life lessons to share with his students. One night in class, many of us were struggling with the Law of Momentum, P=M x V. Dr. Ho jumped in to say that we were making it too hard and helped make the Law of Momentum easier to understand with this definition.

"Life is like flying a 747. All the energy is used at takeoff and landing. Once you get the plane up in the air it takes less energy to keep the momentum going." How simple is that? Get the plane up in the air and keep it in the air. Dr. Ho was a wise man.

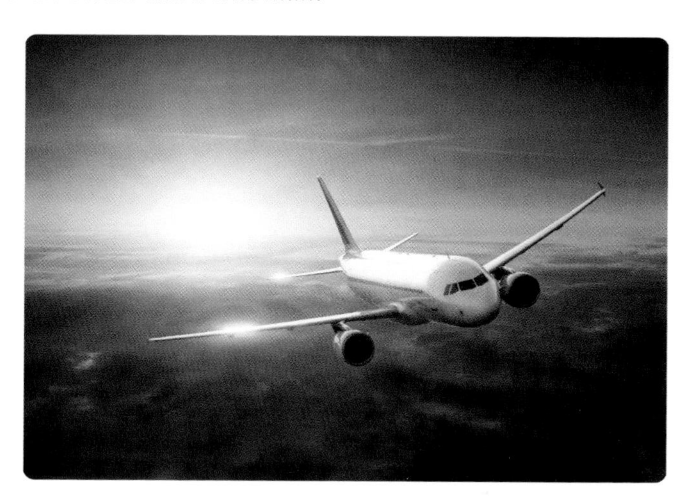

You Have the Power Essentials

Big Picture

- The greatest change occurs when we go from Zero to One.
- There are two types of motivation we all experience: extrinsic and intrinsic.
- A habit is a behavior or action that starts as a choice and then over time becomes an unconscious pattern or habit.
- There are three support systems: personal, social, and environmental.
- Willpower can be strengthened over time.
- Momentum—Keep the rock rolling down the hill.
- Your WHY has to be bigger than your BUT.

Ask Yourself

- How do you stay motivated?
- What types of extrinsic and intrinsic motivation work best for you?
- What new habits have you built?
- What causes you to lose willpower?
- Have you plugged in a few support systems?
- Are you trying new things, making a few mistakes, and learning how to pivot?

Small Steps

- Write down what you want. Be specific.
- Determine the behavior or behaviors that support your goals.
- Add support systems connected to your new habit.
- Write down the last time your willpower was weak and when it was strong.
- Don't be afraid to make mistakes. Learning to pivot is essential for success.
- Surround yourself with ways to stay intrinsically motivated.
- Take a few minutes to dive into your WHY or WHYs.

34 Just Let It Rain

During every journey there comes a time or a place where things may not go as planned and dark clouds may begin to move in. Don't worry, stay the course. These experiences can make life incredibly rich and special.

Let's Make a Deal

One of my favorite game shows growing up was *Let's Make a Deal* created by Stefan Hartos and its host Monty Hall. It was a fun and simple show where audience members dressed up in outrageous costumes. The signature part of the show was when contestants were allowed to choose between Door #1, Door #2, and Door #3. The contestant had no idea what was waiting behind each door. It could be some incredible prize like a new car or an exotic vacation, or they could get "zonked." When a contestant selected the wrong door, they got zonked and received all the junk that was behind that door. It usually included a bunch of gag prizes, such as 500 balloons or a year's supply of toilet paper. The anticipation of what was behind each door made the show incredibly fun to watch.

Now imagine your next visit to the doctor or healthcare professional. They show you three doors to better health: Door #1, #2, and #3. You are given the option to choose which door you want to open and subsequently, the path to follow.

Door #1: The Easy Door

Door #1 is an incredibly easy door to open and the easiest path to take. The sun is shining and the birds are chirping. The wind is at our back. We can still eat and drink whatever our heart desires. We never have to move our body. We can still burn the midnight oil. Choosing Door #1 means we do not have to change one thing. No work is required. Just take a pill and it will all be better.

It is a trick, so buckle up. As time goes on, our journey is going to change. In most cases the change occurs very rapidly. The once smooth road becomes incredibly bumpy and the hills steeper to climb. The direction of the wind has shifted. Our health has begun to deteriorate faster than expected. The medication train has now pulled into the station. Life becomes more and more difficult to navigate. We got zonked! If we had known how difficult this path was going to be over time, would we have opted for Door #1?"

Door #2: The Moderate Door

Door #2 is the moderate path to start out on. Some work is necessary to start down this path, but it allows us to slowly ease into some of our new behaviors. As time goes on, we may want to up our game to help maintain a smooth journey on our quest to feel and be our best. There is nothing wrong with choosing Door # 2, and it may be the best way to start for some. It does not preclude us from choosing Door #3 in the future.

Door #3: The Effort Door

Door #3 is the most difficult door to open in the beginning. The path is bumpy and the road is steep. The wind most likely is in our face. Some heavy lifting is required to start the journey. We must take more time for rest, eat foods closer to the center of the Food Target, and move our body on a daily basis. Our journey may be challenging in the beginning, but as our behavior changes and habits are built, our once difficult path becomes easier to follow. The road is smoother and there are fewer hills to climb. The wind has shifted in our favor. The investment we have made for a better future is becoming abundantly clear.

As has been emphasized multiple times throughout this book, we all have to take more ownership in our greatest asset—our health. It is not fair to our doctors or healthcare professionals to come in with high blood pressure, digestive health problems, anxiety, cholesterol imbalances, or broken sleep, and think we can be fixed during a 12-15-minute office visit.

The next time you have an appointment with your doctor or health professional, and they give you a choice, what door are you going to choose?

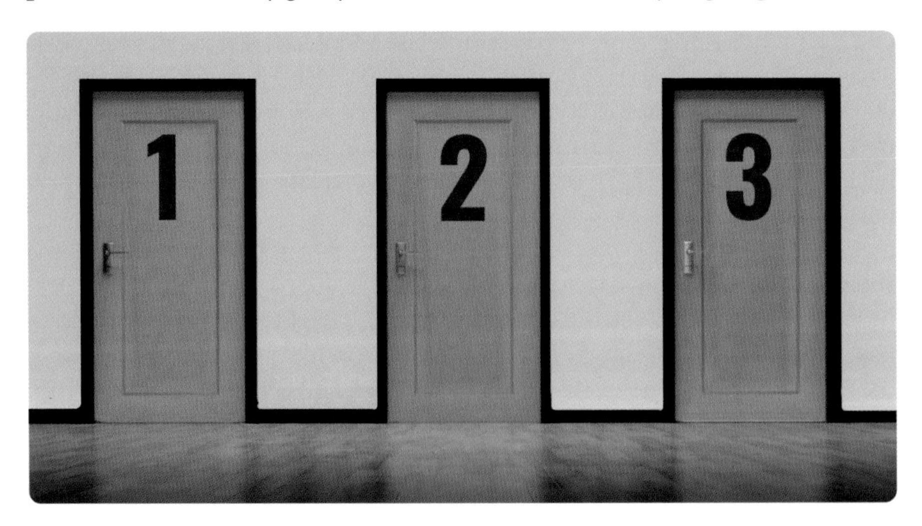

Ducks on a Frozen Pond

We all may begin to make compromises, especially as we age, but are we making compromises prematurely? Have you stopped learning and growing? Are you no longer taking the stairs because it takes more effort than in the past? Have you stopped doing some of the activities you once enjoyed?

Imagine a flock of ducks that decided not to fly south for the winter because it would be too much work and they were comfortable just staying right there in their own pond. Then one day the ducks realize their feet are frozen solid into the pond.

Seasons will change in everyone's life at some point, but we cannot let our feet become frozen into the pond. I have found personally and professionally that most of the good stuff is found in the effort or in the struggle. Don't let yourself get stuck in a frozen pond.

Chinese Bamboo Tree

The Chinese bamboo tree is a story about perseverance, patience, faith, hope, and human potential. What makes a Chinese bamboo tree unique is that it does not grow out of the ground for the first four years after being planted. It needs water, sunlight, love, and nurturing, but for the first four years no visible sign of life or growth can be seen at the surface. Our patience may become tested, and we may begin to wonder if our efforts of caring for the tree will ever be rewarded. But then in year five, the tree pops out of the ground and grows 90 feet in just 90 days. Did the tree lie dormant for four years only to grow exponentially in the fifth year? Was the little tree growing underground, developing a root system strong enough to support its potential for incredible growth in the fifth year and beyond? The answer, of course, is the latter. Had the tree not developed its strong unseen foundation, it could not have sustained its life as it grew so tall.

How many people give up on their dreams or aspirations just when they were about to see a major change start to take shape? Our success may take space, time, patience, and perseverance, but by building a strong foundation we will be able to overcome adversity and challenges along the way. We must stay focused and continue to believe in our plan and process despite not seeing immediate results.

In a culture driven by instant gratification this may be one of our greatest challenges. Maybe you are now prioritizing rest and rejuvenation into your lifestyle. You have started to eat a little better, to drink more water, or move more. Maybe you are not experiencing the results that you had hoped for by now. It is easy to become a little impatient or frustrated. Maybe you have started to lose hope and your confidence is a little shaken. You may start to think that your plan may somehow be flawed.

Listen closely. Stay the course! This is the point in your journey when a habit is on the verge of taking hold. When your habits take hold, they become part of your DNA. This is where the magic begins. Developing habits may take space, time, focus, and energy. Once you have them, they become part of you.

Focus on the Process

I remember my first body building contest back in 1985. In the final 12 weeks before stepping on stage, my nutrition and workouts were dialed in, no stone was left unturned. Unfortunately, after almost 4 weeks of perfect eating and challenging workouts, I was not getting as lean as I thought I should be by this time. By week 6, I was getting nervous. Very little seemed to be happening to my physique. At the time I felt a little like the Chinese bamboo tree. Nothing was happening. I was doing the work, but nothing was coming out of the ground. My confidence was a little shaken. Was my plan and process right?

Then in week 7 my body started to transform almost overnight, and by week 12, I was ready to step up on stage. Just like the Chinese bamboo tree, my body had been changing on the inside from weeks 1-6, but little was visible.

From then on, I have never worried about the outcome. I just stay focused on the process. In the years that followed, every time I competed, I would follow a similar plan and a similar process. I knew that around week 6 to week 7 everything would begin to tighten up. All I had to do was to place all my attention on my behaviors, my habits, my rituals, and most importantly, my process. I could not control the outcome, but I could control the process.

Married to The Process

Learning how to stay married to the process is a powerful mindset to have or develop. Success will come with perseverance, whether in professional sports, entertainment, academics, business, leadership, personal relationships, or your health. Success is attainable once we shift our focus to the process versus the outcome.

Take losing weight as an example. As you have already read throughout this book the weight loss industry is huge with an extremely dismal success rate. People want to lose weight, but unfortunately most or all of the focus is on losing weight, not on the process of losing weight. Even when we focus on the process and do our best, sometimes the outcome may not be exactly what we had in mind. But when we do our best and let the chips fall where they may, it can be extremely freeing and gratifying.

Get married to the process.

If your aspiration is to sleep better, what behavior or tiny habit are you going to focus on to get started?

___

___

If your aspiration is to lose weight, what does your process look like?

___

___

If your aspiration is to improve your fitness level, what are your steps in the process?

___

___

The Climb

As we come to the end, you may be wondering what is next. Consider what you were hoping to learn when you started reading or listening to this book. Have you opened your box of beliefs? What have you learned? Are there small steps that you are willing to start taking? Have your thoughts or aspirations changed along the way?

As discussed earlier, making mistakes is a big part of the learning process. Equally important is maintaining the confidence and trust that we will succeed like so many others before us. We do not need any special talent or skill in order to make the changes we desire. What we do need to do is persevere and learn how to enjoy our journey.

To bring the true hero out in us and to be our best, we must go through struggles during our climb. There may be hurdles to jump, and we may stumble. We may encounter rough waters and bumpy roads along the way. But it is in the pursuit, the experiences, and the journey where we learn the most about ourselves. This is where most of our joy and happiness lives.

You now have the knowledge and a roadmap. Use this book as your guide to help you stay on your path to feeling your best.

Tips to Help You Climb Your Mountain

- Nothing comes from nothing. You have to put in the effort.
- Plant seeds. The seeds you plant today will be your harvest tomorrow.
- Try things. Clarity comes through your experiences.
- Dark clouds may move in when climbing your mountain. Don't give up.
- Develop self-mastery. Joy and happiness come from lifetime pursuits.

Good health is built on the bedrock of Cellular Health, pH Balance and eating from the Source. The journey to optimal health depends on:

REST Relaxation and Rejuvenation reduce stress, improve sleep, and create space.
EAT Let food be your medicine.
MOVE Daily movement is the Fountain of Youth.

Enjoy the simple act of breathing or getting a good night of sleep, cherish the food you eat, and take pleasure in moving your body.

Take time for you and remind yourself that these simple pleasures make the pursuit of health incredibly worthwhile.

You now have to power to feel and be your best. So, when dark clouds begin to move in, don't run for cover. You are ready. Take pleasure when it begins to rain.

Wishing You a Lifetime of Health & Happiness!

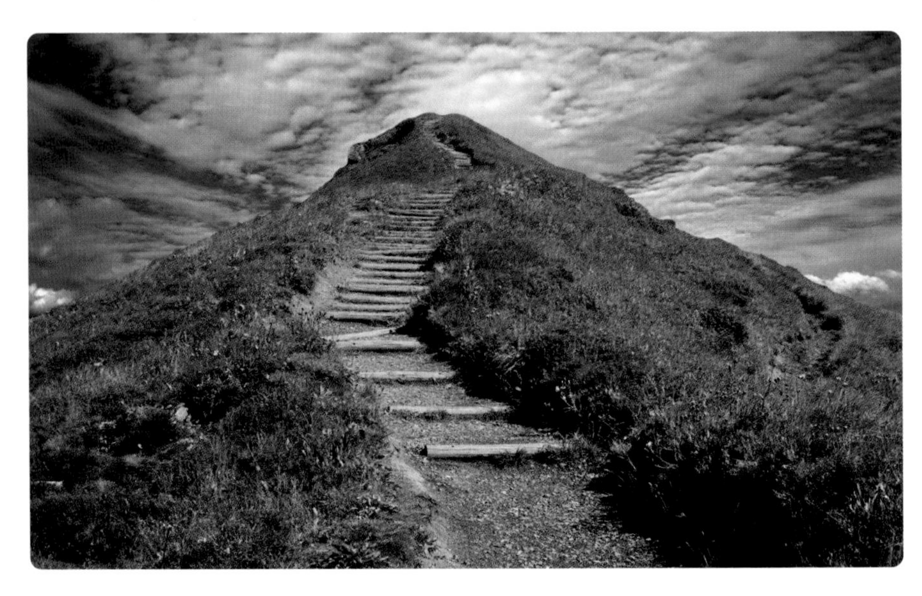

Acknowledgments

There are so many people who have helped and inspired me along my journey that I would like to thank.

I'd like to begin by thanking many of my teachers. To Miss Ellis, my sixth-grade teacher, who told me I could be whoever I wanted to be. To a few of my college professors: Dr. Louis Junker, who opened my eyes to the world of better health and Dr. Kwok Ho, who guided me into the world of prevention.

To our faithful On Target Living clients, readers, and followers, whose phone calls, letters, emails, and testimonials drive me to learn and grow every day—thank you!

To our wonderful team at On Target Living—you are changing lives every day!

To the friends and family who have supported me from the beginning—thank you!

To the team of Bonney, Cindy, and Ida—you all helped to make this book truly come alive!

To my brother and sister—loving siblings are a gift!

To my dad, who taught me how to play, to laugh, and to listen, and to my mom, who taught me how to be gritty and kind—thank you for all your love and support!

And to my wife Paula, my daughter Kristen, son-in-law Sean, my son Matt, daughter-in-law Holly, our grandkids Eze, Hadley, Brady, Karis, and my dog Floyd—may we all continue on our joyous quest to live a Happy & Healthy Life!

Index

D

E

F

G

H

I

J

K

L

M

N

O

P

Q

R

S